Selected Topics in Environmental and Public Health

Volume I

Selected Topics in Environmental and Public Health
Volume I

Edited by **Abby Calvin**

FOSTER ACADEMICS
New Jersey

Published by Foster Academics,
61 Van Reypen Street,
Jersey City, NJ 07306, USA
www.fosteracademics.com

Selected Topics in Environmental and Public Health
Volume I
Edited by Abby Calvin

International Standard Book Number: 978-1-63242-364-1 (Hardback)

Printed in China.

Contents

Preface

The field of studies related to public health and environmental issues is a series of some complex systems. Some of the countries with high income rate and developed scenario, sometimes take many things for granted like availability of clean portable water, low infant mortality rates, control over infectious diseases, etc. and the reason behind this is lack of high functioning systems that require numerous efforts and work. Most of the people notice these issues when the system fails and the problems already take disastrous forms. With the widespread globalization, public health and environment sustainability became a transnational issue. Diseases like H1N1, SARS or any common infection can be transmitted across borders via airplanes in just hours. The biggest reason behind this is lack of planning to prevent such hazards, pollutions and environmental degradation can be controlled in developing countries using recycling techniques and gaining balance in manufacturing processes. Even the non-communicable diseases are transmitted over borders because of global market of tobacco and fast food.

This book covers the key concepts in the field of public health and environmental issues to control these hazards. This book is aimed at the clinicians and scientists who have an interest in public health. My goal is to produce a textbook that can be read and used by practicing environmentalists, whether they are academicians or non-academicians. The second goal was to produce a book that the scientists working in this diverse and divergent field would be able to refer to and read as an authoritative source. And finally, the third goal was to interpret the field for trainees in public health, medicine, resource management, and disease control. My hope is that this book reflects the increasing knowledge within the field of public health treatments and research.

I would like to thank all the contributing authors for their hard work. I would also like to appreciate their adherence to the timelines set for the publication. I also wish to thank the publishing team for their extraordinary support and my family for helping me at every step.

Editor

1

Evaluation of a Bladder Cancer Cluster in a Population of Criminal Investigators with the Bureau of Alcohol, Tobacco, Firearms and Explosives—Part 1: The Cancer Incidence

Susan R. Davis,[1] Xuguang Tao,[2] Edward J. Bernacki,[2] and Amy S. Alfriend[2]

[1] *Federal Occupational Health, Department of Health and Human Services, 4550 Montgomery Avenue, Suite 950, Bethesda, MD 20814, USA*

[2] *Division of Occupational and Environmental Medicine, Department of Medicine, Johns Hopkins University School of Medicine, 615 N. Wolfe Street, Baltimore, MD 21205, USA*

Correspondence should be addressed to Susan R. Davis, sdavis228@comcast.net

Academic Editor: Edward Trapido

This study investigated a bladder cancer cluster in a cohort of employees, predominately criminal investigators, participating in a medical surveillance program with the United States Bureau of Alcohol, Tobacco, Firearms and Explosives (ATF) between 1995 and 2007. Standardized incidence ratios (SIRs) were used to compare cancer incidences in the ATF population and the US reference population. Seven cases of bladder cancer (five cases verified by pathology report at time of analysis) were identified among a total employee population of 3,768 individuals. All cases were white males and criminal investigators. Six of seven cases were in the 30 to 49 age range at the time of diagnosis. The SIRs for white male criminal investigators undergoing examinations were 7.63 (95% confidence interval = 3.70–15.75) for reported cases and 5.45 (2.33–12.76) for verified cases. White male criminal investigators in the ATF population are at statistically significant increased risk for bladder cancer.

1. Introduction

The Bureau of Alcohol, Tobacco, Firearms and Explosives (ATF), a law enforcement agency within the United States Department of Justice, has been in the business of investigating the cause and origin of fires and explosions since the 1970s. ATF typically collaborates with other federal, state, and local authorities to provide this service through several venues. At the local level, criminal investigators with ATF, especially ones holding special designations as certified fire investigators (CFIs), work side-by-side with their state and local counterparts to assist with investigation of post-fire and post-blast scenes. These individuals may also serve on city-based federal arson task forces, in partnership with other federal, state, and local investigators, to address acute arson problems. At the national level, ATF maintains a well-trained national response team (NRT) which provides comprehensive response to assist these other jurisdictions with onsite investigation of major arson and bombing incidents. The NRT is a multispecialty team comprised of criminal investigators with post-fire and post-blast investigation expertise, explosives enforcement specialists, forensic chemists, fire protection engineers, and other technical experts. ATF established the NRT program in 1978 and subsequently instituted a program for certification of criminal investigators as fire investigators (CFIs) in 1986.

In 1995, ATF commenced a voluntary medical surveillance program for members of the NRT to monitor the health of participants working in the potentially hazardous environment of the post-fire/post-blast scene. The agency extended the voluntary program to all CFIs in 1997. By 2000, three white male participants of the program had reported diagnoses of bladder cancer between the years 1994 and 1999. All three individuals were nonsmokers and younger than 50 years of age when diagnosed. This information raised concern that a bladder cancer cluster was occurring among scene investigators. In response to this concern, in 2002 ATF mandated participation in the medical surveillance program for all NRT members, all explosives enforcement specialists, and all criminal investigators, including those not involved in post-fire/post-blast investigations. To facilitate future epidemiologic evaluation of the significance of the apparent cancer cluster, ATF also committed medical surveillance data entry into an electronic database. By 2006, four additional white male program participants had reported diagnoses of bladder cancer between 2001 and 2005. Combined, the seven reported cases ranged in age from 32 to 53 in the year of diagnosis. From a job title perspective, all cases were among criminal investigators, who comprised 96% of the employees participating in the surveillance program. In addition, six of the seven cases reported working post-fire and post-blast scenes while employed with ATF. None of the seven cases reported work histories which involved investigation of such scenes prior to their employment with ATF.

The presence of this cancer cluster generated two questions. First, was this group of employees, predominantly criminal investigators, experiencing a greater than expected incidence of bladder cancer from a demographic perspective? Second, was post-fire/post-blast scene investigation associated with increased risk for bladder cancer? Part 1 of this study addresses the question on cancer incidence and Part 2 addresses the question on cancer risk associated with investigation of these scenes. Analyses for both parts use data collected through the medical surveillance program.

In the United States, bladder cancer is expected to be the sixth most commonly occurring cancer, excluding basal and squamous cell skin cancers, in 2012 [1]. As reported by the American Cancer Society, the estimated number of new bladder cancer cases in 2012 is 73,510, which equates to approximately 4.5% of all new cases of cancer [1]. The demographic characteristics associated with greatest risk for bladder cancer include male gender, white race, and increasing age [2]. According to the surveillance epidemiology and end results (SEER) age-adjusted incidence data for the period 2005–2009, bladder cancer occurs four times more often in men than in women [3]. In this data set, it ranks as the fourth most common cancer among men, but only the twelfth most common cancer among women [3]. The incidence among whites is 1.78 times greater than the incidence among blacks, while the incidence among Hispanics is 0.90 times the incidence among blacks [2, 3]. Bladder cancer incidence is the lowest among Asian/Pacific islanders and American Indian/Alaska natives [3]. The risk of onset increases with age over the age of 40 and is greatest during the ninth decade of life [3]. About 90% of cases occur in individuals over the age of 55, with the average age being 73 at the time of diagnosis [2]. In the ATF cancer cluster, all the cases of bladder cancer represented both the gender and the race with the greatest incidence of bladder cancer, but the ages of the cases at the time of diagnosis were relatively young for bladder cancer as all cases occurred in individuals less than 55 years of age.

Recognized nondemographic risk factors include cigarette smoking, bladder birth defects, chronic bladder inflammation, genetic predisposition, use of herbal remedies containing aristolochic acid, drinking water containing arsenic and chlorination by-products, prior history of bladder cancer, chemotherapy and radiation therapy, and specific industries and occupations with exposures to known or suspect bladder carcinogens [2, 4–13]. Many studies have explored the association of fluid intake and type of fluid intake with risk for bladder cancer, but findings for both total fluids and specific fluids have been inconsistent, likely due to influences of confounding variables such as the presence of bladder carcinogens in tap water [14–24]. Two studies have demonstrated that increased frequency of urination is associated with reduced risk for bladder cancer [18, 21].

Smoking, the number one risk factor for bladder cancer, is estimated to cause approximately 50% of bladder cancer cases in men and 30% of cases in women [6]. Second to smoking, occupational exposures to carcinogens may account for as few as 10% of cases in men and five percent of cases in women to as many as 20–25% of all bladder cancers [6, 11]. Established at risk industries include the manufacturing of products such as synthetic dyes and paints, cables, textiles, leather works, and aluminum and the petrochemical, coal tar, and rubber industries [5–7, 12, 25–30]. A number of specific occupations have also been identified to be associated with increased risk of bladder cancer. These include, but are not limited to, cooks and kitchen workers, electricians, hairdressers, leather workers, machinists, petroleum workers, rubber workers, coal miners, truckers, and vehicle mechanics, as summarized by Schulte et al. [12] in 1987, as well as coke oven workers, roofers, dry cleaners, chimney sweeps, and painters, as addressed by others in more recent literature [5–7, 25, 31–34]. Exposure to both cigarette smoke and occupationally related bladder carcinogens may work synergistically to increase further the risk for bladder cancer [2, 7].

As an occupation, the broad job category of law enforcement is generally not recognized for being at increased risk for bladder cancer. In 1987, Schulte et al. [12] did include protection guards on their summary list of occupations associated with risk for bladder cancer, but acknowledged that the potential etiologic agent was unknown. As the rate of occurrence of bladder cancer is almost five times greater than the associated death rate in the US, with 80% of cases surviving for five or more years after diagnosis [1], cancer incidence is a more sensitive measure of occupational risk for bladder cancer than related mortality and it is important to differentiate between epidemiologic studies looking at cancer incidence and those looking at cancer mortality. Many epidemiologic studies on the association of bladder cancer incidence and occupations have not found police officers, guards, and related categories, such as protective services and government worker inspection/investigation occupations, to be associated with increased risk for bladder cancer [11, 35–46]. One exception was a study by Howe et al. [47] which showed guards and watchmen to have a statistically significant age-adjusted relative risk for bladder cancer of 4.0. In Reulen et al.'s [32] 2009 meta-analysis on the association between bladder cancer incidence and occupation, summary relative risks for bladder cancer were obtained for protective service occupations from the findings of 23 studies and for police officers and guards from the findings of 14 studies. These summary relative risks were only marginally elevated and not statistically significant, at 1.07 (95% confidence interval (CI) 0.96–1.19) for protective services and 1.10 (95% CI 0.95–1.29) for police officers and guards. Three mortality studies on police officer cohorts also did not find statistically significant increases in mortality from bladder cancer overall [48–50]. One of these studies did demonstrate that policemen who were professional drivers had significantly increased bladder cancer-related mortality [48] and another showed a higher than expected mortality rate for police officers with 10–19 years of service [50]. As some, but not all, epidemiology studies have demonstrated an increased risk for bladder cancer in jobs with exposure to diesel or traffic fumes [6, 40, 43, 51, 52] and one meta-analysis has shown increased cancer risk for several types of vehicle drivers [32], the use of broad law enforcement job categories in studies on cancer risk and occupation assumes a degree of uniformity in exposures to potential bladder carcinogens and risk for bladder cancer, which may not always be the case.

Part 1 of this study investigates the statistical significance of the incidence of bladder cancer in the ATF employee population comprised of criminal investigators and members of the NRT.

2. Methods

2.1. Study Time Frame and Study Subjects. The time interval of this study is 1993, the year preceding diagnosis of the first bladder cancer case, through 2007. For this period, a full roster cohort was constructed from the annual staffing rosters provided by ATF for each calendar year from 1993 through 2007. The annual staffing rosters included all criminal investigators, explosives enforcement specialists, forensic chemists, fire protection engineers, and a small number of other specialists typically affiliated with NRT work, regardless of individual membership on the NRT or eligibility for participation in the medical surveillance program, who were currently working for ATF in each respective calendar year. ATF provided the demographic study parameters of gender, race, and age, and the job series and titles for all members of the full roster cohort. Members of the full roster cohort are dispersed throughout the United States and its territories Puerto Rico and Guam and may move around within this geographic area during their employment with ATF.

With the advent of the medical surveillance program in 1995, a subset of the full roster cohort, comprised of employees participating in the program, was created. As explained in the introduction, the program was initially voluntary and offered to members of the NRT, but became mandatory in 2002 for all criminal investigators, explosives enforcement specialists, and members of the NRT. Setup in partnership with Federal Occupational Health (FOH), United States Department of Health and Human Services, the program consisted of an annual evaluation which included a medical history and tobacco use questionnaire, physical examination, and laboratory and ancillary tests. Collection of detailed work history information, including job series and titles, began in 2003 with the institution of a work history questionnaire. The use of FOH's electronic database, the Occupational Health Information Management System (OHIMS), to facilitate future epidemiologic evaluation of the bladder cancer cluster began in 2002. Data for key study variables from pre-2002 exams were retrospectively retrieved and also entered into OHIMS.

For the cohort of employees participating in the medical surveillance program from 1995 to 2007, pertinent data collected with each annual evaluation included the demographic variables, gender, race, and age, as well as cancer history and tobacco use history. Data on job series and titles were also provided by members of the cohort participating in the program between 2003 and 2007. The demographic data and the job series and titles data provided by ATF for the full roster cohort were subsequently cross-referenced with the same data provided by employees participating in the medical surveillance program. Any data inconsistencies between the two sources were resolved by medical record review or phone contact with employees.

2.2. Identification and Verification of Bladder Cancer Cases. As stated in the introduction, all bladder cancer cases were initially identified by employees self-reporting the diagnosis and year of diagnosis at the time of the annual medical surveillance evaluation. The self-reported cases were subsequently contacted by the occupational medicine physician overseeing the medical surveillance program, who informed them of the bladder cancer cluster and of the plans to evaluate the significance of the cluster through epidemiologic analysis and requested their assistance with voluntary provision of a pathology report for verification of case diagnosis. Requests for pathology reports were accompanied by provision of medical release forms for completion by cases.

2.3. Study Design. This is a cohort study in which standardized incidence ratios (SIRs) were calculated for four defined populations of ATF employees to compare the observed bladder cancer case numbers in each ATF population with the expected cancer case numbers based on incidence rate in the US general population, appropriately adjusted for age and stratified by sex and race, as relevant to each of the four ATF populations. The US general population was chosen as the best reference population for analysis due to the nationwide dispersion of ATF employees under study. As all the bladder cancer cases occurred among white male criminal investigators, the populations chosen for analysis included: (1) the full roster cohort comprising all males and females, (2) all white males in the full roster cohort, (3) all white males in the full roster cohort with examinations (cancer and tobacco use histories), and (4) all white males in the full roster cohort with both examinations and work histories who were also criminal investigators. Determination of the expected cancer incidence rate was based on data from the surveillance epidemiology and end results (SEER) program for the US population for the period 1993–2007. The SIR estimates the relative risk of bladder cancer incidence in the ATF population compared to the US population adjusted for age and stratified by race and gender. Computations for each population included determination of the person-year distribution during the study period, which served as the denominator for the respective SIR analysis. One person-year was counted for each year an individual was a member of the cohort. The person-years were arranged by five-year age increments and three five-year time intervals, 1993–1997, 1998–2002, and 2003–2007.

3. Results

3.1. Study Subjects. Table 1 shows the distribution of individuals by gender and race for the full roster cohort, for the subset of employees with surveillance examinations, for the subset of employees with surveillance examinations and work histories, and for the subset of criminal investigators with surveillance exams and work histories. The percent distribution of individuals by gender and race for each of four of these populations is comparable.

The full roster cohort comprised 3,768 individuals (Table 1). Criminal investigators, with job series 1811, accounted for 96% of all employees in the full roster cohort and 96% of all white males in the full roster cohort. Within the full roster cohort, only 18.2% of members were non-white and only 12.6% of members were female.

Of the full roster cohort, 2,712 (72%) members participated in the medical surveillance program between 1995 and 2007 and had data for one or more examinations in the program's electronic database (Table 1). The percentage of full roster cohort members with examinations was not greater than 72% due in part to the medical surveillance program being voluntary and only open to members of the NRT and to CFIs prior to 2002. Since 2002, when the program became mandatory for all criminal investigators, explosives enforcement specialists, and members of the NRT, the percentage of currently employed cohort members who obtained annual examinations ranged from a low of 50% in 2003 to a high of 67% in 2006. Despite this variance in annual rate of participation in the mandatory program, 2697 of 3136 (86%) full roster cohort members who were employed for one or more years between 2002 and 2007 obtained at least one medical exam.

Job history data, collected from employees between 2003 and 2007 at the time of the annual exam, were available for 2549 (68%) members of the full roster cohort. Of these individuals, 2478 (97%) were criminal investigators (Table 1).

3.2. Characteristics of Bladder Cancer Cases. During the study period, seven individuals reported bladder cancer diagnoses. At the time of the analysis, five of the seven cases had provided medical documentation (pathology reports) verifying the diagnosis of bladder cancer and diagnosis year. Another case provided verifying documentation following the completion of the analysis.

As affirmed from review of pathology reports of the urinary bladder biopsies of the five cases verified at the time of the analysis, four of the cases were low grade papillary transitional cell carcinomas and one was transitional cell carcinoma *in situ*. The subsequent sixth case verified after analysis was also low grade papillary transitional cell carcinoma.

The first case was diagnosed in 1994 and the most recent case was diagnosed in 2005. As already known from the medical surveillance program, all bladder cancers occurred in white males and in criminal investigators. Table 1 includes the distribution of reported bladder cancer cases by gender and race for each defined employee population. White males comprised 72% (2723/3768) of the full roster cohort and 69-70% of each of the three subset populations, including criminal investigators with medical surveillance examinations and work histories (69% (1715/2478)). The cases ranged from 32 to 53 years of age the year of diagnosis, with three individuals being in their 30s, three being in their 40s, and one being in his early 50s. Table 2 shows the distribution of the self-reported bladder cancer cases at the time of diagnosis in the same five-year age increments and three five-year time intervals as used to establish the person-year distributions for each SIR analysis. Two cases were diagnosed in 1993–1997, four cases were diagnosed in 1998–2002, and one case was diagnosed in 2003–2007.

3.3. Distribution of Person-Years within the Study Populations Undergoing Incidence Analysis. Table 3 summarizes the total person-years calculated for each of the four study populations undergoing incidence analysis. The number of total person-years ranged from a high of 34,818 for the full roster cohort to a low of 17,976 for the population of white male criminal investigators with exams and work histories. The pattern of distribution of person-years was similar for all four study populations and is illustrated in Table 2 for the population of white males in the full roster cohort. The vast majority of employees for each study population fell within 25 and 54 years of age for each of the five-year time intervals. This distribution pattern reflects ATF's practice of hiring criminal investigators with prior work experience and the mandated retirement age of 57 years for federal criminal investigators.

3.4. Bladder Cancer Incidence Ratios. Table 3 presents the standardized incidence ratios (SIRs) calculated for each of the four defined study populations: the full roster cohort, all white males in the full roster cohort, all white males with examinations (cancer and tobacco use histories), and all white males with examinations and work histories who were also criminal investigators. To access the effect of the two unverified cancer cases on SIR outcomes, SIRs were performed for the scenario with seven reported cancer cases and for the scenario with five verified cases for each of the four study populations.

When computed with all seven cases, the SIR is 2.41 (95% CI 1.17–4.96) for the entire roster cohort, 2.93 (95% CI 1.42–6.07) for the white male cohort, 6.08 (95% CI 2.94–12.54) for white males with exams, and 7.63 (95% CI 3.70–15.75) for white male criminal investigators with exams and work histories (Table 3). When recalculated with only

Table 1: Distribution of self-reported bladder cancers and employees in key ATF study populations by gender and race (1993–2007).

Study population	Males				Females				Total		Percent of full roster
	Whites		Nonwhites		Whites		Nonwhites				
	Cases	Employees (%)	Cases	Employees (%)	Cases	Employees (%)	Cases	Employees (%)	Cases	Employees (%)	
Full roster	7	2723 (72.3%)	0	570 (15.1%)	0	358 (9.5%)	0	117 (3.1%)	7	3768 (100%)	100.00
Examinations	7	1885 (69.5%)	0	467 (17.2%)	0	271 (10.0%)	0	89 (3.3%)	7	2712 (100%)	71.97
Examinations and work histories	7	1771 (69.5%)	0	441 (17.3%)	0	253 (9.9%)	0	84 (3.3%)	7	2549 (100%)	67.65
Criminal investigators with examinations and work histories	7	1715 (69.2%)	0	436 (17.6%)	0	244 (9.8%)	0	83 (3.4%)	7	2478 (100%)	65.76

Table 2: Distribution of self-reported bladder cancer cases and of person-years observed for white males in full roster cohort by calendar period and age group.

Age group	1993–1997		1998–2002		2003–2007		Total	
	Cases	Person-years	Cases	Person-years	Cases	Person-years	Cases	Person-years
0–4	0	0.0	0	0.0	0	0.0	0	0.0
5–9	0	0.0	0	0.0	0	0.0	0	0.0
10–14	0	0.0	0	0.0	0	0.0	0	0.0
15–19	0	0.0	0	0.0	0	0.0	0	0.0
20–24	0	25.1	0	81.6	0	71.3	0	178.0
25–29	0	642.9	0	611.6	0	749.7	0	2004.1
30–34	2	1730.8	0	1593.4	0	1670.6	2	4994.8
35–39	0	1321.5	0	2136.4	1	2125.1	1	5583.0
40–44	0	773.1	2	1329.7	0	2111.9	2	4214.6
45–49	0	1574.9	1	763.0	0	1291.9	1	3629.8
50–54	0	1046.2	1	1083.5	0	571.5	1	2701.1
55–59	0	261.6	0	383.1	0	264.5	0	909.2
60–64	0	12.4	0	113.1	0	95.9	0	221.4
65–69	0	3.9	0	5.7	0	43.3	0	52.9
70–74	0	1.8	0	2.7	0	3.0	0	7.5
75–79	0	0.0	0	0.0	0	0.0	0	0.0
80–84	0	0.0	0	0.0	0	0.0	0	0.0
85–89	0	0.0	0	0.0	0	0.0	0	0.0
Total	2	7394.0	4	8103.8	1	8998.7	7	24496.5

* The one remaining unverified cancer case occurred in the 1998–2002 time frame.

Table 3: Standardized incidence ratios (SIRs) of self-reported and verified urinary bladder cancer cases for the period 1993–2007.

Study population	Employee #	Person-years	Expected cases*	Observed cases	SIR	95% CI	
Entire roster cohort	3,768	34,818.01	2.91	7	2.41	1.17	4.96
Entire roster cohort**	3,768	34,818.01	2.91	5	1.72	0.73	4.02
Roster white males	2,723	24,496.47	2.39	7	2.93	1.42	6.07
Roster white males**	2,723	24,496.47	2.39	5	2.09	0.90	1.91
Exam white males	1,885	19,648.25	1.15	7	6.08	2.94	12.54
Exam white males**	1,885	19,648.25	1.15	5	4.34	1.85	10.16
Job 1811 white males	1,715	17,976.42	0.92	7	7.63	3.70	15.75
Job 1811 white males**	1,715	17,976.42	0.92	5	5.45	2.33	12.76

* Expected number of cases calculated using US incidence rates from SEER for the same period.
** SIRs determined for the five verified cases with pathology reports.

the five verified cases, the SIR is 1.72 (95% CI 0.73–4.02) for the entire roster cohort, 2.09 (95% CI 0.90–1.91) for white males, 4.34 (95% CI 1.85–10.16) for white males with exams, and 5.45 (95% CI 2.33–12.76) for white male criminal investigators with exams and work histories (Table 3). The elevated SIRs are statistically significant for all four of these populations when all seven cases are included in the analysis and remain statistically significant for white males with exams and white male criminal investigators with exams and work histories when only the five verified cases are used.

Age-specific cancer incidence rates in the white male ATF population were greater than the rates for the adjusted U.S. reference SEER population for each age group in which cases occurred (Table 4). This finding is expected since 90% of bladder cancers occur in individuals over the age of 55 and all seven cases in the ATF population were younger than 55 years at the time of diagnosis. The highest age-specific relative risk for bladder cancer in the ATF population compared to the reference population, and the only one of statistical significance, was seen in the 30–34 age group, the youngest age group experiencing bladder cancer within the ATF population.

4. Discussion

Recognition of a bladder cancer cluster among white male criminal investigators participating in an ATF medical surveillance program raised concern that the employee population was experiencing a greater-than-expected incidence of bladder cancer and that post-fire/post-blast scene

TABLE 4: Age-specific white male bladder cancer incidence rates (1/100,000) for ATF and SEER (13 registries), with respective rate ratios, for the period 1993–2007.

Age	ATF	SEER	RR	95% CI-L	95% CI-U
20–24	0.00	0.37	0.00	0.00	0.00
25–29	0.00	0.57	0.00	0.00	0.00
30–34	40.04	1.17	34.32	3.78	124.24
35–39	17.91	2.80	6.40	0.19	35.63
40–44	47.45	5.83	8.13	0.89	29.45
45–49	27.55	13.13	2.10	0.06	11.68
50–54	37.02	25.33	1.46	0.04	8.14
55–59	0.00	50.57	0.00	0.00	0.00
60–64	0.00	88.33	0.00	0.00	0.00
65–69	0.00	145.70	0.00	0.00	0.00
70–74	0.00	209.43	0.00	0.00	0.00
75–79	0.00	275.40	0.00	0.00	0.00
80–84	0.00	327.83	0.00	0.00	0.00
85–89	0.00	353.73	0.00	0.00	0.00

investigation might be associated with increased risk of bladder cancer. Part 1 of this epidemiologic study determined that bladder cancer incidence in the white male study population was significantly elevated statistically for the period 1993–2007.

This study illustrates the twofold utility of using a medical surveillance program to monitor the health of an employee population potentially exposed to hazardous agents and to perform epidemiologic analysis of the significance of cancer occurring within the population. Although the ATF medical surveillance program evolved over time in several ways, which included changing from voluntary to mandatory participation, and despite an annual participation rate of 50–67% after the program became mandatory, the requisite data were sufficient to perform SIRs for the ATF study population which showed white males to be at increased risk for bladder cancer when compared to white males in the US reference population.

All bladder cancer cases in the ATF cohort were reported by white males, who constituted about 72% of the full roster cohort. In the incidence analyses of the two larger ATF populations, the full roster cohort and white males in the full roster cohort, the cancer risk was elevated for analyses performed with both seven reported and five verified cases, but was only statistically significant for the analyses with the seven reported cases. Since these two ATF populations included individuals who had not participated in the medical surveillance program and whose cancer history was unknown, which amounted to 28% of the full roster cohort and 31% of white males in the full roster cohort, the actual number of cases of bladder cancer within these two populations could be greater than the observed seven reported and five verified cases, which would lead to even higher SIRs than the ones calculated with the seven and five cases. With the two smaller ATF populations, white males with exams and white male criminal investigators with exams, the computed SIRs were elevated and statistically significant with both seven reported and five verified cancer cases. The SIRs of the two smaller populations, understandably higher than those of the two larger populations, might best depict the true cancer risk for the ATF cohort as the reported cancer history is known for all individuals in these two smaller populations.

The finding that white male criminal investigators in the ATF population are at increased risk for bladder cancer is in contrast with the findings of prior epidemiologic studies of bladder cancer incidence in law enforcement occupations, in which law enforcement and related job categories were generally found not to be at increased risk for bladder cancer [11, 32, 35–39, 41, 42, 44–46]. In Reulen et al.'s [32] meta-analysis, the summary relative risk was 1.10 (95% CI 0.95–1.29) for police officers and 1.07 (95% CI 0.96–1.19) for protective service occupations. What may make this population of ATF criminal investigators unique from other populations of law enforcement specialists is the presence of a sizable subset of ATF criminal investigators who specialize in investigation of post-fire and post-blast scenes. What we know from the medical surveillance program is that six of the seven bladder cancer cases in the current study had occupational histories of working these scenes while employed with ATF. Thus, the increased incidence of bladder cancer identified among white male criminal investigators in the current study appears to be associated with the performance of post-fire/post-blast investigations. If this is the case, the increased risk for bladder cancer in this subset of specialized criminal investigators is sufficiently strong to influence the bladder cancer risk within the entire ATF study population.

The magnitude of the SIRs computed in this study deserves some discussion. For the population of white male criminal investigators with exams, the SIRs were 7.63 (95% CI 3.70–15.75) for seven reported cases and 5.45 (95% CI 2.33–12.76) for five verified cases, and for the slightly larger population of all white males with exams, the SIRs were 6.08 (95% CI 2.94–12.54) for seven reported cases and 4.34 (95% CI 1.85–10.16) for five verified cases. In individual epidemiologic studies of bladder cancer incidence in other occupations and industries, statistically significant elevations in relative risk have been found with a 1.1-fold to fivefold increase [11, 32, 33, 39, 41–44, 46, 52–54] and even with a sixfold to tenfold increase for some occupations such as chemical workers [41, 47], dye manufacturing [55, 56], railroad workers [47], and physicians [41]. In one epidemiologic study on firefighters, the reported statistically significant odds ratio for bladder cancer was as high as 22.7 [41]. Thus, some epidemiologic studies on other occupations have obtained elevated relative risk for bladder cancer of the same order of magnitude as that found in the present study on criminal investigators. In Reulen et al.'s [32] meta-analysis on the association between bladder cancer and occupations, however, statistically significant summary relative risks which were found for several occupations only fell in the 1.1–1.3 range. These occupations included miners, rubber workers, leather workers, four types of professional drivers, and mechanics, but not chemical workers, firefighters, police officers, protective service occupations, or health care professionals.

The elevated risk for bladder cancer in the current study cohort also approximates the increased risk for bladder cancer seen in smokers compared to nonsmokers, as demonstrated in various epidemiologic studies which show smokers to have a twofold to sixfold increased risk for bladder cancer [1, 6, 57–59]. Further corroborating study is advised to verify the magnitude of the increased risk found among criminal investigators in the current study.

Although the elevated SIRs for the two populations with exams remained statistically significant when analyzed with only the five verified cases, having two of the seven reported cases (28%) unverified at the time of statistical analysis constitutes a weakness of the study and illustrates a limitation of using data from a medical surveillance program to conduct a cancer incidence analysis. With so few total cases, the difference in number between reported and verified cases can impact the significance of study outcomes, as demonstrated by comparing the SIRs computed with both the seven reported and the five verified cases for the full roster cohort and for white males in the full roster cohort. Since the study analysis was completed, ongoing effort to verify the unverified cases was successful in verifying one of the two cases.

Another point to make is that the SIRs on the populations with exams could in actuality be artificially high, as only 72% of individuals in the full roster cohort underwent physical examination and individuals without medical issues may have selectively avoided coming in for exams. Since the institution of the mandatory program in 2002, however, 86% of individuals employed by ATF between 2002 and 2007 obtained at least one exam during this time frame and these 2697 employees accounted for 99% of the 2712 individuals in the full roster cohort with exams. With this level of participation in the mandatory program since 2002, potential for bias due to exam avoidance is likely very limited.

In conclusion, white male members of the ATF cohort experienced statistically significant increased risk for bladder cancer when compared to white males in the US population for the study period 1993–2007. Among white males with exams and white male criminal investigators with exams, the elevated risk was demonstrated for computations with both seven reported and five verified cancer cases. There was no observed bladder cancer risk for nonwhite males and all females in the cohort study.

With six of the seven cases in the bladder cancer cluster, having known histories of investigating post-fire and post-blast scenes while employed with ATF, scene investigation work appeared to be linked with the observed increase in bladder cancer incidence. Part 2 of the study will evaluate the association of post-fire/post-blast scene work history and risk for bladder cancer, while controlling for tobacco use history.

Acknowledgments

The authors thank ATF for funding the epidemiologic study and paper preparation, FOH for providing support for the study, including but not limited to advocating for the medical surveillance program for ATF that discovered the reported bladder cancer cases, performing the examinations and ancillary tests on the employees participating in the program, and providing OHIMS for management of program data, and Bruce Higgins, database manager of OHIMS, for managing the database of the medical surveillance program and assisting with preparation of data for analysis. The opinions in this paper are the authors' and do not necessarily represent the opinions of ATF or of FOH. S. R. Davis, X. Tao, E. J. Bernacki and A. S. Alfriend received funding for this study from the Bureau of Alcohol, Tobacco, Firearms and Explosives, Department of Justice, Washington, DC, USA.

References

[1] American Cancer Society, *Cancer Facts and Figures 2012*, American Cancer Society, Atlanta, Ga, USA, 2012.

[2] American Cancer Society, *Bladder Cancer*, American Cancer Society, Atlanta, Ga, USA, 2012.

[3] N. Howlader, A. M. Noone, M. Krapcho et al., Eds., "SEER Cancer Statistics Review," 1975–2009 (Vintage Populations), Bethesda, Md, USA, National Cancer Institute, 2012, http://seer.cancer.gov/csr/1975_2009_pops09/ based on November 2011 SEER data submission posted to the SEER web site April 2012.

[4] S. M. Cohen, T. Shirai, and G. Steineck, "Epidemiology and etiology of premalignant and malignant urothelial changes," *Scandinavian Journal of Urology and Nephrology, Supplement*, vol. 34, no. 205, pp. 105–115, 2000.

[5] R. W. Clapp, G. Howe, and M. J. Lefevre, *Environmental and Occupational Causes of Cancer, A Review of Recent Scientific Literature*, Lowell Center for Sustainable Production, Lowell, Mass, USA, 2005.

[6] S. M. Olfert, S. A. Felknor, and G. L. Delclos, "An updated review of the literature: risk factors for bladder cancer with focus on occupational exposures," *Southern Medical Journal*, vol. 99, no. 11, pp. 1256–1263, 2006.

[7] R. W. Clapp, M. M. Jacobs, and E. L. Loechler, "Environmental and occupational causes of cancer: new evidence 2005–2007," *Reviews on Environmental Health*, vol. 23, no. 1, pp. 1–37, 2008.

[8] J. L. Nortier, M. C. Martinez, H. H. Schmeiser et al., "Urothelial carcinoma associated with the use of a Chinese herb (Aristolochia fangchi)," *The New England Journal of Medicine*, vol. 342, no. 23, pp. 1686–1692, 2000.

[9] International Agency for Research on Cancer, "Some traditional herbal medicines," *IARC Monographs on the Evaluation of Carcinogenic Risks to Humans*, vol. 82, pp. 69–129, 2002.

[10] A. Lemy, K. M. Wissing, S. Rorive et al., "Late onset of bladder urothelial carcinoma after kidney transplantation for end-stage aristolochic acid nephropathy: a case series with 15-year follow-up," *American Journal of Kidney Diseases*, vol. 51, no. 3, pp. 471–477, 2008.

[11] P. Vineis and L. Simonato, "Estimates of the proportion of bladder cancers attributable to occupation," *Scandinavian Journal of Work, Environment & Health*, vol. 12, no. 1, pp. 55–60, 1986.

[12] P. A. Schulte, K. Ringen, G. P. Hemstreet, and E. Ward, "Occupational cancer of the urinary tract," *Occupational Medicine*, vol. 2, no. 1, pp. 85–107, 1987.

[13] A. L. Golden, S. B. Markowitz, and P. J. Landrigan, "The risk of cancer in firefighters," *Occupational Medicine*, vol. 10, no. 4, pp. 803–820, 1995.

[14] C. M. Lu, S. J. Lan, Y. H. Lee, J. K. Huang, C. H. Huang, and C. C. Hsieh, "Tea consumption: fluid intake and bladder cancer risk in southern Taiwan," *Urology*, vol. 54, no. 5, pp. 823–828, 1999.

[15] D. S. Michaud, D. Spiegelman, S. K. Clinton et al., "Fluid intake and the risk of bladder cancer in men," *The New England Journal of Medicine*, vol. 340, no. 18, pp. 1390–1397, 1999.

[16] M. P. A. Zeegers, E. Dorant, R. A. Goldbohm, and P. A. van den Brandt, "Are coffee, tea, and total fluid consumption associated with bladder cancer risk? Results from the Netherlands cohort study," *Cancer Causes and Control*, vol. 12, no. 3, pp. 231–238, 2001.

[17] B. Geoffroy-Perez and S. Cordier, "Fluid consumption and the risk of bladder cancer: results of a multicenter case-control study," *International Journal of Cancer*, vol. 93, no. 6, pp. 880–887, 2001.

[18] V. Radosavljevic, S. Jankovic, J. Marinkovic J, and M. Djokic, "Fluid intake and bladder cancer. A case control study," *Neoplasma*, vol. 50, no. 3, pp. 234–238, 2003.

[19] M. P. Zeegers, E. Kellen, F. Buntinx, and P. A. van den Brandt, "The association between smoking, beverage consumption, diet and bladder cancer: a systematic literature review," *World Journal of Urology*, vol. 21, no. 6, pp. 392–401, 2004.

[20] D. S. Michaud, M. Kogevinas, K. P. Cantor et al., "Total fluid and water consumption and the joint effect of exposure to disinfection by-products on risk of bladder cancer," *Environmental Health Perspectives*, vol. 115, no. 11, pp. 1569–1572, 2007.

[21] X. Jiang, J. E. Castelao, S. Groshen et al., "Water intake and bladder cancer risk in Los Angeles County," *International Journal of Cancer*, vol. 123, no. 7, pp. 1649–1656, 2008.

[22] M. Hemelt, Z. Hu, Z. Zhong et al., "Fluid intake and the risk of bladder cancer: results from the South and East China case-control study on bladder cancer," *International Journal of Cancer*, vol. 127, no. 3, pp. 638–645, 2010.

[23] M. M. Ros, H. B. Bas Bueno-de-Mesquita, F. L. Büchner et al., "Fluid intake and the risk of urothelial cell carcinomas in the European Prospective Investigation into Cancer and Nutrition (EPIC)," *International Journal of Cancer*, vol. 128, no. 11, pp. 2695–2708, 2011.

[24] C. M. Villanueva, K. P. Cantor, W. D. King et al., "Total and specific fluid consumption as determinants of bladder cancer risk," *International Journal of Cancer*, vol. 118, no. 8, pp. 2040–2047, 2006.

[25] K. Golka, A. Wiese, G. Assennato, and H. M. Bolt, "Occupational exposure and urological cancer," *World Journal of Urology*, vol. 21, no. 6, pp. 382–391, 2004.

[26] N. E. L. Hall and K. D. Rosenman, "Cancer by industry: analysis of a population-based cancer registry with an emphasis on blue-collar workers," *American Journal of Industrial Medicine*, vol. 19, no. 2, pp. 145–159, 1991.

[27] International Agency for Research on Cancer, "Polynuclear aromatic compounds, Part 3: industrial exposures in aluminum production, coal gasification, coke production, and iron and steel founding," *IARC Monographs on the Evaluation of Carcinogenic Risks to Humans*, vol. 34, pp. 1–219, 1984.

[28] International Agency for Research on Cancer, "Overall evaluations of carcinogenicity: an updating of IARC monographs volumes 1 to 42," *IARC Monographs on the Evaluation of Carcinogenic Risks to Humans*, supplement 7, pp. 1–440, 1987.

[29] International Agency for Research on Cancer, "Some non-heterocyclic polycyclic aromatic hydrocarbons and some related compounds," *IARC Monographs on the Evaluation of Carcinogenic Risks to Humans*, vol. 92, pp. 754–759, 2010.

[30] International Agency for Research on Cancer, "Some aromatic amines, organic dyes, and related exposures," *IARC Monographs on the Evaluation of Carcinogenic Risks to Humans*, vol. 99, pp. 1–692, 2010.

[31] P. Gustavsson, A. Gustavsson, and C. Hogstedt, "Excess of cancer in Swedish chimney sweeps," *British Journal of Industrial Medicine*, vol. 45, no. 11, pp. 777–781, 1988.

[32] R. C. Reulen, E. Kellen, F. Buntinx, M. Brinkman, and M. P. Zeegers, "A meta-analysis on the association between bladder cancer and occupation," *Scandinavian Journal of Urology and Nephrology. Supplementum*, no. 218, pp. 64–78, 2008.

[33] E. Pukkala, J. I. Martinsen, E. Lynge et al., "Occupation and cancer follow-up of 15 million people in five Nordic countries," *Acta Oncologica*, vol. 48, no. 5, pp. 646–790, 2009.

[34] International Agency for Research on Cancer, "Painting, firefighting, and shiftwork," *IARC Monographs on the Evaluation of Carcinogenic Risks to Humans*, vol. 98, pp. 43–394, 2010.

[35] P. R. Band, N. D. Le, A. C. MacArthur, R. Fang, and R. P. Gallagher, "Identification of occupational cancer risks in British Columbia: a population-based case-control study of 1129 cases of bladder cancer," *Journal of Occupational and Environmental Medicine*, vol. 47, no. 8, pp. 854–858, 2005.

[36] P. Cole, R. Hoover, and G. H. Friedell, "Occupation and cancer of the lower urinary tract," *Cancer*, vol. 29, no. 5, pp. 1250–1260, 1972.

[37] E. Dryson, A. t' Mannetje, C. Walls et al., "Case-control study of high risk occupations for bladder cancer in New Zealand," *International Journal of Cancer*, vol. 122, no. 6, pp. 1340–1346, 2008.

[38] H. M. Firth, K. R. Cooke, and G. P. Herbison, "Male cancer incidence by occupation: New Zealand, 1972–1984," *International Journal of Epidemiology*, vol. 25, no. 1, pp. 14–21, 1996.

[39] R. R. W. Gaetner, L. TrpeskiL, K. C. Johnson, and Canadian Cancer Registries Epidemiology Research Group, "A case-control study of occupational risk factors for bladder cancer

in Canada," *Cancer Causes and Control*, vol. 15, pp. 1007–1019, 2004.

[40] J. Guo, T. Kauppinen, P. Kyyrönen, P. Heikkilä, M. L. Lindbohm, and E. Pukkala, "Risk of esophageal, ovarian, testicular, kidney and bladder cancers and leukemia among Finnish workers exposed to diesel or gasoline engine exhaust," *International Journal of Cancer*, vol. 111, no. 2, pp. 286–292, 2004.

[41] G. C. Kabat, G. S. Dieck, and E. L. Wynder, "Bladder cancer in nonsmokers," *Cancer*, vol. 57, no. 2, pp. 362–367, 1986.

[42] M. Kogevinas, A. t' Mannetje, S. Cordier et al., "Occupation and bladder cancer among men in Western Europe," *Cancer Causes and Control*, vol. 14, no. 10, pp. 907–914, 2003.

[43] H. A. Risch, J. D. Burch, A. B. Miller, G. B. Hill, R. Steele, and G. R. Howe, "Occupational factors and the incidence of cancer of the bladder in Canada," *British Journal of Industrial Medicine*, vol. 45, no. 6, pp. 361–367, 1988.

[44] R. C. Reulen, E. Kellen, F. Buntinx, and M. P. Zeegers, "Bladder cancer and occupation: a report from the Belgian case-control study on bladder cancer risk," *American Journal of Industrial Medicine*, vol. 50, no. 6, pp. 449–454, 2007.

[45] D. T. Silverman, R. N. Hoover, S. Albert, and K. M. Graff, "Occupation and cancer of the lower urinary tract in Detroit," *Journal of the National Cancer Institute*, vol. 70, no. 2, pp. 237–245, 1983.

[46] K. Teschke, M. S. Morgan, H. Checkoway et al., "Surveillance of nasal and bladder cancer to locate sources of exposure to occupational carcinogens," *Occupational and Environmental Medicine*, vol. 54, no. 6, pp. 443–451, 1997.

[47] G. R. Howe, J. D. Burch, A. B. Miller et al., "Tobacco use, occupation, coffee, various nutrients, and bladder cancer," *Journal of the National Cancer Institute*, vol. 64, no. 4, pp. 701–713, 1980.

[48] F. Forastiere, C. A. Perucci, A. Di Pietro et al., "Mortality among urban policemen in Rome," *American Journal of Industrial Medicine*, vol. 26, no. 6, pp. 785–798, 1994.

[49] J. E. Vena, J. M. Violanti, J. Marshall, and R. C. Fiedler, "Mortality of a municipal worker cohort: III. Police officers," *American Journal of Industrial Medicine*, vol. 10, no. 4, pp. 383–397, 1986.

[50] J. M. Violanti, J. E. Vena, and S. Petralia, "Mortality of a police cohort: 1950–1990," *American Journal of Industrial Medicine*, vol. 33, no. 4, pp. 366–373, 1998.

[51] P. Boffetta, M. Dosemeci, G. Gridley, H. Bath, T. Moradi, and D. Silverman, "Occupational exposure to diesel engine emissions and risk of cancer in Swedish men and women," *Cancer Causes and Control*, vol. 12, no. 4, pp. 365–374, 2001.

[52] K. Richardson, P. R. Band, G. Astrakianakis, and N. D. Le, "Male bladder cancer risk and occupational exposure according to a job-exposure matrix—a case-control study in British Columbia, Canada," *Scandinavian Journal of Work, Environment & Health*, vol. 33, no. 6, pp. 454–464, 2007.

[53] F. Ma, L. E. Fleming, D. J. Lee, E. Trapido, and T. A. Gerace, "Cancer incidence in Florida professional firefighters, 1981 to 1999," *Journal of Occupational and Environmental Medicine*, vol. 48, no. 9, pp. 883–888, 2006.

[54] S. R. Sama, T. R. Martin, L. K. Davis, and D. Kriebel, "Cancer incidence among Massachusetts firefighters, 1982–1986," *American Journal of Industrial Medicine*, vol. 18, no. 2, pp. 47–54, 1990.

[55] H. M. Anthony and G. M. Thomas, "Tumors of the urinary bladder: an analysis of the occupations of 1,030 patients in Leeds, England," *Journal of the National Cancer Institute*, vol. 45, no. 5, pp. 879–895, 1970.

[56] P. Vineis and C. Magnani, "Occupation and bladder cancer in males: a case-control study," *International Journal of Cancer*, vol. 35, no. 5, pp. 599–606, 1985.

[57] A. J. Alberg, A. Kouzis, J. M. Genkinger et al., "A prospective cohort study of bladder cancer risk in relation to active cigarette smoking and household exposure to secondhand cigarette smoke," *American Journal of Epidemiology*, vol. 165, no. 6, pp. 660–666, 2007.

[58] A. J. Alberg and J. R. Hébert, "Cigarette smoking and bladder cancer: a new twist in an old saga?" *Journal of the National Cancer Institute*, vol. 101, no. 22, pp. 1525–1526, 2009.

[59] D. Baris, M. R. Karagas, C. Verrill et al., "A case-control study of smoking and bladder cancer risk: emergent patterns over time," *Journal of the National Cancer Institute*, vol. 101, no. 22, pp. 1553–1561, 2009.

Does Playground Improvement Increase Physical Activity among Children? A Quasi-Experimental Study of a Natural Experiment

Erika E. Bohn-Goldbaum,[1] Philayrath Phongsavan,[1] Dafna Merom,[2] Kris Rogers,[1] Venugopal Kamalesh,[3] and Adrian E. Bauman[1]

[1] *Prevention Research Collaboration, School of Public Health, The University of Sydney, NSW 2006, Australia*
[2] *School of Science and Health, University of Western Sydney, Camperdown Campus, NSW, Australia*
[3] *IMPACT Strategic Research Centre, School of Medicine, Deakin University, VIC, Australia*

Correspondence should be addressed to Erika E. Bohn-Goldbaum; erika.goldbaum@sydney.edu.au

Academic Editor: Pam R. Factor-Litvak

Outdoor recreational spaces have the potential to increase physical activity. This study used a quasi-experimental evaluation design to determine how a playground renovation impacts usage and physical activity of children and whether the visitations correlate with children's physical activity levels and parental impressions of the playground. Observational data and intercept interviews were collected simultaneously on park use and park-based activity among playground visitors at pre- and postrenovation at an intervention and a comparison park during three 2-hour periods each day over two weeks. No detectable difference in use between parks was observed at followup. In the intervention park, attendance increased among boys, but decreased among girls although this (nonsignificant) decline was less marked than in the comparison park. Following renovation, there was no detectable difference between parks in the number of children engaged in MVPA (interaction between park and time: $P = 0.73$). At the intervention park, there was a significant decline in girls engaging in MVPA at followup ($P = 0.04$). Usage was correlated with parental/carer perceptions of playground features but not with physical activity levels. Renovations have limited the potential to increase physical activity until factors influencing usage and physical activity behavior are better understood.

1. Introduction

Regular moderate-intensity physical activity (PA) can confer substantial health benefits for children, including reducing risks for chronic diseases, maintaining healthy body weight, and improving social and mental health [1]. Despite the importance of PA to health, only about one-quarter of the Australian children meet the recommended 60 minutes of moderate to vigorous physical activity (MVPA) daily [2]. Inactive children are at greater risk of being overweight or obese [3–5]. In Australia, about one-quarter of children are either overweight or obese [6, 7].

Structured as well as unstructured activities like walking, cycling, and in particular outdoor active free play have been shown to be associated with children's PA [8, 9]. Neighborhood environments [10] as well as specific aspects, such as park quality and proximity to playgrounds, have also been shown to be associated with numerous psychological and social benefits to adults and children [11, 12] and healthy body mass index in Canadian children [13]. Public parks can also provide recreational spaces for active play to support children's PA participation [12, 14–16].

Among Australian schoolchildren, time spent outdoors is correlated to time spent in MVPA and can predict higher MVPA levels in boys [8]. However, children are more likely to spend outdoor time in home backyards than in playgrounds [17]. To support opportunities for children's PA, particularly in low-income urban environments in which homes have small or no backyards, the provision of quality public outdoor spaces which support PA may be an important public health strategy. Among recreational areas specifically designed to support children's PA, such as playgrounds, swimming pools and playfields, playgrounds are the most frequently used [18]. Also, children are more active in playgrounds than in other park activity areas such as fields [19].

Cross-sectional and qualitative studies of park and playground use by children identified perceptions of quantity and quality of park amenities [20, 21] and park and neighborhood safety to be linked to parents encouraging their child to use playgrounds [13, 16, 20–24] and parks [25]. These studies also highlighted that the distance to parks, which is the strongest determinant of adults' visits [14, 26], is less clear in children's park use and may be secondary to park amenities [22, 23].

Environmental interventions such as park upgrades have the potential to facilitate increased park usage and to provide more opportunities for PA. In school settings, playground improvements increase student's playground usage and PA [27–32]; yet the impact of playground renovations in the community on usage and PA is still unclear. Quigg and colleagues [33] found environmental changes alone to be ineffective in increasing PA. Total daily PA was not significantly different at followup among school-age children living in a community with renovated playgrounds compared to those with unrenovated playgrounds. These results need to be interpreted with caution as only two of six playgrounds in the intervention setting actually underwent renovations, playground usage was not measured, and the type of playgrounds (i.e., "standalone" or within a park) was not described. Tester and Baker [34] found increased visits in a renovated playground among girls but a decline among boys. Thus, the effects of structural changes alone on children's playground usage and PA levels remain unknown.

An opportunity to observe the effects of environmental changes in a children's playground on usage, PA behavior, and users' perceptions arose in a metropolitan area of Sydney, Australia. Using a quasi-experimental design, the aims of the current study were to (1) determine if an urban park renovation that included playground alterations affects usage and PA in children within playgrounds; (2) determine whether playground alterations affects parents' self-report of playground visitation post intervention, in association with proxy reports of children's PA levels; and (3) assess parental impressions of environmental features (e.g., equipment safety) of the renovated playground post intervention.

2. Methods

2.1. Study Setting. The intervention Park A for this study is located in a lower socioeconomic urban neighborhood within the city of Sydney, the council responsible for the central Sydney areas. The comparison park (Park B) was chosen for its similarities to Park A and is located in a nearby urban neighborhood within the city of Sydney. These similarly sized parks each included a playground, a large open area, and a sports field; several small "standalone" playgrounds can be found within a short walk of each of these parks. The neighborhood population of Park B is generally socioeconomically similar to Park A (e.g., percent population identified as Indigenous) though it has a higher employment rate and a higher proportion of English-only speaking households [35, 36].

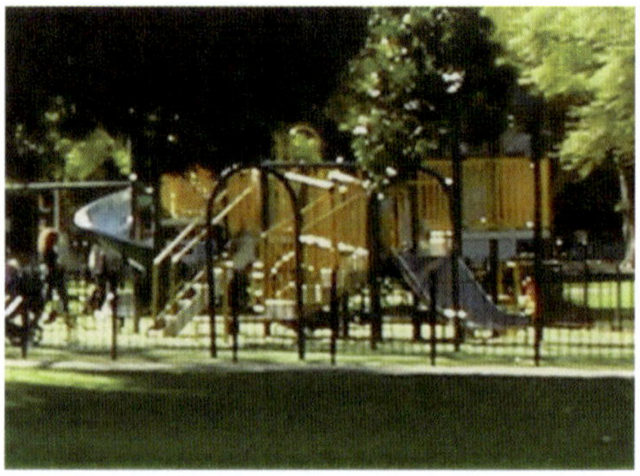

Figure 1: Playground in Park A, prerenovation. The gated playground included a large multifunction apparatus on soft-fall flooring in a gated area in the middle of the park.

2.2. Elements of Park Upgrade. Sydney's recreational strategy aims to "increase participation by residents in physical activity thereby enhancing their health and well-being" [37] and its objectives for this park renovation included provision for recreation and children's play by "amenities to facilitate use and enjoyment . . .including but not limited to children's play equipment" [38]. Specific changes in the park renovation included upgrading paths and adding new greenery, lighting, and facilities (e.g., park furniture). More green space was created by opening the adjacent sports field to public use, thus increasing the accessible park size from 2.2 to 4.6 ha.

Prior to the upgrade, there was one playground located near the center of the park. As shown in Figure 1, the gated playground had soft-fall flooring and included a large multifunction apparatus, multiple swings, slides, and other equipment. The new children's playgrounds are three unfenced areas dispersed throughout the park. The playgrounds incorporate the city of Sydney's design mandate to include public art, an aboriginal theme, and, following community consultation, a water play feature. One area includes two swings and a climbing structure designed for use primarily by young children, with wood chips as flooring. For children up to 7 years old, play sculptures with a soft-fall surface and an interactive water feature on cement were installed in a second area, as shown in Figure 2. A third play area, for older children, is comprised of three climbing poles with wood chips as flooring. As part of the upgrade, a large cement area for basketball and skating was installed adjacent to the poles.

The comparison park was chosen for its similar size (4.2 ha) and type of park. Its playground is similar to the prerenovation playground in Park A: a fenced area with soft-fall flooring and containing multifunction apparatuses, swings, slides, and other equipment as shown in Figure 3. The comparison playground had a shade net and equipment pieces were grouped into toddler and school-age sections.

2.3. Study Design. This study employed a quasi-experimental pre-post evaluation design with a comparison park. Data from two cross-sectional observational and intercept interviews were collected before and after the upgrade. Data collection involved children aged 2–12 years and their parents

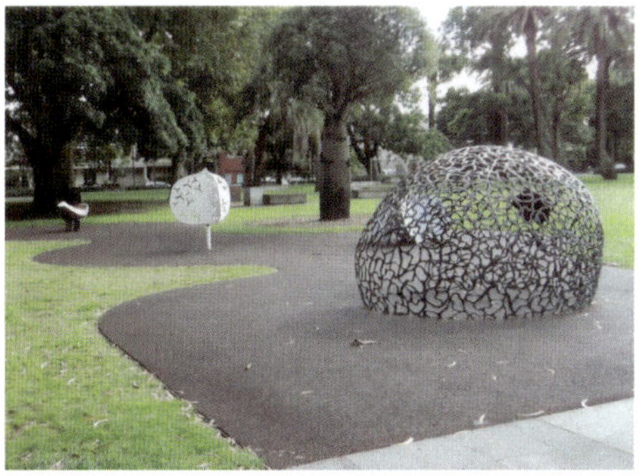

Figure 2: Playground in Park A, postrenovation. Play sculptures on soft-fall flooring were installed in an open area.

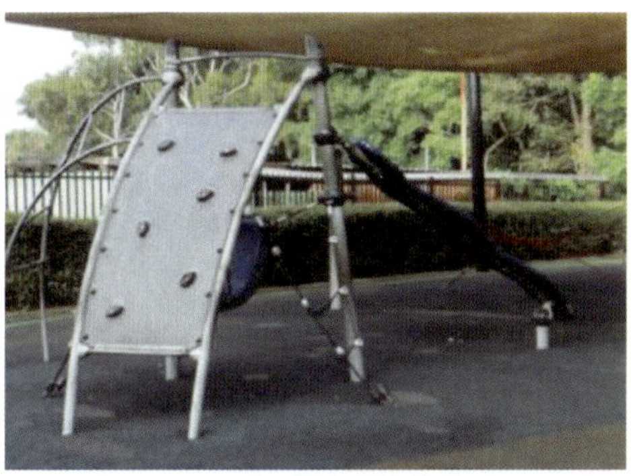

Figure 3: Playground in Park B. The gated and shaded playground featured more traditional style equipment on a soft-fall surface.

or care givers (hereafter referred to as parents) in intervention and comparison parks in May 2007 prior to the upgrade, and nine months after the upgrade completed in May 2009. The study was approved by the University of Sydney Ethics Committee (Ref. no. 04-2007/9905).

2.4. Data Collection

2.4.1. Direct Observation. Systematic observations of playground visitors aged 2–12 years were carried out using the System for Observing Play and Recreation in Communities (SOPARC) [31] adapted for use in Sydney [39]. SOPARC uses momentary time sampling to measure park user characteristics and PA behavior and has been determined to produce acceptable reliability and validity [40].

Each park was divided into target areas for observation. The children's playground was one of four preupgrade observation areas in the intervention park. Due to significant changes in park design and accessible area with the upgrade, the postupgrade observation areas were changed to six areas with the three playground areas each being a unique observation area. At analysis, the data from scans for these three playground observation areas were combined as one scan to provide an accurate picture of total playground usage. In the comparison park, the children's playground was one of four observation areas.

Staff scanned target areas from left to right every thirty minutes during the observation periods and recorded park users' gender, age, activity type, and activity intensity. Activity type included both sedentary and active pursuits. Activity intensity was coded light, moderate, or vigorous.

Direct observation was conducted over a 2-week period during clement weather in May 2007 and May 2009. Observations occurred simultaneously at both parks during 2-hour periods in the morning (7:00–9:00), mid-day (11:30–13:30), and afternoon (15:00–17:00). All field staff including the authors (EB) participated in one full day of data collection training, followed by a half-day field practice in park observation. The interrater tests included nine field staff in 2007 and 13 field staff in 2009. The intraclass coefficients (ICC) in 2007 for total counts, gender, age, and PA intensity (light/sedentary versus MVPA) were 0.67, 0.82, 0.94, and 0.68, respectively. The corresponding ICCs for 2009 were 0.89, 0.92, 0.86, and 0.94, respectively.

2.4.2. Park User Interviews. Postupgrade intercept surveys were conducted with consenting park users aged 16 years or older who were accompanied by children under 13 years of age. Ages were verified verbally with participants. Intercept surveys, brief face-to-face interviews with park users, were conducted in both parks using the Sydney Parks User Interview Survey [39] to measure parent's demographics, PA behavior, and park usage. Postintervention interviews were supplemented with a retrospective question on playground use to capture the intervention context and questions regarding children's playground usage. Perceptions of park features were measured using a 5-point Likert scale, and playground features used a 4-point scale of agreement. These were followed by an open-ended question for additional comments. Respondents were also asked about the PA behavior of their oldest child aged 5–12 years, using questions derived from a state-wide New South Wales Population Health Survey [41]. These questions asked the number of days and hours on weekdays and weekend days a child engaged in PA outside of school hours.

Interviews were conducted by one of the authors (EB) between 10:30 and 17:00 hours on the same days during which direct observation was performed. Interviews were conducted throughout the park space, one interview per target area, rotating through all target areas for each data collection period. In the event of a refusal, another park user within the same area was approached; if no users participated in a given target area, data collection directly continued in the next target area. The researcher (EB) received interview training during the observation training sessions.

Two new pieces of school-age play equipment were installed in Park A in August 2009, and a café in the park grounds opened. Therefore, the intercept survey was repeated on clement days over a two-week period in September 2009.

2.5. Statistical Analyses. The primary outcomes were the daily mean number of children visiting playgrounds, and the proportion of children engaging in MVPA based on observational data. The first set of analyses examined both

TABLE 1: Children's playground usage in intervention Park A and comparison Park B, pre- and postintervention, expressed as mean number of children per 2-hour observation period.

	Boy		Girl		Total children	
	Pre[a]	Post	Pre[a]	Post	Pre[a]	Post
Intervention Park A*	3.95 (4.68)	5.33 (5.92)	5.05 (5.41)	4.62 (6.30)	4.50 (5.03)	4.98 (6.05)
Comparison Park B	7.76 (8.30)	7.71 (6.91)	9.29 (11.59)	5.67 (6.37)	8.52 (9.99)	6.69 (6.64)

Note: Data included observations from scans performed every 30 minutes during three 2-hour periods on 5 weekdays and 2 weekend days; $n = 84$ scans for Park A and Park B (preintervention), and 80 for Park B post intervention. *In Park A at followup, three scan areas included play equipment; these three scans were combined as one for comparison purposes. Means were compared via a generalized linear model, with significance set at $P < 0.05$. [a]A significant difference was found between parks.

playground use and MVPA. Using data from the Bureau of Meteorology, dates from pre- and postintervention were matched for clemency; this resulted in data from five weekdays and two weekend days from each time period being used. Data points concerning infants were omitted. Due to large fluctuations in usage, there was some variation in the number of scans per 2-hour observation periods both within and between parks. To standardize this difference, usage means (observed persons per observation period) were calculated for playground usage for total children and by gender. Overall differences between pre- and postintervention counts of children and children engaged in MVPA were tested using a generalized linear model. An initial examination of the data revealed that both counts were not normally distributed and too dispersed for a Poisson model, so these were modeled with a negative binomial distribution (with log link function) to allow for overdispersion. Deviance (from the "perfect" model) was used to assess the fit of the model. Models were fitted for each count (total children + total in MVPA) with park (Park A versus Park B) and time (pre- and postintervention) and adjusted for gender (as a covariate). The interaction between the park and time variables was used to test if the amount of change within parks from pre- to postintervention was meaningfully different between Park A and Park B.

The second set of analyses examined parent's playground usage profile, their familiarity with Park A's playground prior to renovation, and parent's proxy report of their children's PA levels, based on intercept survey. Survey participation in Park B ($n = 17$ parents) was inadequate for analysis and therefore is not presented here. Chi-square tests were used to test associations between parent usage profile and follow-up study groups at significance level of 0.05. The questions and computation of children's PA levels followed the protocol from the New South Wales Population Health Survey [41]. Parents reported the number of hours on weekdays and weekend days their oldest child between the ages of 5 and 12 years engaged in physical activity outside of school hours. Total physical activity hours per week were summed, and a daily mean was calculated. Sufficient physical activity was defined as meeting or exceeding the recommended daily hour of at least moderate-intensity physical activity.

The third set of analyses examined parent's impressions of environmental features (e.g., equipment safety) of the renovated playground, based on intercept survey. For open-ended questions, answers were grouped according to themes. Statistical analyses were conducted using PASW 19 (IBM-SPSS Inc., 2009) and SAS 9.2 (SAS Institute, Cary, NC, USA).

3. Results

3.1. Playground Use. As shown in Table 1, children's playground usage at baseline was lower in the intervention Park A compared to comparison Park B (likelihood ratio test: $P = 0.03$). This difference could be due to a childcare facility being located next to the comparison park. However, there was no detectable difference between the parks at followup (interaction between park and time: $P = 0.42$), when the mean number of children in the playground in Park A increased by approximately 10% ($P = 0.74$) and decreased by 22% at Park B ($P = 0.42$). There was no difference in usage according to gender ($P = 0.97$) in the use of parks before or after intervention. When analyzed by gender, the playgrounds exhibited similar changes in usage over time in girls but not in boys. Attendance decreased for girls at both parks, but for boys this remained unchanged (Park B) or increased (Park A); however, none of these pre-post renovation changes were statistically significant.

At baseline, fewer children performed MVPA in Park A than in Park B ($P = 0.02$), as shown in Table 2. After the park upgrade, there was no detectable difference between parks in the number of children engaged in MVPA (interaction between park and time: $P = 0.73$); the proportion of physically active children had decreased by 41% at the intervention playground and by 32% at the comparison playground. Boys were slightly more active than girls in both parks at baseline and followup although this difference was not statistically significant ($P = 0.09$). Within the intervention park, there was a significant decline in girls engaging in MVPA at followup ($P = 0.04$).

3.2. Parental Park Use and Physical Activity Level of Children. A total of 140 parents (73% response rate) took part in the postintervention interviews. There were no significant differences in sociodemographic characteristics between the survey participants at the two survey points ($n = 75$ in May and $n = 65$ in September), with the exception of a higher percentage of mothers in September (73.0%) than in May (53.2%, $P < 0.01$).

More than half of the parents visited Park A at least once per week (Table 3). First time visitors accounted for approximately 13% of the respondents. A lower proportion

TABLE 2: Children engaged in MVPA in playground in Intervention Park A and Comparison Park B, preand post intervention, expressed as mean number of children engaged in MVPA per 2-hour observation period.

	Boy		Girl		Total children	
	Pre[a]	Post[a]	Pre[a]	Post[a,b]	Pre[a]	Post[a]
Intervention Park A*	1.19 (2.09)	1.10 (1.51)	1.14 (2.37)	0.24 (0.44)	1.17 (2.21)	0.67 (1.18)
Comparison Park B	3.19 (4.76)	2.38 (3.79)	2.52 (3.03)	1.57 (2.04)	2.86 (3.95)	1.98 (3.03)

Note: Data included observations from scans performed every 30 minutes during three 2-hour periods on 5 weekdays and 2 weekend days; $n = 84$ scans for Park A and Park B (preintervention), and 80 for Park B postintervention. *In Park A at followup, three scan areas included play equipment; these three scans were combined as one for comparison purposes. Means were compared via generalized linear model, with significance set at $P < 0.05$. [a]A significant difference was found between parks. [b]A significant difference was found between pre and postintervention MVPA for girls in Park A.

TABLE 3: Playground use profile of parents in playground of intervention Park A as measured by intercept survey postintervention, percent (number).

	Total ($n = 140$)	May ($n = 75$)	September ($n = 65$)	Chi-square (P value)
Playground visit frequency				
At least once per week	59.4 (79)	57.7 (41)	61.3 (38)	$\chi^2_{(2)} = 1.51$ (0.47)
1-2 per fortnight or less	27.1 (36)	31.0 (22)	22.6 (14)	
First time	13.5 (18)	11.3 (8)	16.1 (10)	
Visited playground before renovation				
Yes	58.6 (82)	66.7 (50)	49.2 (32)	$\chi^2_{(1)} = 4.36$ (0.04)
No	41.4 (58)	33.3 (25)	50.8 (33)	

of survey respondents from September had visited the playground before the renovation (49.2%) than those from May (66.7%, $P = 0.04$). Respondents reported that at least half of the children achieved at least one hour daily PA (Table 4). There was no significant difference with time or by gender. Attainment of sufficient daily PA was not correlated with frequency of park use ($P = 0.23$).

3.3. Park Features. Parents were overwhelmingly positive about the renovated Park A, with 88% agreeing it was well-maintained and 75% finding it attractive. General park safety was rated positively by 68% of parents; of those feeling unsafe, crime (40.4%) and safety (34%) in the park were the main concerns. The majority (61%) felt the park offered social opportunities. Opinions regarding the play equipment characteristics were also mostly positive. Most parents agreed there was a good variety of equipment (64.5%), the equipment was safe and in good condition (83.9%), and it was adventurous or exciting (71.9%). Participants were divided on whether there was sufficient play equipment (49.6% agreement). In general, perceptions of the park and playground were not affected by time of data collection (May versus September; $P > 0.1$ for all variables) or frequency of playground visitation ($P > 0.41$). The two exceptions were that the less frequent (less than once per week) playground visitors were more likely than high frequency (at least once per week) visitors to find the equipment adventurous or exciting ($P < 0.03$) and safe and in good condition ($P < 0.03$).

The majority (69%) of interviewed parents offered one or more remarks when asked for comments regarding the upgraded playground; sociodemographic differences between these parents and the total sample were not statistically significant ($P > 0.07$). Two major themes emerged from these comments: a lack of play equipment and a presence of safety concerns. Forty-nine respondents believed that the playground lacked certain playground equipment, particularly slides and sufficient swings. Comments regarding safety related primarily to concerns about the unfenced toddler play area: its placing close to a road, its lack of fencing, and its woodchip surfacing. Comments regarding the nontraditional play equipment comprised a third theme. Parent's perceptions were mixed, describing these structures as "an art gallery," "style over substance," and "of limited value to kids." Participants' main reason to visit playgrounds was to let children play, and nearly all parents (90%) reported frequenting other playgrounds as well. Their main reason(s) for choosing the other playgrounds included equipment and convenience. Playgrounds which offered a variety of equipment were popular; the amount or type of equipment was important as well. Typical comments included choosing a playground because it offered "lots of equipments," "lots of swings," or "big slides."

4. Discussion

While increasing children's PA levels may not be the primary motivation for playground/park upgrades by local council authorities, cross-sectional evidence to date suggests that using public open spaces involves some level of physical activity. Examining the level of effects following physical environmental changes is, therefore, worth investigating. This evaluation study of a natural experiment provides preliminary evidence on the impact of a playground upgrade on both usage and PA behaviors among children. We found that following playground renovation usage between the intervention and comparison parks did not differ. While usage among

TABLE 4: Physical activity level of children of playground intervention Park A users as measured by parental proxy questionnaire, postintervention.

Physical activity	Total % ($n = 58$)	May % ($n = 34$)	September % ($n = 24$)	Chi-square (P value)
Sufficient activity	55.2 (32)	58.8 (20)	50.0 (12)	$\chi^2_{(1)} = 0.44$ (0.51)
Insufficient activity	44.8 (26)	41.2 (14)	50.0 (12)	

Parents were asked to report the number of hours of physical activity on weekdays and weekend days engaged in by their oldest child between the ages of 5 and 12 years. A daily mean of MVPA was then calculated. Sufficient physical activity was defined as attaining the recommended daily hour of MVPA.

girls decreased at both playgrounds, the (nonsignificant) decline was less marked at the renovated playground. Among boys, usage increased more at the renovated playground, but this was also nonsignificant. This finding is consistent with other studies which found more boys than girls using renovated school playgrounds [28] and at renovated public playfields [34]. Together, these results suggest that structural changes at public playgrounds can influence boys' usage but may be less effective in affecting usage by girls.

This study observed a decline in children's MVPA levels post renovation; this decrease was significant in girls at the renovated playground. Other playground renovation studies have found increases [27, 42] or no difference [28] in activity levels. The conflicting results of those studies with present results may be explained by differences in study setting (school playgrounds) and design. The changes in the playground design which dispersed the play equipment throughout the renovated park likely also impacted the MVPA levels: the resulting playground scan areas now also included amenities (e.g., picnic tables and large open spaces) associated with more sedentary behavior [29, 43, 44].

A unique contribution of the present study is the interviews which were conducted simultaneously with the observational measurements. These interviews elucidate factors which may explain the observed lack of significant positive effect in playground usage and MVPA. We found that although the perception of overall park safety during the day was not related to frequency of usage ($P = 0.49$), perception of the playground equipment safety was a factor, with frequent visitors less inclined to perceive the equipment as safe and in good condition than infrequent visitors ($P < 0.03$). Specific concerns expressed by parents in regards to the safety of fencing and flooring of the renovated playground suggest these safety factors could play a role in the observed usage and MVPA levels in that specific area. Parents are hesitant to endanger children through use of playground equipment perceived as dangerous [45]. If these parents discouraged their children from using the "unsafe" equipment, then the children are left to play in empty spaces, and in such areas children are less active than in areas with play structures [29].

The perception of equipment as "adventurous or exciting" may also be important to stimulate playground usage, at least initially. In this study, there was a trend for increased usage and an increase in the proportion of parents who were new to the renovated playground after additional equipment was added, but a lower proportion of frequent users, compared to infrequent users, agreeing that the equipment was "adventurous or exciting" in character (chi-square test with $P < 0.03$). Thus, the equipment appears to have stimulated attraction but not to play a role in continued playground use. This agrees with a recent study [46] which found unique equipment merely fosters interest in, but not usage of, public playgrounds.

For sustainable and active use, specific types of equipment (e.g., water features and maneuverable equipment) appear to be important. Though parents found the water feature on this renovated playground attractive, what influenced them to visit other local playgrounds was the presence of traditional equipment, like swings or slides, or maneuverable materials like play trucks. Previous studies agree that specific types of equipment (e.g. water features and loose equipment) influence public and school playground use [16, 21, 22, 29]. In this study, the sculptures supported creative play but, by design, were focused on passive use (e.g. sitting and reading) [47], as opposed to providing for a variety of physical activities like hanging and sliding; they were "aesthetic but not functional". Thus, the sculptures' focus possibly explains the observed decline in MVPA in the study playground.

If equipment qualities like safety or functionality are important for supporting playground usage and PA behaviors, could the amount or variety of equipment also play a role? At first glance, usage appears to depend on equipment amount but not variety. In this study, observed usage slightly increased on the renovated playground which had more pieces of equipment but offered less variation in activities compared to preupgrade. This is consistent with a previous finding [48] that usage in renovated playgrounds was related to the number of equipment pieces but not the number of unique types of play offered. However, parent comments in this study and others [16, 21, 22] support the ideas that specific equipment types influence playground usage and diversity of equipment is desirable [23, 49]. Consider also that perceptions of equipment sufficiency and variety in this study remained unchanged following the additions of the basketball courts and skate park. This equipment was designed for older children but tended to be used more by adolescents and young adults and hence may have been perceived by the parents as having no play value. Thus, both the amounts of equipment and perceived play value may be factors in playground usage.

Any relationship between MVPA behavior and the amount or variety of equipment may also have underlying nuances. In this study, MVPA decreased in the renovated playground which had more equipment but less play variety. Previous studies have reported that children's PA levels were directly correlated to the number of equipment pieces on school playgrounds [50, 51]; however, MVPA levels were not correlated with the total number or number of unique equipment types in a separate study [48]. The key to supporting children's PA attainment may instead relate to functional aspects of the play equipment (play affordances) [29, 49]. Additionally, these affordances may vary with gender in terms of preferred equipment, types of play [27, 45, 52], and PA levels: girls' PA levels were higher in renovated playground areas with swings, play equipment, and fields and lower in renovated hard surface areas such as basketball courts than in control playgrounds [27]. In this study, the observed decrease in girls' MVPA levels following the renovation which reduced the number of swings and other active play equipment supports the idea that specific play affordances are critical to fostering PA, particularly in girls.

Further, this study found no correlation between playground usage and the level of children's daily PA. Other research noted that children obtain less than 2% of their PA in public parks [53]. This can mean that either playground use does not lead to overall daily PA levels among children, or that more could be done to maximize playgrounds (and parks) as an affordable setting to get children to be more active, particularly in low-income neighborhoods.

There are a number of limitations in this study. Firstly, the generalizability is limited because the findings relate to one intervention and comparison park. Secondly, changes in playground layout resulted in observation scan areas at followup that include both play equipment and other park amenities. This complicated the comparison of playground usage and PA levels. While the observation periods occurred at predetermined times throughout the day totaling six hours per day for 14 days, this period may neither be representative of total playground use nor capture secular variations in usage and PA. Our inter-rater agreement for PA levels (sedentary/light versus MVPA) was lower than that reported in a previous study which used a similar tool [40], but also higher at followup. This could be because more people were doing light/sedentary activities at followup; there were relatively few PA observations classified at MVPA level. Alternatively, there may be a greater error in our baseline survey in relation to MVPA assessment, and so our findings for decline may be biased. Furthermore, this was a short-term followup post renovation; a long-term followup might result in increased usage or other changes. The study estimates, however, do provide a snapshot of playground use by gender and PA level.

In addition, no intercept survey of parents was conducted prior to the upgrade, thus limiting the ability to infer change from baseline to followup. Due to the small sample size of those completing intercept surveys in the comparison park, we were unable to compare parental views between intervention and comparison parks. The intercept surveys relied on parental proxy reports of their children's PA, which could result in biased reporting.

Despite its limitations, this study contributes some initial evidence on the relationship between the built environment and PA of children, in particular examining children's usage of and PA levels in playgrounds following an upgrade to an inner city park in Sydney. In addition, this study presents findings of parental preferences for play equipment and playground design in the same areas and at the same time as the direct observation of the children was conducted.

5. Conclusions

In this study playground renovations did not translate to an increase in observed MVPA among children. Parental perceptions of playground equipment may explain attendance and PA levels. This study adds to the growing evidence that there are many factors influencing playground usage and PA behavior. Future research should investigate the relationship between specific play equipment characteristics, children's usage, and PA behavior in playgrounds so that the health benefits of environmental changes are maximized. Determining whether such relationships are influenced by playground setting (e.g. in school or in public parks) and other features (e.g. presence of other activity areas) can help guide policies which promote sustained active usage of playgrounds.

Conflict of Interests

The authors declare that they have no conflict of interests.

Authors' Contribution

Erika E. Bohn-Goldbaum conducted data collection, data analysis and drafted the paper; Philayrath Phongsavan conceived study design, developed data collection instruments, contributed to analysis protocol and results interpretation, and contributed to drafting the paper; Dafna Merom conceived study design, developed data collection instruments, contributed to analysis protocol, data analysis, and results interpretation, and contributed to drafting the paper; Kris Rogers and Venugopal Kamalesh conducted data analyses and contributed to paper drafts; Adrian E. Bauman contributed to study design, results interpretation, and commented on paper drafts. All authors read and approved the final paper.

Acknowledgments

The authors wish to thank the city of Sydney for enabling the study to be undertaken; the Prevention Research Collaboration project officers, Bronwyn McGill and Belinda Von Hofe, for day-to-day management of the study; field staff for data collection; and study parents and children for taking part in the interviews. This study was funded by the Cluster for Physical Activity and Health, Prevention Research Collaboration, School of Public Health, the University of Sydney.

References

[1] I. Janssen and A. G. LeBlanc, "Systematic review of the health benefits of physical activity and fitness in school-aged children and youth," *International Journal of Behavioral Nutrition and Physical Activity*, vol. 7, article 40, 2010.

[2] Centre for Epidemiology and Research, *2008 Summary Report on Adult Health from the New South Wales Population Health Survey*, NSW Department of Health, Sydney, Australia, 2009.

[3] J. A. O'Dea, "Why do kids eat healthful food? Perceived benefits of and barriers to healthful eating and physical activity among children and adolescents," *Journal of the American Dietetic Association*, vol. 103, no. 4, pp. 497–501, 2003.

[4] World Health Organization, "Childhood overweight and obesity," World Health Organization, Geneva, Switzerland, 2011, http://www.who.int/dietphysicalactivity/childhood/en/index.html.

[5] World Health Organization, "Activity and young people," Geneva, 2011, http://www.who.int/dietphysicalactivity/factsheet_young_people/en/index.html.

[6] Australian Bureau of Statistics, "National Health Survey: summary of results, 2007-08 (Reissue), risk factors," 2009, http://www.abs.gov.au/.

[7] M. Booth, A. Okely, E. Denney-Wilson, L. Hardy, B. Yang, and T. Dobbins, *New South Wales Schools Physical Activity and Nutrition Survey (SPANS) 2004: Self Reported Activity*, New South Wales Department of Health, Sydney, Australia, 2006.

[8] V. Cleland, D. Crawford, L. A. Baur, C. Hume, A. Timperio, and J. Salmon, "A prospective examination of children's time spent outdoors, objectively measured physical activity and overweight," *International Journal of Obesity*, vol. 32, no. 11, pp. 1685–1693, 2008.

[9] J. F. Sallis, J. J. Prochaska, and W. C. Taylor, "A review of correlates of physical activity of children and adolescents," *Medicine and Science in Sports and Exercise*, vol. 32, no. 5, pp. 963–975, 2000.

[10] G. de Bruijn, S. P. J. Kremers, G. Lensvelt-Mulders, H. de Vries, W. van Mechelen, and J. Brug, "Modeling individual and physical environmental factors with adolescent physical activity," *American Journal of Preventive Medicine*, vol. 30, no. 6, pp. 507–512, 2006.

[11] S. E. Coen and N. A. Ross, "Exploring the material basis for health: characteristics of parks in Montreal neighborhoods with contrasting health outcomes," *Health and Place*, vol. 12, no. 4, pp. 361–371, 2006.

[12] A. L. Bedimo-Rung, A. J. Mowen, and D. A. Cohen, "The significance of parks to physical activity and public health: a conceptual model," *American Journal of Preventive Medicine*, vol. 28, no. 2, pp. 159–168, 2005.

[13] L. R. Potwarka, A. T. Kaczynski, and A. L. Flack, "Places to play: association of park space and facilities with healthy weight status among children," *Journal of Community Health*, vol. 33, no. 5, pp. 344–350, 2008.

[14] D. A. Cohen, T. L. McKenzie, A. Sehgal, S. Williamson, D. Golinelli, and N. Lurie, "Contribution of public parks to physical activity," *American Journal of Public Health*, vol. 97, no. 3, pp. 509–514, 2007.

[15] B. Giles-Corti and R. J. Donovan, "The relative influence of individual, social and physical environment determinants of physical activity," *Social Science and Medicine*, vol. 54, no. 12, pp. 1793–1812, 2002.

[16] J. Veitch, J. Salmon, and K. Ball, "Children's perceptions of the use of public open spaces for active free-play," *Children's Geographies*, vol. 5, no. 4, pp. 409–422, 2007.

[17] J. Veitch, J. Salmon, and K. Ball, "Children's active free play in local neighborhoods: a behavioral mapping study," *Health Education Research*, vol. 23, no. 5, pp. 870–879, 2008.

[18] J. A. Reed and S. P. Hooker, "Where are youth physically active? A descriptive examination of 45 parks in a southeastern community," *Childhood Obesity*, vol. 8, no. 2, pp. 124–131, 2012.

[19] J. O. Spengler, M. F. Floyd, J. E. Maddock, P. H. Gobster, L. J. Suau, and G. J. Norman, "Correlates of park-based physical activity among children in diverse communities: results from an observational study in two cities," *American Journal of Health Promotion*, vol. 25, no. 5, pp. e1–e9, 2011.

[20] R. Miles, "Neighborhood disorder, perceived safety, and readiness to encourage use of local playgrounds," *American Journal of Preventive Medicine*, vol. 34, no. 4, pp. 275–281, 2008.

[21] A. Pearce, C. Kirk, S. Cummins et al., "Gaining children's perspectives: a multiple method approach to explore environmental influences on healthy eating and physical activity," *Health and Place*, vol. 15, no. 2, pp. 614–621, 2009.

[22] P. Tucker, J. Gilliland, and J. D. Irwin, "Splashpads, swings, and shade: parents' preferences for neighbourhood parks," *Canadian Journal of Public Health*, vol. 98, no. 3, pp. 198–202, 2007.

[23] J. Veitch, S. Bagley, K. Ball, and J. Salmon, "Where do children usually play? A qualitative study of parents' perceptions of influences on children's active free-play," *Health and Place*, vol. 12, no. 4, pp. 383–393, 2006.

[24] L. A. Weir, D. Etelson, and D. A. Brand, "Parents' perceptions of neighborhood safety and children's physical activity," *Preventive Medicine*, vol. 43, no. 3, pp. 212–217, 2006.

[25] N. Christie, H. Ward, R. Kimberlee, E. Towner, and J. Sleney, "Understanding high traffic injury risks for children in low socioeconomic areas: a qualitative study of parents' views," *Injury Prevention*, vol. 13, no. 6, pp. 394–397, 2007.

[26] A. Mowen, E. Orsega-Smith, L. Payne, B. Ainsworth, and G. Godbey, "The role of park proximity and social support in shaping park visitation, physical activity, and perceived health among older adults," *Journal of Physical Activity & Health*, vol. 4, no. 2, pp. 167–179, 2007.

[27] L. A. Brink, C. R. Nigg, S. M. R. Lampe, B. A. Kingston, A. L. Mootz, and W. Van Vliet, "Influence of schoolyard renovations on children's physical activity: the learning landscapes program," *American Journal of Public Health*, vol. 100, no. 9, pp. 1672–1678, 2010.

[28] N. Colabianchi, A. E. Kinsella, C. J. Coulton, and S. M. Moore, "Utilization and physical activity levels at renovated and unrenovated school playgrounds," *Preventive Medicine*, vol. 48, no. 2, pp. 140–143, 2009.

[29] T. A. Farley, R. A. Meriwether, E. T. Baker, J. C. Rice, and L. S. Webber, "Where do the children play? The influence of playground equipment on physical activity of children in free play," *Journal of Physical Activity and Health*, vol. 5, no. 2, pp. 319–331, 2008.

[30] T. A. Farley, R. A. Meriwether, E. T. Baker, L. T. Watkins, C. C. Johnson, and L. S. Webber, "Safe play spaces to promote physical activity in inner-city children: results from a pilot study of an environmental intervention," *American Journal of Public Health*, vol. 97, no. 9, pp. 1625–1631, 2007.

[31] T. L. McKenzie, S. J. Marshall, J. F. Sallis, and T. L. Conway, "Leisure-time physical activity in school environments: an observational study using SOPLAY," *Preventive Medicine*, vol. 30, no. 1, pp. 70–77, 2000.

[32] N. D. Ridgers, M. Tóth, and M. Uvacsek, "Physical activity levels of Hungarian children during school recess," *Preventive Medicine*, vol. 49, no. 5, pp. 410–412, 2009.

[33] R. Quigg, A. I. Reeder, A. Gray, A. Holt, and D. Waters, "The effectiveness of a community playground intervention," *Journal of Urban Health*, vol. 89, no. 1, pp. 171–184, 2012.

[34] J. Tester and R. Baker, "Making the playfields even: evaluating the impact of an environmental intervention on park use and physical activity," *Preventive Medicine*, vol. 48, no. 4, pp. 316–320, 2009.

[35] Australian Bureau of Statistics, *Erskineville (State Suburb) Community Profile*, 2006.

[36] Australian Bureau of Statistics, Redfern (State Suburb) Community Profile, 2006, http://www.censusdata.abs.gov.au/.

[37] Stratcorp CPL, "Open space and recreation needs study," Sydney, 2006.

[38] City of Sydney, "Redfern park draft plan of management (attachment B)," City of Sydney, 2006.

[39] P. Phongsavan, D. Merom, and H. Bowles, "SOPARC (system for observing play and recreation in communities) description and procedures manual," Training Manual adapted from original protocol prepared by T. L. McKenzie and D. A. Cohen for the Sydney Parks Study, 2007.

[40] T. L. McKenzie, D. A. Cohen, A. Sehgal, S. Williamson, and D. Golinelli, "System for observing play and recreation in communities (SOPARC): reliability and feasibility measures," *Journal of Physical Activity & Health*, vol. 3, supplement 1, pp. S208–S222, 2006.

[41] Centre for Epidemiology and Research, *2005-2006 Report on Child Health from the New South Wales Population Health Survey*, NSW Department of Health, Sydney, Australia, 2008.

[42] G. Stratton and E. Mullan, "The effect of multicolor playground markings on children's physical activity level during recess," *Preventive Medicine*, vol. 41, no. 5-6, pp. 828–833, 2005.

[43] M. F. Floyd, J. O. Spengler, J. E. Maddock, P. H. Gobster, and L. J. Suau, "Park-based physical activity in diverse communities of two U.S. cities. An observational study," *American Journal of Preventive Medicine*, vol. 34, no. 4, pp. 299–305, 2008.

[44] K. A. Shores and S. T. West, "The relationship between built park environments and physical activity in four park locations," *Journal of Public Health Management and Practice*, vol. 14, no. 3, pp. E9–E16, 2008.

[45] M. B. Ferré, A. O. Guitart, and M. P. Ferret, "Children and playgrounds in Mediterranean cities," *Children's Geographies*, vol. 4, no. 2, pp. 173–183, 2006.

[46] M. Jansson, "Attractive playgrounds: some factors affecting user interest and visiting patterns," *Landscape Research*, vol. 35, no. 1, pp. 63–81, 2010.

[47] F. Foley, "Urban art projects," Attachment A: Redfern Park Upgrade Intuitive Play Elements Presentation, in Environment and Heritage Committee 30 July 2007 Meeting Notes, City of Sydney, 2007.

[48] N. Colabianchi, A. L. Maslow, and K. Swayampakala, "Features and amenities of school playgrounds: a direct observation study of utilization and physical activity levels outside of school time," *International Journal of Behavioral Nutrition and Physical Activity*, vol. 8, article 32, 2011.

[49] L. J. Willenberg, R. Ashbolt, D. Holland et al., "Increasing school playground physical activity: a mixed methods study combining environmental measures and children's perspectives," *Journal of Science and Medicine in Sport*, vol. 13, no. 2, pp. 210–216, 2010.

[50] G. Nielsen, A. Bugge, B. Hermansen, J. Svensson, and L. B. Andersen, "School playground facilities as a determinant of children's daily activity: a cross-sectional study of Danish primary school children," *Journal of Physical Activity and Health*, vol. 9, no. 1, pp. 104–114, 2012.

[51] G. Nielsen, R. Taylor, S. Williams, and J. Mann, "Permanent play facilities in school playgrounds as a determinant of children's activity," *Journal of Physical Activity and Health*, vol. 7, no. 4, pp. 490–496, 2010.

[52] L. Karsten, "Children's use of public space: the gendered world of the playground," *Childhood*, vol. 10, no. 4, pp. 457–473, 2003.

[53] R. Quigg, A. Gray, A. I. Reeder, A. Holt, and D. L. Waters, "Using accelerometers and GPS units to identify the proportion of daily physical activity located in parks with playgrounds in New Zealand children," *Preventive Medicine*, vol. 50, no. 5-6, pp. 235–240, 2010.

3

A Pilot Study of Increasing Nonpurposeful Movement Breaks at Work as a Means of Reducing Prolonged Sitting

Dean Cooley and Scott Pedersen

University of Tasmania, Faculty of Education, Launceston, TAS 7248, Australia

Correspondence should be addressed to Dean Cooley; dean.cooley@utas.edu.au

Academic Editor: Li Ming Wen

There is a plethora of workplace physical activity interventions designed to increase purposeful movement, yet few are designed to alleviate prolonged occupational sitting time. A pilot study was conducted to test the feasibility of a workplace e-health intervention based on a passive approach to increase nonpurposeful movement as a means of reducing sitting time. The study was trialled in a professional workplace with forty-six participants (33 females and 13 males) for a period of twenty-six weeks. Participants in the first thirteen weeks received a passive prompt every 45 minutes on their computer screen reminding them to stand and engage in nonpurposeful activity throughout their workday. After thirteen weeks, the prompt was disabled, and participants were then free to voluntary engage the software. Results demonstrated that when employees were exposed to a passive prompt, as opposed to an active prompt, they were five times more likely to fully adhere to completing a movement break every hour of the workday. Based on this pilot study, we suggest that the notion that people are willing to participate in a coercive workplace e-health intervention is promising, and there is a need for further investigation.

1. Introduction

Increasing purposeful, or voluntary, physical activity both during leisure and work time is advocated as a means of reducing the risk of cardiovascular disease (CVD) [1–3]. In response workplace physical activity interventions have been designed to increase participation in purposeful physical activity programs during scheduled breaks in work time [4]. Yet the effectiveness of such interventions is mixed because of problems with sustainability and adherence [5]. Moreover, it appears that an increase in purposeful physical activity does not alleviate the CVD risk associated with prolonged periods of sitting (>4 hrs) [6–11]. Changes to the built environment, such as increases in technology, have resulted in prolonged occupational sitting time in excess of 6 hours [12], with concomitant decreases in energy expenditure for desk-based workers (>300 calories/per/day) [13, 14]. Guidelines for increasing cardiorespiratory fitness have changed over the years to reflect a growing understanding of the role of dose and frequency [15]. Recent evidence suggests short bouts of physical activity both purposeful and nonpurposeful (i.e., chores, standing up) are positively associated with cardiorespiratory fitness [15] and may buffer against issues of adherence to workplace health and wellbeing programs [4]. Moreover increasing nonpurposeful activity as part of an intervention may also ameliorate the health risks posed by prolonged sitting.

Research shows that short bursts of physical activity (<10 minutes) result in a reduction of CVD risk factors [16, 17]. For example, a cross-sectional analysis of the Framingham Heart Study Third Generation participants showed that accruing physical activity bouts of <10 minutes resulted in favourable changes to CVD risk [17]. There is evidence of the feasibility of these results being transferred to workplace interventions. For example, successful interventions may include a 10-minute flexibility and strength program [18], a single 10-minute bout of physical activity [19], mixed program for 30 minutes [20], or group physical activity classes [4]. Moreover, it appears that sustainability and adherence rates may be superior to those reported for purpose-based exercise interventions. In one study, average monthly attendance ranged from 76 to 86 percent over six months [4]. Given these results it would appear that short bursts of nonpurposeful activity may be suitable for worksites interventions.

Purposeful activities are effective in improving cardiorespiratory fitness, but increases may not ameliorate the risks associated with prolonged sitting because the activities only occur once a day [21], and the seated position needs to be regularly interrupted throughout the day. A number of studies have shown that regularly breaking a seated position results in positive changes to glucose and lipid profiles [16], lipoprotein lipase [22], and metabolic risk [23]. Consequently, there is support for an increase in nonpurposeful movement into desk-based work [14, 24, 25]. One strategy for increasing nonpurposeful activity is changing the built environment by including ergonomic equipment that affords movement [13, 14]. In one study [26] middle-aged men who were either overweight or obese participated in three separate daily sitting schedules with a break of six days between each of the days. In the first trial condition, each participant sat for five hours with no break. In the second experiment, they walked on a treadmill desk at a light-intensity pace for two minutes every 20 minutes, and in the third trial condition they walked on a treadmill desk at moderate-intensity pace for 2 minutes every 20 minutes. Results revealed that light-intensity movement, such as standing up and moving regularly throughout the workday yielded health benefits. Nonetheless, despite promising results there is little data to suggest that installation of treadmill desks will result in people changing their prolonged sitting periods because their use reflects planned behaviour, and subsequently such a strategy may suffer from the same problems as other purposive movement interventions. Moreover, sitting for desk-based work reflects a habit rather than a planned behaviour, and therefore interventions may be better informed by theory of habits [27].

Sitting for desk-based work is a habit because it is a learned act that is automatically performed in the presence of situational cues [27, 28]. Initially, the decision to sit at work is likely to be under the control of constructs as described by the theory of planned behaviour [29]. Within the workplace employees are faced with a limited choice of built environment (i.e., chairs and fixed height desks), prevailing workplace attitudes towards what is required to complete the daily tasks, and social pressures to sit while working. These factors are likely to create a perception that one has little control to execute an alternative to sitting [30]. Nonetheless, developing a new habit is more complex than substituting a new behaviour for the existing behaviour, especially if the behaviour is complex such as those that require multiple decisions to be made in short periods of time.

Sitting for desk-based workers is a complex behaviour because it typically involves more than one action. For example, the worker has to turn on the computer, select an appropriate chair, acquire the necessary equipment for a job task on the desk, complete multiple tasks within short time frames, and decide upon the sequence of these tasks. The sequence of behaviours could be described as a habitual pattern [31], but it may contain semiautomatic responses [32, 33] or behavioural scripts [34], which require some level of conscious thought. Yet preexisting habits may cause a breakdown of the intention-behaviour relationship by overriding the intention to perform an alternative behaviour [27]. When an individual intends to perform a new behaviour but engages in an old behaviour it is described as a slip or action switch and is evidence of a strong habit intrusion [35]. The performance of counter-habitual goal-directed actions (e.g., standing while taking a telephone call instead of sitting) requires conscious attention to interrupt the habit. If attentional resources are absorbed by other tasks and the intention to perform an alternative course of action is not capable of "over-ruling" the activation of a habitual programme [35–37], an action slip may result. For example, a desk-based worker under a high stress load because of attending to multiple tasks in a short time frame may find that when the phone rings, rather than stand as they have been instructed to do to break prolonged occupational sitting time (alternative course of action) they find themselves maintaining the old habit of sitting. The issue for interventions designed to break prolonged sitting is how to increase the odds of people performing an alternative behaviour.

One mechanism for counteracting the effect of an existing habit on a new habit is through the use of prompts at the point of decision [27, 28, 38]. Prompts at points of decision include a wide range of mechanisms including signs, emails, text messages, or telephone calls [39]. The rationale is the prompt presents a situation whereby the individual is able to reevaluate behavioural choices [38]. There is research that supports the efficacy of prompts to help people decide to participate in alternative health behaviour. These changes typically involve the use of electronic prompts and reminders to encourage people to engage in a particular behaviour [40]. For example, one study showed that a simple message at the point of decision extoling the health benefits of taking the stairs over the escalator resulted in an increase in stair use over baseline measures [38]. In terms of the efficacy of prompting to change prolonged sitting one study [41] showed that participants who received a computer-based prompt significantly reduced their sitting times compared to their counterparts who received education only about the health effects associated with prolonged sitting. Nonetheless, the effect was observed only over a 5-day period within a clinically controlled environment.

Despite the promising results for interventions to reduce prolonged sitting thus far, there are some limitations to consider. Changes to the built environment, such as having workers use treadmill desks, may result in an increase in work errors [42]. Second, the assessment of efficacy of ergonomic posture equipment is restricted to clinical studies, with no data available from field-based research to provide an understanding of how such changes to the built environment might work or be implemented in a workplace. Thus the applicability and sustainability of such equipment in workplaces to break prolonged sitting is unknown. Moreover, the financial costs associated with ergonomic workplace equipment may be prohibitive to small organisations. Finally, the efficacy of prompts is also mixed, with numerous variables influencing their effectiveness [39, 43]. Further, no field studies have reported the sustainability of such an intervention to break prolonged sitting in the workplace.

Although prompts at points of decision alert individuals about alternative behaviours, the individual can either consciously or unconsciously (i.e., action slip) ignore the prompt. This is a common occurrence in other health habits such as seat-belt wearing [44] and cell phone use while driving a car [45]. Thus, strategies should go beyond the usual range of education, rehabilitation, punishment, reward, and disincentive schemes to change individual attitude and belief about health behaviour [32] and environmental modifications to achieve significant behavioural changes among the target population [46]. We believe that it is timely to revisit some of the notions within a communitarian model of health promotion [47–49], in particular the active-passive approach for individual behaviour and preventative health interventions. Within this model when individuals voluntarily performing a preventative health action (e.g., regularly breaking sitting posture during the workday) it is considered an active prevention strategy. Thus, only individuals who choose to engage in the behaviour would gain the protective health benefit associated with that of regular standing, whereas passive prevention strategies remove some or all of the decision making process from the individual (e.g., only having water available in the drink machines). To assess this model we utilised a workplace e-health program that allowed us to manipulate the delivery of passive and active prompts in an effort to have desk-based employees engage in nonpurposeful movements throughout the workday as a means of reducing their prolonged occupational sitting time.

For health interventions there are a number of benefits in adopting a more passive approach. Health interventions that are passive have higher compliance levels and therefore greater efficiencies [44, 49–53]. Of note is the use of persuasive systems, which are computerised software systems designed to change or shape attitudes or behaviours [52, 53]. Noncoercive [52] and coercive [53] persuasive systems have been successful in changing health behaviours. Given the less than successful outcomes of purposeful physical activity interventions in the workplace which have relied on an active approach to preventive health [5], we hoped to learn if desk-based employees would tolerate a coercive, passive-prompting e-health intervention. We were also interested in differences between passive-based and active-based prompts for maintaining adherence to the health behaviour designed to increase nonpurposeful movement throughout the workday. We hypothesised that a passive prompt, compared to an active prompt, would significantly increase the odds of participants complying with seven periods of non-purposive movement during a workday. Noncompliance to the prompting conditions was defined as recording between one and six activities per workday. This number was based on the maximum number of prompts that a participant could receive during an eight-hour shift with a one-hour lunch break.

2. Methods

2.1. Sample. Participants were randomly selected from approximately 460 desk-based employees to take part in a field-based, sequential intervention study within a professional workplace across multiple sites (Project PAUSE). Given the lack of previous studies to guide power analysis and the pilot nature of this study, we chose a relative wide precision estimate of 28% with 95% confidence intervals, which indicated that a sample size of 50 was needed. Participants were randomly recruited through a computerised random draw. Eligibility criteria for inclusion into the study were (a) full-time desk-based employment, (b) clear of any medical health issues, and (c) daily desktop computer access to the internet.

In terms of the sample frame, the organisation's full-time desk-based workers were largely composed of females (67%); so, for parsimony, we chose a 1/3 split for our sample. Four participants withdrew from the study because of personal reasons two days before the induction and were not replaced, as replacements could not attend the induction at short notice. So the study proceeded with a reduced sample ($N = 46$). Participants had a range of work roles including receptionists, forensic analysis, administrative support, call center, sworn duties, and media/community liaison. Approximately 80 percent of participants worked in urban-based offices. Workplace configurations included open plan worksites, single offices, and shared office spaces. All participants completed the Exercise Stages of Change questionnaire [54], which assesses individual motivation to participate in exercise. Participants (females = 33, male = 13) all reported being in one of the first three stages of exercise participation (i.e., precontemplation (23%), contemplation (58%), or preparation (19%)), with no participant indicating that they had started or had been involved in a regular exercise program for the previous six months. Before data collection participants provided informed consent in accordance with granted university ethics committee procedures (H10875). Demographic characteristics of the sample are presented in Table 1.

2.2. Procedures. All participants first attended an induction session to inform them about the protocol of the study. The sequence of the session was the collection of demographic baseline data (30 minutes), an educational session on the negative health effects associated with prolonged sitting (15 minutes), general instructions on the recommended dose of movement to alleviate the adverse effects of prolonged sitting (20 minutes), and an informational session on using the e-health software (30 minutes). Participants were instructed that the length of the study would be 26 weeks and were reminded that their involvement in the study was strictly voluntary and they could withdraw at any time. At the completion of this induction session, all participants had the e-health software installed onto their computers. Participants were not blinded to other participants' involvement because of the nature of some worksites, and all attended the one induction session.

2.3. Intervention. The intervention was an e-health software program designed to passively prompt employees to break prolonged sitting periods by increasing nonpurposeful workday movement. The software has two distinct phases. It contains a set timed prompt that reminds employees to break their sitting time by engaging in nonpurposeful movement throughout the workday. The software provides employees a choice of 60 office-appropriate activities (i.e., walking, taking the stairs, and retrieving the photocopies). As the aim of the intervention was to increase nonpurposeful movement during the workday, participants were free to choose the

TABLE 1: Demographic characteristics of the sample. Values are means standard deviations.

Variable	Before	After
Age (years)		
Female	41.53 (12.1)	
Male	46.10 (6.3)	
Height (cm)		
Female	164.61 (6.74)	
Male	176.76 (6.85)	
Weight (kg)		
Female	71.91 (13.45)	70.87 (11.88)
Male	96.31 (17.96)	95.46 (17.28)
BMI		
Female	26.55 (4.36)	26.19 (3.96)
Male	30.81 (5.17)	30.52 (4.90)

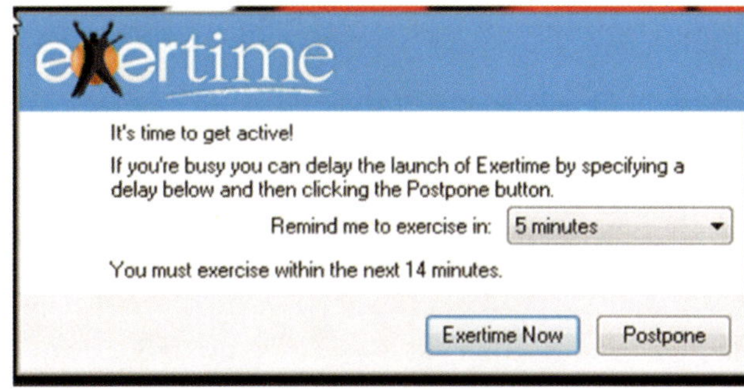

FIGURE 1: Prompting message seen by participants on their computer screens.

activity, duration, and intensity. This e-health program was tested through passive and active prompting strategies.

2.4. Passive Prompt Condition. The passive prompting condition was initiated during the first 13 weeks of the study. During this period, participants were exposed to a prompt that did not allow them to ignore the request to engage in the recommended behaviour. This was achieved through two mechanisms that were occurred in the following sequence. First, a small icon appeared on the taskbar. After 45 minutes the small icon automatically enlarged into a coloured pop-up prompt (5 cm × 3 cm) onto the bottom right hand side of participants' screens. The prompt contained a message alerting participants that the movement sequence was about to start (Figure 1).

Second, after the prompt appeared, a countdown clock started, and after 60 seconds, participants' screens were deactivated, and a cover screen appeared revealing the e-health software interface. At this point of decision, participants could select to complete a movement activity. Participants had freedom of choice over which activity to perform and the frequency or duration of participation. When participants completed their chosen activities, they were then prompted to record their progress. These activities were time stamped and stored on a remote server so that we were able to calculate the total number of logged activities for each day. Logged activities served as our dependent variable of compliance. Once data were recorded, the sequence terminated, and the participants regained access to their original computer screen at the point of deactivation. The prompt would then reinitiate after 45 minutes.

The dependent variable was determined by calculating the total number of days with seven or more logged activities and the total number of days with one to six logged activities. We set the criteria for compliance at seven or more activities per day because this indicated that participants were regularly breaking their prolonged sitting every hour as indicated by the Australian national guidelines [55]. We excluded days where no activity was logged because this may have reflected that the participant was out of their office, on leave, or working at other worksites with no computer. As this was a self-report measure, participants received a phone call from the researchers once throughout the study period to remind participants about the necessity to accurately report their activities.

2.5. Active Prompted Condition. After 13 weeks of the passive prompting condition, the researchers disabled the timed prompt for a further 13-week period. During this phase, if the participants wanted to engage with the e-health software, they needed to do so under their own volition. Participants could still view the icon on their taskbar and could still use the e-health software but had to voluntarily initiate the program by clicking on the icon. Once voluntarily initiated, the sequence remained the same as that for the passive prompting condition, and the dependent variable of logged activity frequency to determine compliance was used in the same manner.

2.6. Data Analysis. Using commercially available software [56] odds within conditions (compliance/noncompliance), odds ratio (OR), and 95 percent confidence intervals for the OR were generated using a 2 (compliance/noncompliance) × 2 (passive prompt/active prompt) contingency table. For each prompt condition, total number of days compliant and noncompliant for the 26-week experimental period were calculated and used as the frequency measure. A test of the hypothesis (OR = 1) was assessed using a chi-square statistic.

3. Results

All participants ($N = 46$) maintained the software on their desktop computers for the 26 weeks of the study and recorded activities through the study. Participants recorded a total of 2893 days out of a possible 5980 days where at least one activity was logged for the day across the 26-week study period. Participants recorded using a wide variety of movement-based activities, with the most popular activities being stair climbing, walking, and chair squats. Most days of recorded activity (Table 2) were associated with the passive prompted condition ($n = 2321$ days). Similarly, the highest number of activities recorded for a day by an individual was 23 in the passive prompt condition compared to 16 activities for the active prompt condition. For the passive prompt

TABLE 2: Total number of days for compliance and noncompliance in each prompt condition.

	Passive prompt	Active prompt
Compliance	1216	108
Noncompliance	1104	465

condition, nine activities in a day were the most frequent count (12%) compared to one logged activity per day for the active condition (37%).

In terms of each prompting condition, results showed that odds of compliance were greater in the passive condition (Odds = 1.1) compared to the active condition (Odds = 0.23). In terms of comparing the two conditions, a passive prompt improved the odds of desk-based workers complying to participate in nonpurposeful movement every hour seven times a day nearly five times more compared to the active condition (OR = 4.78, 95%CI = 3.78–5.93, and $P < 0.05$). Therefore, participants who were automatically reminded and forced to make a decision about moving were significantly more likely to engage in nonpurposeful physical activity seven times a day compared to when they were left to spontaneously stand throughout the workday on their own accord.

4. Discussion

The first finding of this study was that the employees in our sample were willing to accept a passive-based workplace e-health intervention [48] that was predicated on the principles of introducing nonpurposeful movement. No participant withdrew from the study during the 26-week study, although not all participants achieved our rigid criteria of full compliance by completing seven nonpurposeful movement breaks throughout the workday. Given that CVD is a major health issue [1–3] and the widening of guidelines for physical activity dose and frequency [15], these results are encouraging. Adherence to purposeful physical activity intervention are a constant problem. One cause of low adherence and compliance rates is some recruits to purposeful-based physical activity interventions cannot meet the high dose and frequency rates set for increases in cardiorespiratory fitness because of a variety of factors. Our results give an indication that people who do not exercise regularly and are willing and capable of increasing nonpurposeful movement activities that were associated with their work if regularly prompted to do so. Given the number of people who are not regularly participating in purposeful physical activity [5], CVD risk could be somewhat addressed through workplace physical activity interventions based on increasing compulsory nonpurposeful movement.

Our second finding was the enhanced benefit of using a passive prompt compared to an active prompt to achieve increase adherence to new health behaviour. A workplace e-health intervention underpinned by a passive prompt increased compliance by nearly five times to increasing nonpurposeful movement during the workday compared to when employees were left to their own free will to comply with the intervention. Within the context of passive versus active approaches to interventions [48] we believe this is the first field-based report of desk-based employees accepting a coercive persuasive system within a preventative health intervention designed to increase nonpurposeful movement at work. Given the low compliance rates for the active condition, which occurred after the passive condition for all participants, it could be assumed that the new behaviour of participating in hourly nonpurposeful movement had not become habitual. Despite the best intentions of health professionals, interventions designed to increase purposeful activity (e.g., walking, running, and strength training) have returned mixed results [5]. Our results provide preliminary evidence for the use of coercive persuasive systems to ameliorate low compliance rates may work with other health preventative initiatives.

Finally, the compliance results in the active condition, which followed the passive condition for all participants in our sample, highlight issues with sustainability of workplace physical activity-based interventions. The difficulty health professionals have in establishing new behaviours is well documented in the literature [57]. It would appear that 13 weeks of exposure to a coercive prompt is insufficient time to establish the nonpurposeful movement as a new behaviour. Sitting at work is a complex behaviour that involves many subroutines, and thus longer periods of exposure to the passive prompt may be needed to develop the new habit of regularly breaking sitting posture to move. Or as others have [58] argued, an insistent and obtrusive reminder might well be effective in the short run, but the effect reduces significantly over time. We would advocate that future research investigates a multiple strategy approach for changing workplace health behaviours to include changes to the built environment, such as treadmill or standing desks, coupled with a passive prompt to encourage workers to become less sedentary during the workday.

Our results have several possible implications. Coercing people to comply with health recommendations has the potential to reduce wastage of personal and monetary resources, help improve the efficacy of health and wellbeing interventions, and, most importantly, potentially reduce mortality and morbidity associated with preventable diseases such as CVD. Yet, the palatability of using passive approaches for individual preventative health interventions, such as increasing physical activity levels, has yet to be fully tested by researchers. Further, to date, despite the widespread knowledge of the effect of base levels of exercise (e.g., walking 30 minutes per day) on health and wellbeing, health researchers lament the low adherence rates within the population to recommended dose levels yet remain largely silent and inactive in recommending and prescribing nonpurposeful movement as an alternative or an adjunct strategy.

Nonetheless, there were several limitations to this study. This was a pilot study to test the feasibility of the e-health software and the efficacy of applying a passive persuasive system to a workplace e-health intervention. We did not measure habit strength and thus are unable to determine if participants' nonpurposeful movement habits had fully developed by the end of passive prompt condition. Hence, the poor compliance rates during the active condition may reflect that the behaviour had not become habitual. Second, in the active condition, the small number of reports for both compliance and noncompliance may lead to an under-estimation and hence alter the final odds ratio calculation. Third, we are unable to establish if participants may have chosen to simply stand to break their sitting time and elected not to complete a period of nonpurposeful activity in either condition. Finally, the measure of compliance was based on self-report. It is possible that participants simply became annoyed with the prompts or software and chose to record a false activity or no activity because of time and work pressure. Follow-up studies should incorporate a larger sample size and use more direct measures of compliance, such as accelerometers, in conjunction with e-health, passive-prompting software programs. Moreover, there is scope to determine the saliency of the coercive approach with other health behaviours.

5. Conclusion

Results from this study found that desk-based workers who received information about the health effects of prolonged sitting and who subsequently participated in a workplace e-health intervention based on a passive approach model had significantly higher compliance levels to participate in non-purposeful movement compared to voluntary engagement in the same program. Further research is needed to rigorously test the efficacy of a such an approach in terms of sustainability, as well as what conditions employees are willing to be coerced into changing their health behaviours while at work. We plan to conduct further studies on a larger sample of desk-based workers across multiple worksites to help understand how health can be positively influenced within the workplace in an effort to reduce the risks associated with CVD.

Acknowledgments

This study was partly funded through a Healthy@Work Grant supplied by the Tasmanian government.

References

[1] O. H. Franco, C. De Laet, A. Peeters, J. Jonker, J. Mackenbach, and W. Nusselder, "Effects of physical activity on life expectancy with cardiovascular disease," *Archives of Internal Medicine*, vol. 165, no. 20, pp. 2355–2360, 2005.

[2] I. M. Lee, E. J. Shiroma, F. Lobelo, P. Puska, S. N. Blair, and P. T. Katzmarzyk, "Effect of physical inactivity on major non-communicable diseases worldwide: an analysis of burden of disease and life expectancy," *The Lancet*, vol. 380, no. 9838, pp. 219–229, 2012.

[3] C. E. Matthews, S. M. George, S. C. Moore et al., "Amount of time spent in sedentary behaviors and cause-specific mortality in US adults," *American Journal of Clinical Nutrition*, vol. 5, no. 2, pp. 437–445, 2012.

[4] W. C. Taylor, R. Shegog, V. Chen et al., "The Booster Break program: description and feasibility test of a worksite physical activity daily practice," *Work*, vol. 37, no. 4, pp. 433–443, 2010.

[5] V. S. Conn, A. R. Hafdahl, P. S. Cooper, L. M. Brown, and S. L. Lusk, "Meta-analysis of workplace physical activity interventions," *American Journal of Preventive Medicine*, vol. 37, no. 4, pp. 330–339, 2009.

[6] D. W. Dunstan, J. Salmon, N. Owen et al., "Physical activity and television viewing in relation to risk of undiagnosed abnormal glucose metabolism in adults," *Diabetes Care*, vol. 27, no. 11, pp. 2603–2609, 2004.

[7] D. W. Dunstan, B. Howard, G. Healy, and N. Owen, "Too much sitting—a health hazard," *Diabetes Research and Clinical Practice*, vol. 97, no. 3, pp. 368–376, 2012.

[8] D. W. Dunstan, J. Salmon, G. N. Healy et al., "Association of television viewing with fasting and 2-h postchallenge plasma glucose levels in adults without diagnosed diabetes," *Diabetes Care*, vol. 30, no. 3, pp. 516–522, 2007.

[9] D. W. Dunstan, A. A. Thorp, and G. N. Healy, "Prolonged sitting: is it a distinct coronary heart disease risk factor?" *Current Opinion in Cardiology*, vol. 26, no. 5, pp. 412–419, 2011.

[10] M. T. Hamilton, G. Healy, D. W. Dunstan, T. W. Zderic, and N. Owen, "Too little exercise and too much sitting: inactivity physiology and the need for new recommendations on sedentary behaviour," *Current Cardiovascular Risk Report*, vol. 2, pp. 292–298, 2008.

[11] G. Hu, P. Jousilahti, R. Antikainen, and J. Tuomilehto, "Occupational, commuting, and leisure-time physical activity in relation to total and cardiovascular mortality among Finnish subjects with hypertension," *American Journal of Hypertension*, vol. 20, no. 12, pp. 1242–1250, 2007.

[12] A. A. Thorp, D. W. Dunstan, B. Clark et al., *Stand Up Australia: Sedentary Behaviour in Workers, Report for Medibank Private Limited*, Melbourne, Australia, 2009.

[13] J. Levine, E. L. Melanson, K. R. Westerterp, and J. O. Hill, "Measurement of the components of nonexercise activity thermogenesis," *American Journal of Physiology*, vol. 281, no. 4, pp. E670–E675, 2001.

[14] J. A. Levine and J. M. Miller, "The energy expenditure of using a "walk-and-work" desk for office workers with obesity," *British Journal of Sports Medicine*, vol. 41, no. 9, pp. 558–561, 2007.

[15] R. Ross and A. McGuire, "Incidental physical activity is positively associated with cardiorespiratory fitness," *Medicine & Science in Sports & Exercise*, vol. 44, no. 3, pp. 2189–2194, 2012.

[16] F. B. Hu, T. Y. Li, G. A. Colditz, W. C. Willett, and J. E. Manson, "Television watching and other sedentary behaviors in relation to risk of obesity and type 2 diabetes mellitus in women," *Journal of the American Medical Association*, vol. 289, no. 14, pp. 1785–1791, 2003.

[17] N. L. Glazer, A. Lyass, D. W. Esliger et al., "Sustained and shorter bouts of physical activity are related to cardiovascular health," *Medicine & Science in Sports & Exercise*, vol. 45, no. 1, pp. 109–115, 2013.

[18] S. J. Pronk, N. P. Pronk, A. Sisco, D. S. Ingalls, and C. Ochoa, "Impact of a daily 10-minute strength and flexibility program in a manufacturing plant," *American Journal of Health Promotion*, vol. 9, no. 3, pp. 175–178, 1995.

[19] A. K. Yancey, W. J. McCarthy, W. C. Taylor et al., "The Los Angeles Lift Off: a sociocultural environmental change intervention to integrate physical activity into the workplace," *Preventive Medicine*, vol. 38, no. 6, pp. 848–856, 2004.

[20] A. Lara, A. K. Yancey, R. Tapia-Conye et al., "Pausa para tu Salud: reduction of weight and waistlines by integrating exercise breaks into workplace organizational routine," *Preventing Chronic Disease*, vol. 5, no. 1, p. A12, 2008.

[21] J. Y. Chau, H. P. V. der Ploeg, J. G. Z. van Uffelen et al., "Are workplace interventions to reduce sitting effective? A systematic review," *Preventive Medicine*, vol. 51, no. 5, pp. 352–356, 2010.

[22] M. T. Hamilton, D. G. Hamilton, and T. W. Zderic, "Exercise physiology versus inactivity physiology: an essential concept for understanding lipoprotein lipase regulation," *Exercise and Sport Sciences Reviews*, vol. 32, no. 4, pp. 161–166, 2004.

[23] G. N. Healy, D. W. Dunstan, J. Salmon et al., "Breaks in sedentary time: beneficial associations with metabolic risk," *Diabetes Care*, vol. 31, no. 4, pp. 661–666, 2008.

[24] S. N. Blair, "The expert weights in," in *Obesity Management*, pp. 92–95, 2008.

[25] N. Owen, P. B. Sparling, G. N. Healy, D. W. Dunstan, and C. E. Matthews, "Sedentary behavior: emerging evidence for a new health risk," *Mayo Foundation for Medical Education and Research*, vol. 85, no. 12, pp. 1138–1141, 2010.

[26] D. W. Dunstan, B. A. Kingwell, R. Larsen et al., "Breaking up prolonged sitting reduces postprandial glucose and insulin responses," *Diabetes Care*, vol. 35, no. 5, pp. 976–983, 2012.

[27] H. Aarts and A. Dijksterhuis, "The automatic activation of goal-directed behaviour: the case of travel habit," *Journal of Environmental Psychology*, vol. 20, no. 1, pp. 75–82, 2000.

[28] H. Aarts and A. Dijksterhuis, "Habits as knowledge structures: automaticity in goal-directed behavior," *Journal of Personality and Social Psychology*, vol. 78, no. 1, pp. 53–63, 2000.

[29] I. Ajzen, "The theory of planned behavior," *Organizational Behavior and Human Decision Processes*, vol. 50, no. 2, pp. 179–211, 1991.

[30] I. Ajzen and M. Fishbein, *Understanding Attitudes and Predicting Social Behavior*, Prentice-Hall, Englewood Cliffs, NJ, USA, 1980.

[31] B. Verplanken, H. Aarts, A. van Knippenberg, and A. Moonen, "Habit versus planned behaviour: a field experiment," *British Journal of Social Psychology*, vol. 37, pp. 111–128, 1998.

[32] I. Ajzen, "Residual effects of past on later behavior: habituation and reasoned action perspectives," *Personality and Social Psychology Review*, vol. 6, no. 2, pp. 107–122, 2002.

[33] J. A. Bargh, "The four horsemen of automaticity: awareness, intention, efficiency, and control in social cognition," in *Handbook of Social Cognition*, R. S. Wyer and T. K. Srull, Eds., pp. 1–40, Hillsdale, NJ, USA, Lawrence Erlbaum Associates, 1994.

[34] C. A. Klöckner and E. Matthies, "How habits interfere with norm-directed behaviour: a normative decision-making model for travel mode choice," *Journal of Environmental Psychology*, vol. 24, no. 3, pp. 319–327, 2004.

[35] H. Heckhausen and J. Beckmann, "Intentional action and action slips," *Psychological Review*, vol. 97, no. 1, pp. 36–48, 1990.

[36] P. Norman, M. Conner, and R. Bell, "The theory of planned behaviour and exercise: evidence for the moderating role of past behaviour," *British Journal of Health Psychology*, vol. 5, no. 3, pp. 249–261, 2000.

[37] J. T. Reason, "Actions not as planned: the price of automatization," in *Aspects of Consciousness*, G. Underwood and R. Stevens, Eds., pp. 67–89, Academic Press, London, UK, 1979.

[38] H. Aarts and A. Dijksterhuis, "The automatic activation of goal-directed behaviour: the case of travel habit," *Journal of Environmental Psychology*, vol. 20, no. 1, pp. 75–82, 2000.

[39] J. P. Fry and R. A. Neff, "Periodic prompts and reminders in health promotion and health behavior interventions: systematic review," *Journal of Medical Internet Research*, vol. 11, no. 2, article e16, 2009.

[40] P. Krebs, J. O. Prochaska, and J. S. Rossi, "A meta-analysis of computer-tailored interventions for health behaviour change," *Journal of Preventive Medicine*, vol. 51, pp. 214–221, 2010.

[41] R. E. Evans, H. O Fawole, S. A. Sheriff, P. M. Dall, P. M. Grant, and C. G. Ryan, "Point-of-choice prompts to reduce sitting time at work: a randomized trial," *American Journal of Preventative Medicine*, vol. 43, no. 3, pp. 293–297, 2012.

[42] L. Straker, J. Levine, and A. Campbell, "The effects of walking and cycling computer workstations on keyboard and mouse performance," *Human Factors*, vol. 51, no. 6, pp. 831–844, 2009.

[43] P. D. Cooley, S. J. Foley, and C. G. Magnussen, "Increasing stair usage in a professional workplace: a test of the efficacy of positive and negative message prompts to change pedestrian choices," *Health Promotion Journal of Australia*, vol. 19, no. 1, pp. 64–67, 2008.

[44] A. F. Williams, J. K. Wells, A. T. McCartt, and D. F. Preusser, "Buckle Up NOW! An enforcement program to achieve high belt use," *Journal of Safety Research*, vol. 31, no. 4, pp. 93–99, 2000.

[45] M. Clayton, B. Helms, and C. Simpson, "Active prompting to decrease cell phone use and increase seat belt use while driving," *Journal of Applied Behavior Analysis*, vol. 39, no. 3, pp. 341–349, 2006.

[46] L. H. Engbers, M. N. M. van Poppel, M. J. M. Chin A Paw, and W. van Mechelen, "Worksite health promotion programs with environmental changes: a systematic review," *American Journal of Preventive Medicine*, vol. 29, no. 1, pp. 61–70, 2005.

[47] J. Forster, "A communitarian ethical model for public health interventions: an alternative to individual behavior change strategies," *Journal of Public Health Policy*, vol. 3, no. 2, pp. 150–163, 1982.

[48] M. C. Roberts, "Public health and health psychology: two cats of Kilkenny?" *Professional Psychology: Research and Practice*, vol. 18, no. 2, pp. 145–149, 1987.

[49] A. F. Williams, "Passive and active measures for controlling disease and injury: the role of health psychologists," *Health Psychology*, vol. 1, no. 4, pp. 399–409, 1982.

[50] K. Real, "Information seeking and workplace safety: a field application of the risk perception attitude framework," *Journal of Applied Communication Research*, vol. 36, no. 3, pp. 339–359, 2008.

[51] J. E. Bauer, A. Hyland, Q. Li, C. Steger, and K. M. Cummings, "A longitudinal assessment of the impact of smoke-free worksite policies on tobacco use," *American Journal of Public Health*, vol. 95, no. 6, pp. 1024–1029, 2005.

[52] H. Oinas-Kukkonen, P. Hasle, M. Harjumaa, K. Segerståhl, and P. Øhrstrøm, Eds., *Persuasive*, vol. 5033, Springer, Heidelberg, Germany, 2008.

[53] S. Langrial and H. Oinas-Kukkonen, "Less fizzy drinks: a multimethod study of persuasive reminders," in *Persuasive*, M. Bang and E. L. Ragnemalan, Eds., pp. 256–261, 2012.

[54] B. H. Marcus, V. C. Selby, R. S. Niaura, and J. S. Rossi, "Self-efficacy and the stages of exercise behavior change," *Research Quarterly for Exercise and Sport*, vol. 63, no. 1, pp. 60–66, 1992.

[55] Worksafe Australia, "Guidance note for the prevention of Occupational Overuse Syndrome in keyboard employment," in *National Occupational Health and Safety Commission*, National Government Publishing Service, Canberra, Australia, 1996.

[56] *Medicalc Software, Medicalc, Version 12*, Medicalc Software, Mariakeric, Belgium, 2012.

[57] P. Lally, C. H. M. van Jaarsveld, H. W. W. Potts, and J. Wardle, "How are habits formed: modelling habit formation in the real world," *European Journal of Social Psychology*, vol. 40, no. 6, pp. 998–1009, 2010.

[58] T. Bickmore, D. Mauer, F. Crespo, and T. Brown, "Persuasion, task interruption and health regimen adherence," in *Persuasive*, Y. A. W. de Kort, W. A. IJsselsteijn, C. Midden, B. Eggen, and B. J. Fogg, Eds., vol. 4744, pp. 1–11, Springer, Heidelberg, Germany, 2007.

4

A Review of Exposure Assessment Methods in Epidemiological Studies on Incinerators

Michele Cordioli,[1,2] Andrea Ranzi,[2] Giulio A. De Leo,[3] and Paolo Lauriola[2]

[1] *Department of Bio-Sciences, University of Parma, Parco Area delle Scienze 11/a, 43124 Parma, Italy*
[2] *Regional Reference Centre Environment & Health, Regional Agency for Environmental Protection in Emilia-Romagna, Via Begarelli 13, 41121 Modena, Italy*
[3] *Hopkins Marine Station and Woods Institute for the Environment, Stanford University, 120 Oceanview Boulevard, Pacific Grove, CA 93950, USA*

Correspondence should be addressed to Michele Cordioli; mik.cordioli@gmail.com

Academic Editor: Roberto Pasetto

Incineration is a common technology for waste disposal, and there is public concern for the health impact deriving from incinerators. Poor exposure assessment has been claimed as one of the main causes of inconsistency in the epidemiological literature. We reviewed 41 studies on incinerators published between 1984 and January 2013 and classified them on the basis of exposure assessment approach. Moreover, we performed a simulation study to explore how the different exposure metrics may influence the exposure levels used in epidemiological studies. 19 studies used linear distance as a measure of exposure to incinerators, 11 studies atmospheric dispersion models, and the remaining 11 studies a qualitative variable such as presence/absence of the source. All reviewed studies utilized residence as a proxy for population exposure, although residence location was evaluated with different precision (e.g., municipality, census block, or exact address). Only one study reconstructed temporal variability in exposure. Our simulation study showed a notable degree of exposure misclassification caused by the use of distance compared to dispersion modelling. We suggest that future studies (i) make full use of pollution dispersion models; (ii) localize population on a fine-scale; and (iii) explicitly account for the presence of potential environmental and socioeconomic confounding.

1. Introduction

Incineration is one of the most common technologies for waste disposal [1]. The number of incineration plants in Europe has been constantly rising in the last years, in the effort to manage and treat an ever-increasing waste production according to the EU directives and minimizing landfill disposal [2]. As waste incineration releases in the atmosphere chemicals that are potentially toxic [3], there is increasing public concern about the possible adverse effects on human health caused by this waste management technology [4, 5].

The literature on health effects of waste incinerators is extensive and can be essentially classified into two groups: observational studies (i.e., epidemiological analyses) and simulation studies (i.e., health risk assessment). The first group includes studies that make use of a variety of statistical techniques to describe the potential relationship between the *observed* health status of the population and the exposure level from incinerators. The second group includes studies aimed at estimating the *expected* impact, in terms of health risk and/or number of sanitary cases, of a measured or simulated exposure to environmental contaminants [6–8].

Available epidemiological studies have been well reviewed in many published papers [9–11] and reports published by international agencies [12, 13]. However, the lack of a common framework for study designs makes the results of the different investigations on the health impacts hardly comparable and thus inconclusive. Poor exposure assessment is claimed as one of the main reasons of inconsistency of results in published studies [3, 9, 10, 13].

Exposure is generally defined as the contact between a stressor and a receptor and can be characterized either by direct (e.g., personal monitoring and biological markers) or indirect methods (e.g., environmental monitoring, modelling, and questionnaires) [14]. Although direct measures of exposure can be considered the best measures for assessing the effect of a specific substance on the target population, indirect measures of exposure (e.g., simulations of atmospheric dispersion) have greater utility for source emission assessment and control, since they are capable of linking population health to specific pollution emission sources [14]. These indirect methods have rapidly evolved in the last years [15], especially due to the increasing diffusion of the use of Geographical Information Systems (GIS) [16] and computer models to simulate atmospheric dispersion [17].

The aims of the present work were twofold: first, we wanted to investigate what methods and approaches are commonly used in the published literature to characterize exposure levels from waste incinerators; second, we wanted to assess, through a computer simulation study, how the classification of the expected exposure level may change as a function of the method used to estimate it.

The analysis was performed by using the literature database gathered within a project supported by the Emilia Romagna Region (North Italy) between 2007 and 2012 (MONITER Project) [18], to standardize environmental monitoring and health surveillance methods in areas characterized by the presence of incinerators and to evaluate the health status of populations around the eight incinerators of the region.

Although the focus of the present work was on waste incinerators, the results of our analysis can be extended to any point source of atmospheric pollution [19] or more generally to contaminated sites, where the presence of multiple sources has to be taken into proper account.

2. Material and Methods

2.1. Literature Review. We analyzed papers referenced in previously published reviews on incinerator health effects [9–13, 20] and, additionally, searched for further references on MEDLINE, PubMed, Scopus, and Google Scholar by using a number of keywords combinations (e.g., "epidemiology," "incinerator," "adverse effect," etc.). We focused our analysis only on observational epidemiological studies. Human biomonitoring [21, 22] and risk assessment studies [7, 8, 23] were not considered here. We excluded also studies on incinerator's workers [9] as the exposure pathway and levels can be completely different from those experienced by the population living around the incinerator plants.

The studies reviewed, rather than defining a relationship between environmental pollution and human health, aimed at evaluating the possible association with a specific industrial source of pollution (i.e., incinerators). The conceptual model for the emission-exposure pathways is sketched in Figure 1. Waste incineration epidemiological studies usually focus on gas stack emissions from the combustion process, while other possible sources of pollution (water discharges, ashes, smell emission, traffic, etc.) are not generally investigated [3]. After the emission from the incineration stack, pollutants dispersion in the atmosphere depends upon a number of physical and environmental variables such as stack height,

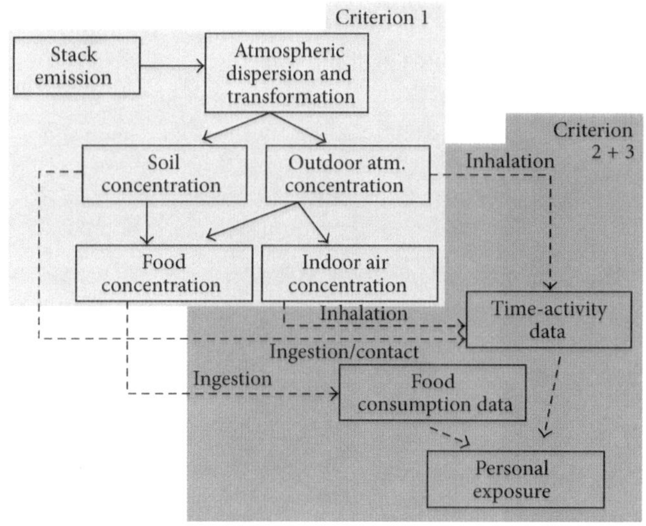

Figure 1: Conceptual model representing the principal impact pathways that determine exposure to atmospheric emissions from an incinerator. Contamination of drinking water is not represented.

wind speed and direction, temperature, and atmospheric stability. Some gases may undergo various chemical transformations, and part of the contaminants may eventually settle down on a variety of surfaces such as soil, vegetation, and water. Concentrations in the atmosphere and in soil may be either directly inhaled, ingested, or absorbed through dermal contacts or they can enter the agricultural food chain [24]. The actual exposure to potentially hazardous contaminants is thus determined by the time spent by various sectors of the population in different environments (outdoor, indoor at home, or at work) and could be due to inhalation, ingestion of contaminated water or food, and dermal contact with contaminated vectors (e.g., soil, water) [25]. Since incinerators are potential sources of persistent pollutants (e.g., dioxins, heavy metals, etc.) [3], ingestion can represent a relevant exposure pathway.

Exposure to pollutants has conceptually at least three dimensions, namely, (i) the intensity of exposure, which depends among the other things upon the concentration level of contaminants in different media; (ii) space, as both population density and concentration of contaminants are spatially heterogeneous; (iii) time, which is the duration and variability of exposure, as this determines the total amount of contaminant that has been eventually ingested, inhaled, or absorbed through dermal contacts [14]. Exposure assessment reconstructs the relationship between receptors and locations and between locations and the presence and amount of a certain risk factor. Accordingly, we reviewed the selected literature focusing only on the approaches used to define the exposure level and classifying them on the basis of three criteria (Table 1):

(1) the approach used to define the intensity of exposure to the emission source (3 categories);

(2) the scale at which the spatial distribution of the exposed population was accounted for (3 categories);

TABLE 1: Classification of exposure assessment methods.

Category	Description
	Criterion 1: definition of exposure intensity
1	Qualitative (e.g., presence/absence of the source/contamination in an area)
2	Distance from the source (e.g., linear distance)
3	Dispersion models (e.g., average annual atmospheric concentration)
	Criterion 2: definition of population distribution
1	Municipality/community/postcode sector
2	Census unit/full postcode
3	Exact residential address location
	Criterion 3: temporal variability
1	Time-invariable (i.e., fixed) exposure
2	Time-variable exposure (e.g., residential history and/or variability in emissions from the source)

(3) whether temporal variability in exposure was considered or not in the published study (2 categories).

The combination of all categories can result in a total of 18 possible methods of exposure assessment and was hereafter referred to as "$x.y.z$," where x represents the method used to estimate expected intensity, y the method used to estimate population distribution, and z whether the exposure was variable or not in time. For example, a published study classified as "2.3.1" means that the exposure level was evaluated as a function of the distance from the source, population distribution in the territory was assessed by using exact residential address location, and exposure was fixed in time.

Exposure assessment methods were categorized only on the basis of the exposure variables actually used in the epidemiological model. As discussed afterward, some studies reported additional information (such as measured concentrations of pollutants in various media) useful to interpret or support exposure model outcomes, even though this information was not used in statistical calculations.

Another important element of the exposure assessment process is the control of confounding factors, that is, variables that may hide or enhance the measure of effect [26, 27]. These factors can be socioeconomic (e.g., people living in industrial areas near incinerators may be more deprived) or environmental (e.g., frequently incinerators are located in areas with high pollution from other industrial sources and traffic).

For each reviewed study we analysed also whether and how confounding factors were accounted for. Since evaluation of confounding factors can follow a variety of approaches, we decided not to include this aspect as a fourth criterion in our classification scheme. Nevertheless we thoroughly comment on the role of confounding factors as well as their importance in epidemiological studies in the discussion.

2.2. Case Study: Parma. To understand how the choice of one or another approach of Table 1 may ultimately affect the estimated exposure, we run a simulation case study based on real data from an epidemiological surveillance program for a new incinerator that is under construction in the city of Parma (Italy).

The data used to simulate the effect of alternative methods of exposure assessment were as follows:

(i) location of the stack of the incinerator;

(ii) exact location of the address of residence for 31,019 people living around the incinerator (circle of 4 km of radius);

(iii) boundaries of the 2001 Italian census blocks for the area, as defined by the Italian National Institute of Statistics;

(iv) the results of an atmospheric dispersion model for PM_{10} emitted from the incinerator.

Geographic coordinates of addresses were provided by the local registry office. Atmospheric dispersion was simulated using the ADMS Urban model [28], a second generation quasi-Gaussian model already employed in other studies on health effects of incinerators [29–31]. Since the study area is located in a flat plane, this model was judged suitable to compute long-term average concentration and deposition [32].

We used PM_{10} as a tracer for the complex mix of pollutants emitted by the incinerator, after a test on various types of pollutant. The aim of the simulation was to determine a geographic gradient of exposure inside the study area: this spatial gradient is mainly determined by the incinerator's characteristics and atmospheric conditions, while it is only poorly dependent on the pollutant's properties.

We used five years of hourly meteorological data (2005–2010) from the nearest meteorological station (about 4 km from the plant) and source characteristics from the authorized project (i.e., stack height: 70 m; gas temperature: 150°C; PM_{10} emission flux: 231 mg s^{-1}) to calculate average hourly concentrations at ground level (ng m^{-3}) and average hourly deposition (ng m^{-2} h^{-1}) of PM_{10} over the period 2005–2010 on a regular 200 m receptor grid. Calculated concentrations were interpolated (using quadratic inverse distance weighting) to obtain continuous maps (Figure 3).

For each individual, we evaluated residential time-invariant exposure to the incinerator using the following methods:

(1) distance between census block centroid and incinerator (CBDI, method 2.2.1);

(2) distance between exact address location and incinerator (ADDI, method 2.3.1);

(3) average concentration and deposition inside the census block of each address (CBCO and CBDE, method 3.2.1);

(4) concentration and deposition at the address location (ADCO and ADDE, method 3.3.1).

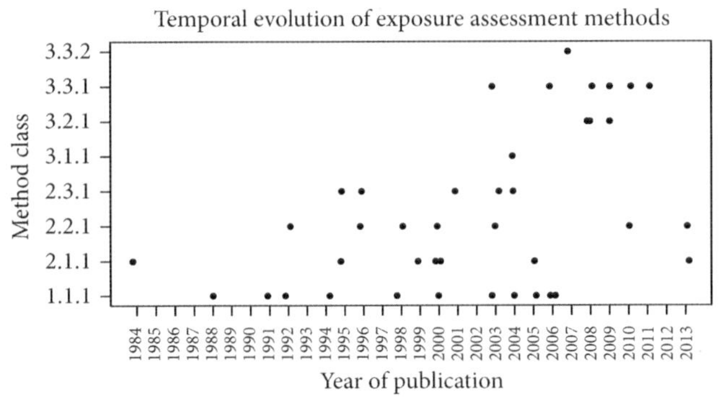

FIGURE 2: Temporal evolution of exposure assessment methods. Methods are classified according to Table 1 and sorted in the y-axis from the less precise to the best one.

We then contrasted the results of using alternative approaches for the assessment of the exposure level for each individual in the sample. Exposure variables were categorized in 5 classes (i.e., 1: lowest exposure, 5: highest exposure) using quintiles of each variable distribution. Thus, each exposure class contain approximately the same number of subjects. Only for address distance from the incinerator we defined also a second categorization using regular buffers, as done in the majority of published studies [33–35].

Concentration and deposition estimates based on dispersion models are affected by their own degree of uncertainty and should be possibly ground trued with field measurements and/or experiments. A previous validation study conducted in France [32] demonstrated that this kind of models provide a reliable proxy for incinerator exposure in simple terrain such as the area under study: we here assumed that simulated concentrations represent the closest estimate to the actual exposure.

Therefore we evaluated the degree of exposure misclassification using two-way tables and Cohen's kappa test of agreement [36, 37]. Cohen's kappa was calculated using quadratic weighting to assign less importance to misclassification between adjacent classes and higher importance to other misclassifications.

3. Results

3.1. Literature Review. A total of 41 studies published between 1984 and January 2013 were identified by the literature search. Table S1 in Supplementary Material available online at http://dx.doi.org/10.1155/2013/129470 (Supplementary Information) reports the resulting categorization of exposure methods and other relevant information for each study. The column "covariates" lists the confounding factors that were evaluated in each study.

Figure 2 represents the evolution of methodologies in time, based on the year of publication. Methods on the y-axis are sorted from the less precise to the best one.

With reference to the first classification criterion, that is, method used to assess exposure intensity, 19 studies (46%) used a measure of distance, both on a continuous scale and more commonly by defining concentric areas with arbitrary radius. In some cases [38–41] also wind direction was used to introduce some spatial anisotropy in exposure. Lee and Shy [42] used distance to define exposed communities but developed also a longitudinal study using daily PM_{10} measurement from fixed air monitors. One study [43] analysed spatial clustering of disease cases: since the analysis was based on the position of the community of residence, we classified this method as 2.1.1. One study [41] presented multiple assessment methods: presence/absence of the incinerator, distance from the plant, and an exposure index based on distance, wind direction, and time spent outdoor by people.

11 studies (27%) used atmospheric dispersion models to define population exposure. Generally models were used to estimate long-term average atmospheric concentrations at ground level, although one study used cumulated depositions [44]. Two studies [29, 45] used also heavy metals as indicator of exposure, while all the others used dioxins.

The remaining 11 studies (28%) used a qualitative definition of exposure to contrast the health status of communities/municipalities with and without incinerators. One study [46] developed quantitative indicators to classify municipalities, using emission inventories for dioxin from incinerators.

All the published studies used the residence as the place where exposure to atmospheric pollution occurs (criterion no.2). Nevertheless, different levels of detail were used in defining residence location. The majority of the papers (n = 19, 46%) considered the municipality or community of residence (e.g., postcode sector, school, hospital, etc.), 12 studies (29%) used the exact geographic coordinates of the address of residence, and 10 (24%) used the full postcode or census unit.

Finally, all the published literature, with one exception [47], defined exposure proxies that did not account for temporal variability in population spatial distribution and incinerators' emissions (criterion 3) that is, they considered the residence at the time of diagnosis, at enrolment, or the longest residence of the subject. Residential histories and changes in exposure intensity (e.g., as a consequence of changes in combustion and gas depuration technologies) were not accounted for in the other examined studies.

Overall, Figure 2 shows a trend of improvement in the quality of exposure assessment during the examined years, although three studies published after 2010 still used linear distance as the exposure proxy.

3.2. Results of the Simulation Case Study in Parma. Figure 3 reports the map of the census blocks around the incinerator under construction in Parma, its location (the star), the location of the sample of resident people used in the present study (small black dots), the expected PM_{10} concentration as simulated with the ADMS model, and the regular, 800 m wide, circular buffers around the emission source. Figure 4 contrasts the results of alternative approaches to assess exposure level in terms of intensity (simulated concentration versus distance from the emission sources) and accuracy in residence location.

TABLE 2: Evaluation of the agreement between concentration maps and other exposure assessment methods. Quadratic weighted Cohen's kappa and percentages of subjects classified in the same exposure class or in different classes.

Comparison exposure	Weighted kappa[a]	Matching subjects	Misclassification in adjacent categories	Misclassification in >1 class apart
ADCO versus ADDE	0.91	69.6%	29.3%	1.1%
ADCO versus CBCO	0.97	89.2%	10.5%	0.3%
ADCO versus CBDE	0.90	70.0%	27.8%	2.2%
ADCO versus $ADDI_1$	0.61	38.9%	45.1%	16.0%
ADCO versus CBDI	0.60	40.2%	44.5%	15.3%
ADCO versus $ADDI_2$	0.35	25.4%	39.8%	34.8%

ADCO: address concentration (quintiles), ADDE: address deposition (quintiles), CBCO: census block concentration (quintiles), CBDE: census block deposition (quintiles), $ADDI_1$: address distance (quintiles), $ADDI_2$: address distance (regular 800 m buffers), CBDI: distance between census block centroid and incinerator. [a]all kappa with $P < 0.001$.

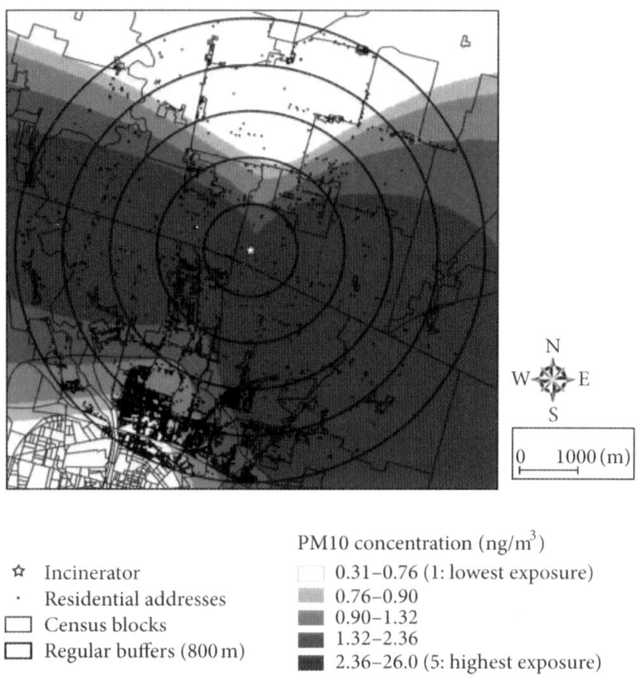

FIGURE 3: Representation of the area considered in the case study of Parma.

Table 2 shows Cohen's kappa indices of agreement between concentration maps and other exposure assessment methods. The table reports also the share of individuals over the 31,019 samples assigned to the same class of exposure, the share of individuals classified in an adjacent exposure class, and that of individuals classified into two or more classes apart. High kappa values are encountered when concentrations and depositions are considered, while comparison between concentration and distance approaches gave worst results when distance is categorized on regular concentric circles.

4. Discussion

4.1. Evaluation of Exposure Intensity (Criterion 1). The majority of the papers reviewed in the present study appear to suffer from poor exposure characterization. A relevant part of these papers (28%) used qualitative definitions of exposure (e.g., presence/absence of the source or anecdotic presence of pollution). These methods cannot account for the complexity of impact pathways described in Figure 1 nor for the heterogeneity in the exposure level that is normallyv expected as a consequence of the uneven distribution of the resident population and of the anisotropic dispersal of pollutants in the atmosphere. For instance, in the simulation case study we ran in Parma, the use of method 1.1.1 (presence of the incinerator in the municipality) would not allow us to discriminate between different levels of exposure and, therefore, all the 30,019 people in our sample (as well as the remaining 158,660 inhabitants of Parma) would be all classified as highly exposed, which would probably not be the case.

Epidemiological analyses carried out on a significant number of municipalities still represent a valuable instrument for public health tracking since they can evidence disease clusters in some regions that must be studied further. Even though any departure of disease incidence in large communities from background levels has to be taken very seriously, it is very difficult to use this type of evidence to infer about the role of specific emission sources (i.e., an incinerator), as many other potential confounding factors might exert a significant effect, particularly in highly urbanized areas. Moreover, the risk of false positive and, to a greater extent, false negative results, common to all exposure assessment methods, can be exacerbated when epidemiological data are averaged out on a vast territory with large internal differences in the exposure levels, as in method 1.1.1.

Almost half of the studies used distance to measure exposure. This is certainly a substantial improvement with respect to just an absence/presence evaluation, as contamination from an atmospheric emission source (e.g., air, soil, and locally produced food) is generally expected to decrease with distance. However, the assumption of isotropy in atmospheric dispersion of contaminants could lead to remarkable errors in exposure assessment. Many features of the emission source (e.g., stack height, gas flow temperature and velocity, and pollutant concentration) and of the local environment (e.g., local meteorology, topography, and land use) determine where and how far stack emissions disperse and how ultimately enter different environmental compartments.

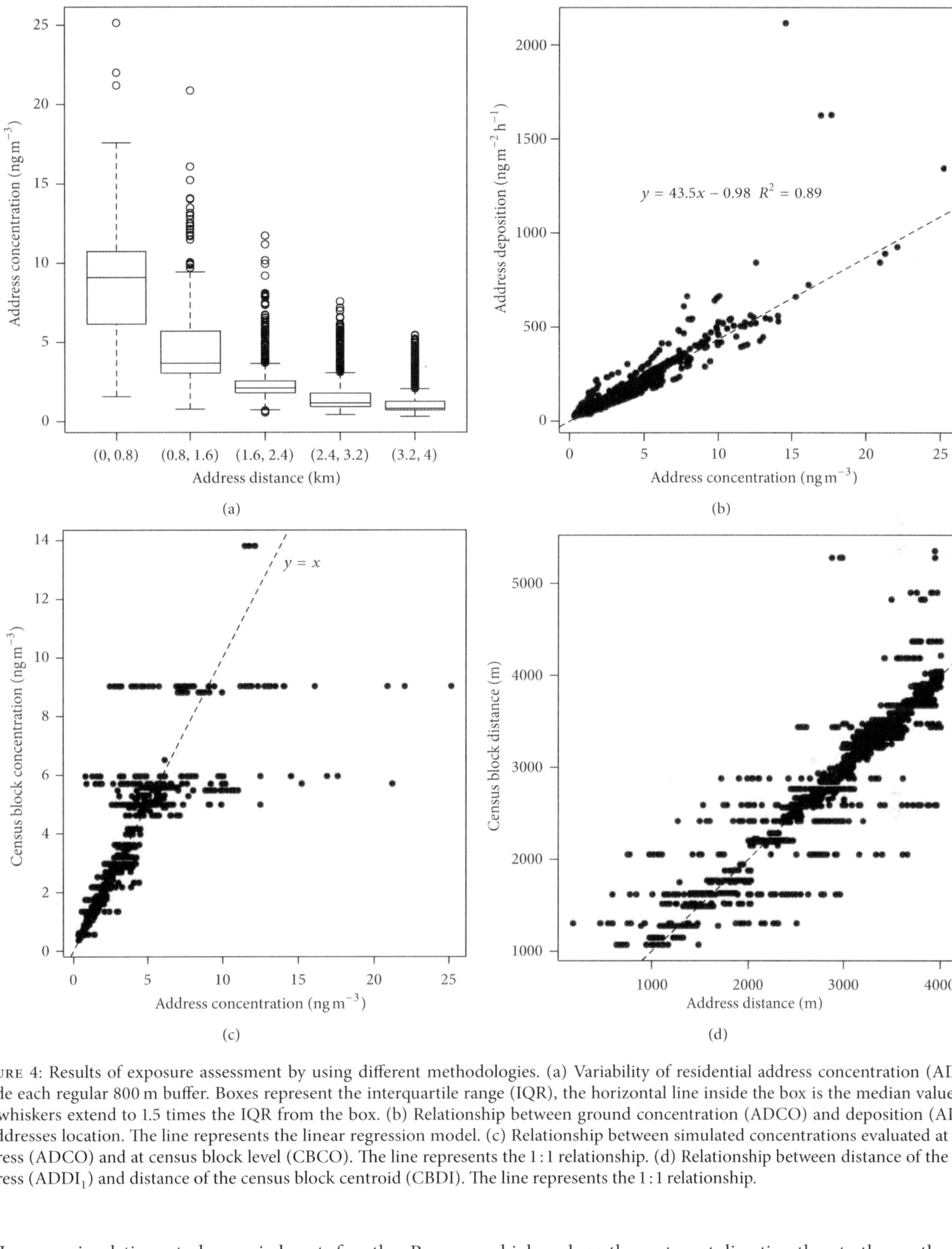

FIGURE 4: Results of exposure assessment by using different methodologies. (a) Variability of residential address concentration (ADCO) inside each regular 800 m buffer. Boxes represent the interquartile range (IQR), the horizontal line inside the box is the median value, and the whiskers extend to 1.5 times the IQR from the box. (b) Relationship between ground concentration (ADCO) and deposition (ADDE) at addresses location. The line represents the linear regression model. (c) Relationship between simulated concentrations evaluated at exact address (ADCO) and at census block level (CBCO). The line represents the 1 : 1 relationship. (d) Relationship between distance of the exact address ($ADDI_1$) and distance of the census block centroid (CBDI). The line represents the 1 : 1 relationship.

In our simulation study carried out for the Parma incinerator, the distance method assigns the same exposure level to people resident in the northern and eastern parts of the territory around the emission stack, even though simulations showed that concentrations are expected to be higher along the east-west direction than to the north-south one (Figure 3).

Because of the anisotropic dispersion of pollutants in the atmosphere, the expected PM_{10} concentrations at the residence address vary wildly inside each 800 m wide buffer around the incinerator (Figure 4(a)). Consequently, the use of distance from the emission source as a proxy of actual concentrations could cause a high degree of misclassification (Table 2).

The use of well-tuned atmospheric dispersion models allows a substantial improvement in the estimation of exposure level, especially if carried out along with a fine scale estimation of the spatial distribution of the vulnerable population. Anyway, atmospheric pollution models are themselves affected by a considerable level of uncertainty [48] depending upon assumptions on actual atmospheric conditions, reconstruction of wind fields, and type of dispersion processes, including the possibility of simulating chemical transformation which are known to be highly relevant for the formation of tropospheric ozone and secondary fine particulate matter.

A significant number of the published papers analysed in the present study provided only a limited information on the atmospheric model: generally there was no discussion about the type of model used, the type and source of meteorological data, model adequacy to represent complex morphological natural or urban landscape and/or wind calms, and the assumptions made about pollutant's emission rates and physical-chemical properties.

Only few studies explicitly acknowledged limitations in the modelling approach used. For example, instead of adopting a different dispersion model as suggested by the same authors in a previous study [32], in Viel et al.'s [49] a part of the study area was excluded because dispersion model results were judged unreliable in that area. Another study [50] used maps of ground level concentrations estimated on the basis of emissions and meteorological data, but no dispersion model was cited. Almost all the studies used dioxins as an impact indicator: dioxins represent a family of 210 congeners, each one with different physical-chemical characteristics: no study clearly explained how these chemicals were treated in the model (e.g., using 2,3,7,8-TCDD congener properties). Moreover, some studies did not report a clear definition even of the most basic variables used to measure exposure, that is; averaging time for concentrations [31, 45, 51] or distinction between concentrations and depositions to ground [31]. As shown in our case study ground level atmospheric PM_{10} concentrations and depositions from a point source have very similar patterns with some significant departure, nevertheless the choice of one or the other measure of exposure should be at least discussed, related to the main route of exposure considered. All these pieces of information are important to judge the quality of the exposure assessment process, its uncertainties, and to allow comparability and reproducibility of methods.

Regardless of how detailed, accurate and advanced the model to simulate atmospheric dispersion is, it is still only a part of the impact pathways described in Figure 1. All the studies implicitly assumed that inhalation represents the principal exposure pathway, while no published literature measured or modelled the possible exposure through ingestion of contaminated food or contact with contaminated soil.

No study used measured levels of pollution in different media (e.g., atmosphere, soil, and food) as the exposure variable in the epidemiological model, except for one work [42] that used also measured 24 h average PM_{10} concentrations in each community as a predictor for pulmonary function, although there were no differences in average levels between communities defined *a priori* as exposed and not exposed. Many studies presented information on measured levels of pollution [43, 52–54], but these data were not included in the statistical model. This is not surprising, as it is very difficult to discriminate the contribution of single-point sources to the observed concentrations levels. The latter, in fact, invariably depend the contribution of several other confounding emission sources [55, 56], especially if they are located in urbanized areas with intense traffic or industrial activities. Thus, indirect measures of exposure obtained through modelling represent a valid alternative useful to identify the possible role of a specific emission source.

4.2. Evaluation of Receptor's Exposure (Criteria 2 and 3). The actual exposure of an individual to the pollutants emitted by an incinerator may occur in different environments and last a variable amount of time. All published studies used the residence as the place where exposure to atmospheric pollution occurs (criterion 2). Notably, one study [57] considered also the location of workplace of studied subjects.

Residence location can be determined with various degrees of precision. The majority of revised studies (48%) used community level to determine residence location (i.e., town, municipality, postcode sector, and school). In this way the same exposure level is assigned to large groups of population, but this assumption was rarely discussed and no measures of exposure variability inside groups were reported. Thus, it was impossible to evaluate the degree of ecological bias [58] that is, how well the variation in risk between groups with different average exposure applies to the variation in risk between individuals.

Some studies used census block or full postcode for determining residence position. The dimension of these blocks may vary greatly depending on the location: normally these blocks are smaller in populated areas but may become very large in other rural zones. Moreover, no information was generally given about blocks extension, and it was difficult to compare very different blocks types like Small Area Health Statistic Unit (SAHSU) [35], UK census postcode system [59], or UK Lower Layer Super Output Areas (LSOA) [60]. In our case study census blocks had an average area of $0.4\,km^2$ (min: $968.4\,m^2$; max: $6.3\,km^2$) and contained on average 26 addresses (min: 1; max: 130): both address distances and concentrations vary widely inside some census blocks (Figures 4(c) and 4(d)). This was true especially for more exposed areas, since the incinerator is located in a less densely populated area with large census blocks. This aspect could lead to different degree of errors in exposure assignment, that increase with the level of pollutant or proximity to the incinerator.

The most precise way to locate residences is to address geocoding: this procedure assigns a couple of geographic coordinates to each address. Errors in address positioning depend on the quality of the database used but is generally in the order of tens to hundreds meters [61, 62], thus small in comparison with the use of census blocks or full postcode.

In future studies maximum disaggregation of data, to maximise information and minimize potentially differential ecological biases [63], is thus recommended.

The use of residence as exposure location is a very common assumption in environmental epidemiology since it is easily derived and there is evidence that people normally spend a great part of their time inside their residences, for example, on average 69% [64] and 80% [65]. Nevertheless, home location may not well represent total exposure because people may experience shorter but more intense exposures outside home, and residence is a proxy only for inhalation exposure and does not account for indirect pathways [66] (Figure 1). Although this technique has well-known limitations, it is often the only method available, particularly for large populations or for reconstructing historical exposures.

Temporal variability in exposure is an issue rarely explored in the reviewed studies. Temporal variability may result both from changes in source emissions over time or from residential mobility of the population and may be a cause of incorrect exposure assignment [67, 68]. Only one published study [47] explicitly accounts for historical exposure variability by reconstructing residential histories and evolution of dioxin emissions from the sources considered. However the exposure indicator chosen (i.e., the average exposure over time) may introduce some bias: since emissions from the sources considered were progressively reduced starting from the 1990s, the average exposure value decreases with the increase of exposure duration. A better indicator could have been cumulative exposure, that is, the sum of the annual exposure concentration over the exposure duration. One study [29] considered the modification of incinerator emissions over time indirectly, without considering changes in the final statistical model, but evaluating how the morphology of fallout maps was similar in time.

Although difficult to achieve because of data unavailability, especially for studies on old incinerators, in future studies efforts should be developed in reconstructing residential histories and variability in incinerator's emission over time, at least as a sensitivity analysis for the model.

4.3. Exposure Misclassification and Confounding Factors. Almost all papers used categorical definitions of exposure (i.e., exposure classes). One issue rarely discussed is the rationale behind the choice of cut-off values used to classify continuous variables. In the absence of toxicological reference values for this type of exposure, in our case study we used a criterion expected to make the results of the statistical analysis more stable and reliable, that is, having roughly the same number of exposed individuals in each class. In reviewed studies *a priori* cutoffs of exposure were generally chosen without an explicit justification [33–35, 51].

When categorical exposure variables are measured with error, they are said to be misclassified. Misclassification can be differential or nondifferential with respect to disease status of an individual person [26], the latter being more probable in reviewed studies and generally leading to risk estimations biased toward the null. Nevertheless, in presence of more than two exposure categories, non-differential misclassification can move estimates of risk away from null and disrupt exposure-response trends [69].

Our case study showed that

(i) for exposure measures based on distance a relevant part of the population may be classified in the wrong exposure category (assuming that dispersion model better represents real exposure), with relevant percentages of subjects moving by more than one category;

(ii) the use of census blocks to identify the residence may introduce a certain degree of differential misclassification since the error is higher in more exposed areas and lower for less exposed.

Both these factors may bias risk estimates away from the null or modify exposure-response trends.

Sometimes, the degree of error in exposure assessment can be evaluated with a validation study [70], that is, comparing modelled exposure with "gold-standard" measurement of exposure collected for a random subsample of the population, such as direct measurement of individual exposure. In practice, since no such gold standard is generally available, we recommend researchers to conduct sensitivity analyses on exposure assessment [71] and discuss the magnitude of error that may be present in their data.

Another issue that is only partially dealt with in reviewed literature is confounding. Confounding occurs when a risk factor different from the exposure variable under study causes bias in the estimation of association between exposure and disease, due to its differential distribution in exposed and non exposed groups [72]. Various confounding factors may affect a study on incinerators' health effects, that is, socioeconomic differences (e.g., poverty, occupation), personal lifestyles (e.g., alcohol, smoke), and presence of other sources of pollution.

Many reviewed studies did not account for any confounder in the epidemiological model [33, 47, 59, 73–77]. Some studies collected information about personal lifestyles or socio-economic status directly through questionnaires [38–40, 51, 78, 79]. Unfortunately the use of questionnaires and surveys is unfeasible for large populations; thus a large part of the studies did not consider personal lifestyles but included socio-economic indicators (e.g., deprivation indexes) evaluated at municipality/census block of residence [29, 30, 35, 44, 45, 49, 80, 81]. These indexes are generally constructed based on census statistics.

Of particular concern is the general lack of information about environmental confounding. Many of the pathologies under study have been associated with various atmospheric pollutants (e.g., PM_{10}, NO_x, etc.) or specific anthropogenic sources (e.g., road traffic, industrial emissions). Often, waste incinerators are located inside industrial areas or near other major sources of pollution. In our case study, for example, the incinerator is located inside the industrial area of Parma, at about 200 m from a national highway that crosses the study area east-west (i.e., the prevalent wind directions). As a result, most exposed subjects, as identified by the dispersion model, were also more exposed to other sources of pollution. It will be difficult to correctly identify the possible health effect of this incinerator, unless we have some information about the difference in population exposure to other sources between the exposed and nonexposed groups. Only few studies included information about environmental confounders. Biggeri et al. [79] used measured particulate depositions from the nearest monitoring station, Cordier et al. [45] used proxies for the presence of industrial activities and road traffic at community level, and two studies [31, 44] used proxies for traffic and industrial pollution at census block level. Notably, one recent study [29] used atmospheric dispersion models to estimate pollution concentrations at the address of residence from other local sources of atmospheric pollution (road traffic, industrial plants, and heating). This represents a notable improvement since the confounding factor was evaluated with the same spatial resolution as exposure to the incinerator.

As the quantitative contribution of well-managed modern incinerators to total pollution levels in a study area and to baseline health risks is expected to be low, we suggest to draw a careful attention to other local sources of pollution and to implement multisite studies on large populations where feasible.

5. Conclusions

We reviewed 41 articles from the literature with the main aim of retrieving information for the definition of an exposure assessment protocol to be used in a large study on health effects of pollution due to incinerators (MONITER project).

Overall, our analysis showed a trend of improvement in exposure assessment quality over time, with a massive use of dispersion models in exposure assessment after year 2003.

Nevertheless, the lack of a common framework for exposure assessment is demonstrated by the use of a variety of methods, also in recent papers, with different quality of epidemiological findings and difficulties in comparisons of results.

In most of the selected studies the characterization of exposure can be significantly improved by using more detailed data for population residency and better simulation models. Recent development of informative systems and high availability of environmental and demographic data suggest the use of dispersion models of pollutants emitted from a source, combined with precise methods of geographic localizations of people under study, as the state of the art method to assess exposure of population in epidemiological studies. Considerations about residential mobility, temporal variations in pollution emissions, latency period of investigated diseases, and treatment of environmental and sociodemographic confounders can improve exposure assessment accuracy.

All these aspects of exposure assessment are particularly relevant as most of environmental conflicts usually arise from the evaluation of the contribution of the various pollution sources to the overall contamination.

Acknowledgments

The present work has been carried out within the activities of the Project Line no.3 of the MONITER Project. The project was funded by the Health and Environmental Assessorships of the Emilia-Romagna Region. The authors thank Dr. Paola Angelini and all project participants.

References

[1] Eurostat, "Eurostat statistical books. Environmental statistics and accounts in Europe 2010. 2010 Edition," European Union, 2010.

[2] D. Saner, Y. B. Blumer, D. J. Lang, and A. Koehler, "Scenarios for the implementation of EU waste legislation at national level and their consequences for emissions from municipal waste incineration," *Resources, Conservation and Recycling*, vol. 57, pp. 67–77, 2011.

[3] M. F. Reis, "Solid waste incinerators: health impacts," in *Encyclopaedia of Environmental Health*, pp. 162–217, 2011.

[4] M. Allsopp, P. Costner, and P. Johnston, "Incineration and human health: state of knowledge of the impacts of waste incinerators on human health (executive summary)," *Environmental Science and Pollution Research*, vol. 8, no. 2, pp. 141–145, 2001.

[5] British Society for Ecological Medicine, *The Health Effects of Waste Incinerators 4th Report of the British Cociety for Ecological Medicine*, 2nd edition, 2008.

[6] F. Forastiere, C. Badaloni, K. De Hoogh et al., "Health impact assessment of waste management facilities in three European countries," *Environmental Health*, vol. 10, no. 1, article 53, 2011.

[7] R. J. Roberts and M. Chen, "Waste incineration—how big is the health risk? A quantitative method to allow comparison with other health risks," *Journal of Public Health*, vol. 28, no. 3, pp. 261–266, 2006.

[8] M. Cordioli, S. Vincenzi, and G. A. Delleo, "Effects of heat recovery for district heating on waste incineration health impact: a simulation study in Northern Italy," *Science of the Total Environment*, vol. 444, pp. 369–380, 2013.

[9] D. Porta, S. Milani, A. I. Lazzarino, C. A. Perucci, and F. Forastiere, "Systematic review of epidemiological studies on health effects associated with management of solid waste," *Environmental Health*, vol. 8, no. 1, article 60, 2009.

[10] M. Franchini, M. Rial, E. Buiatti, and F. Bianchi, "Health effects of exposure to waste incinerator emissions: a review of epidemiological studies," *Annali dell'Istituto Superiore di Sanita*, vol. 40, no. 1, pp. 101–115, 2004.

[11] S.-W. Hu and C. M. Shy, "Health effects of waste incineration: a review of epidemiologic studies," *Journal of the Air and Waste Management Association*, vol. 51, no. 7, pp. 1100–1109, 2001.

[12] U. K. Defra, Review of Environmental and Health Effects of Waste Management: Municipal Solid Waste and Similar Wastes, 2004.

[13] WHO Europe, *Population Health and Waste Management: Scientific Data and Policy Options*, Copenhagen, Denmark, 2007.

[14] Committee oh Human and Environmental Exposure in the 21st entury, *Exposure Science in the 21st Century. A Vision and a StrAtegy*, National Acedemy of Sciences, 2012.

[15] M. Nieuwenhuijsen, D. Paustenbach, and R. Duarte-Davidson, "New developments in exposure assessment: the impact on the

practice of health risk assessment and epidemiological studies," *Environment International*, vol. 32, no. 8, pp. 996–1009, 2006.

[16] J. R. Nuckols, M. H. Ward, and L. Jarup, "Using geographic information systems for exposure assessment in environmental epidemiology studies," *Environmental Health Perspectives*, vol. 112, no. 9, pp. 1007–1015, 2004.

[17] B. Zou, J. G. Wilson, F. B. Zhan, and Y. Zeng, "Air pollution exposure assessment methods utilized in epidemiological studies," *Journal of Environmental Monitoring*, vol. 11, no. 3, pp. 475–490, 2009.

[18] Emilia Romagna Region, "The MONITER project," 2012, http://www.arpa.emr.it/moniter/index.asp .

[19] A. Kibble and R. Harrison, "Point sources of air pollution," *Occupational Medicine*, vol. 55, no. 6, pp. 425–431, 2005.

[20] L. Giusti, "A review of waste management practices and their impact on human health," *Waste Management*, vol. 29, no. 8, pp. 2227–2239, 2009.

[21] H. L. Chen, H. J. Su, P. C. Liao, C. H. Chen, and C. C. Lee, "Serum PCDD/F concentration distribution in residents living in the vicinity of an incinerator and its association with predicted ambient dioxin exposure," *Chemosphere*, vol. 54, no. 10, pp. 1421–1429, 2004.

[22] M. F. Reis, C. Sampaio, P. Aguiar, J. Maurício Melim, J. Pereira Miguel, and O. Päpke, "Biomonitoring of PCDD/Fs in populations living near portuguese solid waste incinerators: levels in human milk," *Chemosphere*, vol. 67, no. 9, pp. S231–S237, 2007.

[23] M. Schuhmacher, J. L. Domingo, and J. Garreta, "Pollutants emitted by a cement plant: health risks for the population living in the neighborhood," *Environmental Research*, vol. 95, no. 2, pp. 198–206, 2004.

[24] M. Schuhmacher, K. C. Jones, and J. L. Domingo, "Air-vegetation transfer of PCDD/PCDFs: an assessment of field data and implications for modeling," *Environmental Pollution*, vol. 142, no. 1, pp. 143–150, 2006.

[25] EPA, "Human health risk assessment protocol for hazardous waste combustion facilities," Tech. Rep. EPA530-R-05-006, 2005.

[26] A. Blair, P. Stewart, J. H. Lubin, and F. Forastiere, "Methodological issues regarding confounding and exposure misclassification in epidemiological studies of occupational exposures," *American Journal of Industrial Medicine*, vol. 50, no. 3, pp. 199–207, 2007.

[27] L. Sheppard, R. T. Burnett, A. A. Szpiro et al., "Confounding and exposure measurement error in air pollution epidemiology," *Air Quality, Atmosphere and Health*, vol. 5, no. 2, pp. 203–216, 2011.

[28] Cambridge Environmental Research Consultants Ltd, ADMS URban technical specification, 2001.

[29] A. Ranzi, V. Fano, L. Erspamer, P. Lauriola, C. A. Perucci, and F. Forastiere, "Mortality and morbidity among people living close to incinerators: a cohort study based on dispersion modeling for exposure assessment," *Environmental Health*, vol. 10, no. 1, article 22, 2011.

[30] S. Cordier, A. Lehébel, E. Amar et al., "Maternal residence near municipal waste incinerators and the risk of urinary tract birth defects," *Occupational and Environmental Medicine*, vol. 67, no. 7, pp. 493–499, 2010.

[31] J.-F. Viel, C. Daniau, S. Goria et al., "Risk for non Hodgkin's lymphoma in the vicinity of French municipal solid waste incinerators," *Environmental Health*, vol. 7, article 51, 2008.

[32] N. Floret, J.-F. Viel, E. Lucot et al., "Dispersion modeling as a dioxin exposure indicator in the vicinity of a municipal solid waste incinerator: a validation study," *Environmental Science and Technology*, vol. 40, no. 7, pp. 2149–2155, 2006.

[33] P. Comba, V. Ascoli, S. Belli et al., "Risk of soft tissue sarcomas and residence in the neighbourhood of an incinerator of industrial wastes," *Occupational and Environmental Medicine*, vol. 60, no. 9, pp. 680–683, 2003.

[34] P. Michelozzi, D. Fusco, F. Forastiere, C. Ancona, V. Dell'Orco, and C. A. Perucci, "Small area study of mortality among people living near multiple sources of air pollution," *Occupational and Environmental Medicine*, vol. 55, no. 9, pp. 611–615, 1998.

[35] P. Elliott, G. Shaddick, I. Kleinschmidt et al., "Cancer incidence near municipal solid waste incinerators in Great Britain," *British Journal of Cancer*, vol. 73, no. 5, pp. 702–710, 1996.

[36] S. Peters, R. Vermeulen, A. Cassidy et al., "Comparison of exposure assessment methods for occupational carcinogens in a multi-centre lung cancer case—control study," *Occupational and Environmental Medicine*, vol. 68, no. 2, pp. 148–153, 2011.

[37] C. Eriksson, M. E. Nilsson, D. Stenkvist, T. Bellander, and G. Pershagen, "Residential traffic noise exposure assessment: application and evaluation of European Environmental Noise Directive maps," *Journal of Exposure Science and Environmental Epidemiology*, 2012.

[38] F. Barbone, M. Bovenzi, A. Biggeri, C. Lagazio, F. Cavallieri, and G. Stanta, "Comparison of epidemiologic methods in a case-control study of lung cancer and air pollution in Trieste, Italy," *Epidemiologia e Prevenzione*, vol. 19, no. 63, pp. 193–205, 1995.

[39] C. M. Shy, D. Degnan, D. I. Fox et al., "Do waste incinerators induce adverse respiratory effects? An air quality and epidemiological study of six communities," *Environmental Health Perspectives*, vol. 103, no. 7-8, pp. 714–724, 1995.

[40] A. K. Mohan, D. Degnan, C. E. Feigley et al., "Comparison of respiratory symptoms among community residents near waste disposal incinerators," *International Journal of Environmental Health Research*, vol. 10, no. 1, pp. 63–75, 2000.

[41] S.-W. Hu, M. Hazucha, and C. M. Shy, "Waste incineration and pulmonary function: an epidemiologic study of six communities," *Journal of the Air and Waste Management Association*, vol. 51, no. 8, pp. 1185–1194, 2001.

[42] J.-T. Lee and C. M. Shy, "Respiratory function as measured by peak expiratory flow rate and PM10: six communities study," *Journal of Exposure Analysis and Environmental Epidemiology*, vol. 9, no. 4, pp. 293–299, 1999.

[43] J.-F. Viel, P. Arveux, J. Baverel, and J.-Y. Cahn, "Soft-tissue sarcoma and non-Hodgkin's lymphoma clusters around a municipal solid waste incinerator with high dioxin emission levels," *American Journal of Epidemiology*, vol. 152, no. 1, pp. 13–19, 2000.

[44] S. Goria, C. Daniau, P. De Crouy-Chanel et al., "Risk of cancer in the vicinity of municipal solid waste incinerators: importance of using a flexible modelling strategy," *International Journal of Health Geographics*, vol. 8, no. 1, article 31, 2009.

[45] S. Cordier, C. Chevrier, E. Robert-Gnansia, C. Lorente, P. Brula, and M. Hours, "Risk of congenital anomalies in the vicinity of municipal solid waste incinerators," *Occupational and Environmental Medicine*, vol. 61, no. 1, pp. 8–15, 2004.

[46] Y. Fukuda, K. Nakamura, and T. Takano, "Dioxins released from incineration plants and mortality from major diseases: an analysis of statistical data by municipalities," *Journal of Medical and Dental Sciences*, vol. 50, no. 4, pp. 249–255, 2003.

[47] P. Zambon, P. Ricci, E. Bovo et al., "Sarcoma risk and dioxin emissions from incinerators and industrial plants: a population-based case-control study (Italy)," *Environmental Health*, vol. 6, article 19, 2007.

[48] K. S. Rao, "Uncertainty analysis in atmospheric dispersion modeling," *Pure and Applied Geophysics*, vol. 162, no. 10, pp. 1893–1917, 2005.

[49] J.-F. Viel, M.-C. Clément, M. Hägi, S. Grandjean, B. Challier, and A. Danzon, "Dioxin emissions from a municipal solid waste incinerator and risk of invasive breast cancer: a population-based case-control study with GIS-derived exposure," *International Journal of Health Geographics*, vol. 7, article 4, 2008.

[50] R. Tessari, C. Canova, F. Canal et al., "Environmental pollution from dioxins and soft tissue sarcomas in the population of Venice and Mestre: an example of the use of current electronic information sources," *Epidemiologia e Prevenzione*, vol. 30, no. 3, pp. 191–198, 2006.

[51] N. Floret, F. Mauny, B. Challier, P. Arveux, J.-Y. Cahn, and J.-F. Viel, "Dioxin emissions from a solid waste incinerator and risk of non-Hodgkin lymphoma," *Epidemiology*, vol. 14, no. 4, pp. 392–398, 2003.

[52] S. Parodi, R. Baldi, C. Benco et al., "Lung cancer mortality in a district of La Spezia (Italy) exposed to air pollution from industrial plants," *Tumori*, vol. 90, no. 2, pp. 181–185, 2004.

[53] T. Tango, T. Fujita, T. Tanihata et al., "Risk of adverse reproductive outcomes associated with proximity to municipal solid waste incinerators with high dioxin emission levels in Japan," *Journal of Epidemiology*, vol. 14, no. 3, pp. 83–93, 2004.

[54] E. J. Gray, J. K. Peat, C. M. Mellis, J. Harrington, and A. J. Woolcock, "Asthma severity and morbidity in a population sample of Sydney school children: part I—prevalence and effect of air pollutants in coastal regions," *Australian and New Zealand Journal of Medicine*, vol. 24, no. 2, pp. 168–175, 1994.

[55] S. Caserini, S. Cernuschi, M. Giugliano, M. Grosso, G. Lonati, and P. Mattaini, "Air and soil dioxin levels at three sites in Italy in proximity to MSW incineration plants," *Chemosphere*, vol. 54, no. 9, pp. 1279–1287, 2004.

[56] M. Nadal, M. C. Agramunt, M. Schuhmacher, and J. L. Domingo, "PCDD/PCDF congener profiles in soil and herbage samples collected in the vicinity of a municipal waste incinerator before and after pronounced reductions of PCDD/PCDF emissions from the facility," *Chemosphere*, vol. 49, no. 2, pp. 153–159, 2002.

[57] M. Vinceti, C. Malagoli, S. Teggi et al., "Adverse pregnancy outcomes in a population exposed to the emissions of a municipal waste incinerator," *Science of the Total Environment*, vol. 407, no. 1, pp. 116–121, 2008.

[58] G. Shaddick, D. Lee, and J. Wakefield, "Ecological bias in studies of the short-term effects of air pollution on health," *International Journal of Applied Earth Observation and Geoinformation*, vol. 22, pp. 65–74, 2013.

[59] F. L. R. Williams, A. B. Lawson, and O. L. Lloyd, "Low sex ratios of births in areas at risk from air pollution from incinerators, as shown by geographical analysis and 3-dimensional mapping," *International Journal of Epidemiology*, vol. 21, no. 2, pp. 311–319, 1992.

[60] N. F. Reeve, T. R. Fanshawe, T. J. Keegan, A. G. Stewart, and P. J. Diggle, "Spatial analysis of health effects of large industrial incinerators in England, 1998–2008: a study using matched case-control areas," *BMJ Open*, vol. 3, Article ID e001847, 2013.

[61] P. A. Zandbergen, "Geocoding quality and implications for spatial analysis," *Geography Compass*, vol. 3, no. 2, pp. 647–680, 2009.

[62] D. T. Duncan, M. C. Castro, J. C. Blossom, G. G. Bennett, and L. G. G. G. Steven, "Evaluation of the positional difference between two common geocoding methods," *Geospatial Health*, vol. 5, no. 2, pp. 265–273, 2011.

[63] P. Diggle and P. Elliott, "Disease risk near point sources: statistical issues for analyses using individual or spatially aggregated data," *Journal of Epidemiology and Community Health*, vol. 49, no. 2, pp. S20–S27, 1995.

[64] N. E. Klepeis, W. C. Nelson, W. R. Ott et al., "The National Human Activity Pattern Survey (NHAPS): a resource for assessing exposure to environmental pollutants," *Journal of Exposure Analysis and Environmental Epidemiology*, vol. 11, no. 3, pp. 231–252, 2001.

[65] X. Wu, D. H. Bennett, K. Lee, D. L. Cassady, B. Ritz, and I. Hertz-Picciotto, "Longitudinal variability of time-location/activity patterns of population at different ages: a longitudinal study in California," *Environmental Health*, vol. 10, no. 1, article 80, 2011.

[66] Y.-L. Huang and S. Batterman, "Residence location as a measure of environmental exposure: a review of air pollution epidemiology studies," *Journal of Exposure Analysis and Environmental Epidemiology*, vol. 10, no. 1, pp. 66–85, 2000.

[67] M. A. Canfield, T. A. Ramadhani, P. H. Langlois, and D. K. Waller, "Residential mobility patterns and exposure misclassification in epidemiologic studies of birth defects," *Journal of Exposure Science and Environmental Epidemiology*, vol. 16, no. 6, pp. 538–543, 2006.

[68] J. R. Meliker, M. J. Slotnick, G. A. AvRuskin, A. Kaufmann, G. M. Jacquez, and J. O. Nriagu, "Improving exposure assessment in environmental epidemiology: application of spatio-temporal visualization tools," *Journal of Geographical Systems*, vol. 7, no. 1, pp. 49–66, 2005.

[69] M. Dosemeci, S. Wacholder, and J. H. Lubin, "Does nondifferential misclassification of exposure always bias a true effect toward the null value?" *American Journal of Epidemiology*, vol. 132, no. 4, pp. 746–748, 1990.

[70] C. A. Holcroft and D. Spiegelman, "Design of validation studies for estimating the odds ratio of exposure- disease relationships when exposure is misclassified," *Biometrics*, vol. 55, no. 4, pp. 1193–1201, 1999.

[71] D. Spiegelman, "Approaches to uncertainty in exposure assessment in environmental epidemiology," *Annual Review of Public Health*, vol. 31, pp. 149–163, 2010.

[72] R. McNamee, "Confounding and confounders," *Occupational and Environmental Medicine*, vol. 60, no. 3, pp. 227–234, 2003.

[73] H. Rydhstroem, "No obvious spatial clustering of twin births in sweden between 1973 and 1990," *Environmental Research*, vol. 76, no. 1, pp. 27–31, 1998.

[74] G. W. Ten Tusscher, G. A. Stam, and J. G. Koppe, "Open chemical combustions resulting in a local increased incidence of orofacial clefts," *Chemosphere*, vol. 40, no. 9-11, pp. 1263–1270, 2000.

[75] A. Biggeri and D. Catelan, "Mortality for non-Hodgkin lymphoma and soft-tissue sarcoma in the surrounding area of an urban waste incinerator. Campi Bisenzio (Tuscany, Italy) 1981–2001," *Epidemiologia e Prevenzione*, vol. 29, no. 3-4, pp. 156–159, 2005.

[76] A. Biggeri and D. Catelan, "Mortalità per linfomi non Hodgkin nei comuni della Regione Toscana dove sono stati attivi

inceneritori di rifiuti solidi urbani nel periodo 1970–1989," *Epidemiologia & Prevenzione*, vol. 1, pp. 14–15, 2006.

[77] F. Bianchi and F. Minichilli, "Mortalità per linfomi non Hodgkin nel periodo 1981–2001 in comuni italiani con inceneritori di rifiuti solidi urbani," *Epidemiologia & Prevenzione*, vol. 2, pp. 80–81, 2006.

[78] T.-R. Hsiue, S.-S. Lee, and H.-I. Chen, "Effects of air pollution resulting from wire reclamation incineration on pulmonary function in children," *Chest*, vol. 100, no. 3, pp. 698–702, 1991.

[79] A. Biggeri, F. Barbone, C. Lagazio, M. Bovenzi, and G. Stanta, "Air pollution and lung cancer in Trieste, Italy: spatial analysis of risk as a function of distance from sources," *Environmental Health Perspectives*, vol. 104, no. 7, pp. 750–754, 1996.

[80] P. Elliott, M. Hills, J. Beresford et al., "Incidence of cancers of the larynx and lung near incinerators of waste solvents and oils in Great Britain," *The Lancet*, vol. 339, no. 8797, pp. 854–858, 1992.

[81] M. Federico, M. Pirani, I. Rashid, N. Caranci, and C. Cirilli, "Cancer incidence in people with residential exposure to a municipal waste incinerator: an ecological study in Modena (Italy), 1991–2005," *Waste Management*, vol. 30, no. 7, pp. 1362–1370, 2010.

5

Particulate Emissions: Health Effects and Labour Market Consequences

Marie Kruse,[1,2] Bjørn Sætterstrøm,[1] Jakob Bønløkke,[3] Henrik Brønnum-Hansen,[4] Esben Meulengracht Flachs,[5] and Jan Sørensen[1]

[1] *Centre for Applied Health Technology Assessment, University of Southern Denmark, J.B. Winsløwsvej 9B 1, 5000 Odense C, Denmark*
[2] *The Danish Institute for Health Services Research, Dampfærgevej 27–29, 2100 Copenhagen, Denmark*
[3] *Section of Environmental and Occupational Health, Institute of Public Health, Aarhus University, Bartholins Allé 2, 8000 Aarhus C, Denmark*
[4] *Institute of Public Health, University of Copenhagen, Øster Farimagsgade 5, 1014 Copenhagen, Denmark*
[5] *National Institute of Public Health, University of Southern Denmark, Øster Farimagsgade 5, 1014 Copenhagen, Denmark*

Correspondence should be addressed to Marie Kruse, mkr@dsi.dk

Academic Editor: Abul Hasnat Milton

The objective of this study was to analyse the productivity cost savings associated with mitigation of particulate emissions, as an input to a cost-benefit analysis. Reduced emissions of particulate matter ($PM_{2.5}$) may reduce the incidence of diseases related to air pollution and potentially increase productivity as a result of better health. Based on data from epidemiological studies, we modelled the impact of air pollution on four different diseases: coronary heart disease, stroke, lung cancer, and chronic obstructive pulmonary disease. We identified individuals with these diseases and modelled changes in disease incidence as an expression of exposure. The labour market affiliation and development in wages over time for exposed individuals was compared to that of a reference group of individuals matched on a number of sociodemographic variables, comorbidity, and predicted smoking status. We identified a productivity cost of about 1.8 million EURO per 100,000 population aged 50–70 in the first year, following an increase in $PM_{2.5}$ emissions. We have illustrated how the potential impact of air pollution may influence social production by application of a matched study design that renders a study population similar to that of a trial. The result suggests that there may be a productivity gain associated with mitigation efforts.

1. Introduction

Pollution has wide-ranging consequences, for health as well as in other sectors [1]. Following a Health Impact Assessment of particulate matter emissions [2], this study aims to quantify the labour market consequences of particulate emissions as part of a cost-benefit analysis of mitigation efforts.

What are the costs and benefits of air pollution mitigation? The costs include the actual mitigation costs as well as the disutility (and costs) of those who are forced to reduce their emissions, while the benefits include the utility of a cleaner air as well as the benefits associated with lower levels of pollution. Among the benefits from reduced air pollution are the economic gains related to improved health. This study focuses on some of these gains, namely, the productivity gains from lower pollution-related morbidity and mortality. For practical reasons, the gains are quantified by means of assessing their opposite measure: the costs of increased pollution.

Air pollution impacts on health through increased incidence and mortality of a number of diseases [2]. In this analysis, we focus on the increase in incidence of coronary heart disease, stroke, lung cancer, and chronic obstructive pulmonary disease (COPD), all of which are associated with increased levels of fine particulate ($PM_{2.5}$) emissions. Miller et al. [3] found that women who were exposed to an increase in the level of $PM_{2.5}$ by 10 microgram per m^3 had a relative risk (RR) of 1.21 (95% CI: 1.04–1.42) of experiencing a coronary heart disease event and 1.35 (95% CI: 1.08–1.68) of experiencing an episode of stroke. Similarly, Pope III et al. [4] found a RR of 1.14 (95% CI: 1.04–1.23) for lung cancer in both genders when particulate emissions increased by 10 micrograms per m^3. The RR for COPD related to particulate emissions was also 1.14 for a similar increase in both genders [5].

Based on findings on mortality related to particulate emissions [4, 6], we assumed that the RR for cardiovascular events following exposure to particulate emissions for men was lower than that for women. Tentatively, therefore, we assumed that the RR of cardiovascular disease in exposed men was 1.29 and the RR for coronary heart disease in men exposed to particulate emissions was 1.175. We had no reason to assume a similar gender difference for pulmonary diseases. Instead we applied similar RR estimates for the two genders relating to pulmonary diseases.

When analysing health or social consequences of a risk factor such as air pollution in an epidemiological framework, it is necessary to identify exposed and nonexposed individuals. However, when examining the labour market consequences of air pollution, such an approach may not be feasible since all individuals in industrialised countries are exposed to some degree of air pollution. The health effects and the associated labour market consequences are often described in a dose-response relationship. Also, exposure may be related to transport habits and other parameters that are not easily measured at population level. Our approach to measuring exposure was therefore to express exposure to air pollution as the health effects of air pollution. More precisely, we developed a framework where the labour market consequences of diseases were assessed based on assumptions of the RR of disease incidence when exposed to air pollution. Basically, we considered the measurable health effects of air pollution as being an expression of overall exposure to air pollution.

We focused on incidence instead of prevalence because we wished to capture the effects of particulate emission-related disease on both morbidity and mortality. Merely focusing on prevalence would underestimate the mortality impact, because survivors make up a relatively larger share of the prevalent population, compared to their share of the incident population. This applies to any disease study, as simple mathematics dictate that since mortality is often higher in severe cases of a given disease, the prevalent population can be construed as relatively healthier than the incident population.

The aim of this paper was to quantify potential productivity gains due to improved health following a mitigation of air pollution through reduction of small particulate ($PM_{2.5}$) emissions. Practically, we have approached this task by quantifying the productivity costs of health consequences of existing particulate emissions and assumed that this present cost can be saved when mitigation succeeds. In this study, we have applied known health effects of pollution on labour market behaviour. Health effects on labour market behaviour was either productivity costs due to death or early retirement, or relative wage losses, that is, workers with a disease or reduced health will receive a lesser wage increase.

The productivity costs due to mortality and premature departure from the labour market constitute the societal costs of disease, while the wage loss expresses a loss to the individual worker. A cost-benefit analysis will from a societal perspective include both cost components.

2. Materials and Methods

2.1. Selection of Study Population. We assessed the labour market consequences of the four diseases in a register-based analysis. We used disease as an expression of exposure and thus identified a patient group as "the exposed" and a control group as "the nonexposed." The control group was identified such that they were as comparable to the patient group as possible. The difference in labour market affiliation and wage developments were considered as being attributable to disease and thus air pollution. In calculations of changes in costs, we assumed an increase in $PM_{2.5}$ of 10 microgram/m^3.

Patients with at least one hospital admission caused by coronary heart disease (ICD10 diagnoses I20–25), stroke (ICD10: I60–69), lung cancer (ICD10: C33-34), or COPD (ICD10: J41–44) were identified in the Danish National Hospital Register. In addition, individuals that had died from these diseases but had not been hospitalised for the disease while alive were identified in the National Causes of Death Register. The identified patients were matched with a reference group of nonpatients, henceforth called the control group. Both groups were followed for a period of 10 years, with 1998 being the baseline year and 1999 the year of first hospital contact for coronary heart disease patients, lung cancer patients, and stroke patients. Due to hospitalisation occurring late in the disease history for COPD patients, we defined two groups of COPD patients, the first having their first hospitalisation in 1999, like the three other diseases, and the second having their first hospitalisation in 2006. The baseline year for both groups was 1998. We adopted a wash-out period of 5 years (1994–98) during which patients could not have had any health care contacts related to the analysed disease. The rationale of the wash-out period was to ensure that cases were in fact incident and had not been hospitalised for their disease previously.

For each disease, we selected a control group amongst the entire adult Danish population, using individual, nearest neighbour matching by propensity scores [7, 8] comprising age in one-year intervals, comorbidities (a Charlson index [9] excluding the analysed disease), marital status, national origin, length of education, socioeconomic status, and area of residence. Matching was conducted in five-year age strata and gender. There were five controls per case. Controls with the analysed disease occurring before or after 1999 were excluded. For both patients and controls, we obtained data for annual, gross wages, and labour market affiliation from the national registers at Statistics Denmark. These register data were linked to health data via the social security number. Most labour market data reflects the labour market status of

Table 1: Data structure.

Variable	Levels	Application in analysis
Ds: disease	1 if incident disease (first time event of CHD, stroke, or lung cancer in 1999 or COPD hospitalisation in 2006)	Main explanatory variable
Age	1-year age group	Included in propensity score
5-year age intervals	5-year age group	Used for stratification of matching procedure
Gender	0 if man; 1 if woman	Used for stratification of matching procedure
CMI: comorbidities	Diseases weigh from 1 to 6 (modified Charlson index)	Included in propensity score
Married: marital status	1 if married or cohabiting, 0 otherwise	Included in propensity score
Origin: national origin	0 if Danish; 1 if not Danish	Included in propensity score
Edu: length of education	1–8, where 8 is university degree	Included in propensity score
Socio: socioeconomic status at baseline (1998) People outside the labour market were excluded from this analysis	(1) Self-employed (2) White collar (3) Blue collar (4) Unemployed	Included in propensity score
Residence	Regional code used as a proxy for urban/rural	Included in propensity score
LM: labour market affiliation	1 if employed or unemployed, 0 if retired or dead	Outcome variable
Wage	Continuous variable expressing the difference between wage in 2000 and wage in 1998	Outcome variable

Table 2: Risk of leaving the labour market earlier for patients compared to controls, by diagnosis.

Disease	Hazard ratio of leaving the labour market	95 percent confidence interval for hazard ratio
Coronary heart disease	**1.129**	(1.124–1.133)
Stroke	**1.122**	(1.117–1.127)
Lung cancer	**1.355**	(1.342–1.37)
COPD	**1.14**	(1.134–1.147)

Hazard ratios that were statistically significant at $\alpha = 0.05$ are indicated in bold.

a person in November. Data allows, however, for adjustment for unemployment spells during the year.

We used the variables displayed in Table 1 for analysis.

2.2. Labour Market Affiliation. For those patients that were in the labour market at baseline (1998), labour market affiliation was analysed using duration analysis (Cox regression). Individuals were considered to be in the labour market when they were employed, self-employed, or unemployed. If they deceased or received age pension, disability pension, or early retirement, they were considered outside the labour market. Other categories, such as students, were excluded.

The duration model estimated the excess risk of leaving the labour market for patients compared to controls by modelling LM (labour market affiliation) as a function of Ds (disease) (see Table 1 for abbreviations of variables).

The resulting hazard ratio (HR) for the Ds parameter expresses the increased risk of leaving the labour market due to mortality or morbidity among patients, when compared to controls. Since confounding factors have been taken into account in the matching procedure, there is no need to apply adjustment in the model. Indeed, further adjustment would cause overadjustment for the covariates by including their effect twice.

We tested whether the proportional hazards assumption was sustained, using the proportionality test option in PROC PHREG of SAS.

2.3. Wage Consequences. Wage consequences were analysed using a difference-in-difference approach. For each patient, the wage development from 1998 to 2000 was recorded and compared to the wage development for the matched controls, using the same period. Only individuals with a labour market income in both years were included in this analysis. Hence, pensioners and others having only a nonlabour market income were excluded from this analysis of wage development. Also people leaving the labour market due to pension (or death) were excluded.

The crude wage development over the period 1998–2000 was compared between patients and controls. The wage loss related to disease was quantified as

$$\begin{aligned}\mathrm{WL}_{\text{disease}} = {} & \left(\mathrm{Wage}_{\text{control}}2000 - \mathrm{Wage}_{\text{control}}1998\right) \\ & - \left(\mathrm{Wage}_{\text{patient}}2000 - \mathrm{Wage}_{\text{patient}}1998\right). \end{aligned} \tag{i}$$

TABLE 3: Average wage development 1998–2000, EURO-2000 price level.

Disease	Control group			Patient group			Difference in average wage development
	N 2000	Average wage 1998	Average wage 2000	N 2000	Average wage 1998	Average wage 2000	
Coronary heart disease	17,219	28,930	29,913	2,898	28,197	29,100	80
Stroke	8,609	27,956	28,737	1,298	31,434	31,257	958
Lung cancer	2,571	26,706	27,154	110	25,746	27,816	−1,622
COPD	5,034	25,682	26,258	794	25,041	25,527	89

2.4. Productivity Costs of $PM_{2.5}$. The increased risk of leaving the labour market due to disease, multiplied by the annual wage of a control person, constitutes the average productivity cost of leaving the labour market too soon due to disease. Similarly, the wage loss computed via (ii) relates to the total wage loss due to disease. The productivity costs of particulate emission relating to both the labour market withdrawal and the wage loss are computed by multiplying the two with the elevated risk of disease due to particulate emission, that is, RR-1. The particulate emission related productivity costs per person are transformed to population-based figures using incidence of disease. For incidence, we have used data on first-ever hospital admissions and causes of death figures for individuals aged 50–70 years.

The productivity cost ($PC_{\text{pollution}}$) of disease was estimated by multiplying the excess risk of disease incidence (RR-1) with the excess risk of leaving the labour market (HR-1) and the average wage of patients in 2000, being the first calendar year after the event:

$$PC_{\text{pollution}} = (RR - 1) * (HR - 1) * \text{Wage}_{\text{patients}} 2000. \quad \text{(ii)}$$

Similarly for wage differences,

$$WL_{\text{pollution}} = (RR - 1) * WL_{\text{disease}}. \quad \text{(iii)}$$

Equations (ii) and (iii) express labour market consequences per patient. In order to arrive at the socioeconomic gain of mitigation of particulate emissions, the labour market consequences per patient should be related to incidence as shown in the following:

$$\begin{aligned} \text{number of saved cases} &= \text{incidence before} - \text{incidence after} \\ &= \text{incidence before} - \left(\frac{1}{RR}\right) \\ &\quad * \text{incidence before} = \left(\frac{1\text{-}1}{RR}\right) \\ &\quad * \text{incidence before}, \end{aligned} \quad \text{(iv)}$$

where RR is the relative risk of disease incidence when exposed to particulate emissions. Incidence figures are related to the age group 50–70, and results should therefore be interpreted as savings per 100,000 population aged 50–70. We computed the gain for one year and also accumulated the cost over a ten-year period. The results for the ten-year period were computed, considering that a smaller share of the population is in the labour market each year, due to labour market withdrawal in the preceding years. Also, future costs were discounted by 3 per cent per year in order to obtain the net present value. Cost figures are expressed in 2000-EURO's using an exchange rate of €1 = 7.5 DKK.

We used SAS v. 9.2 for all analyses. Individual data were stored at Statistics Denmark which ensured full compliance with all confidentiality laws and regulations.

3. Results

For all four diseases, there was a statistically significant higher risk of leaving the labour market for patients with the four diseases in comparison with nondiseased controls. Table 2 displays the estimated hazard ratios for leaving the labour market early.

The impact of disease on labour market affiliation shown in Table 2 indicates that there is a productivity loss associated with these diseases.

Table 3 displays wages at baseline (1998) and two years later (in 2000). Wage developments were used for calculation of difference-in-difference: did controls experience a better development in wages than patients? All wages were converted to 2000-fixed prices. From Table 3, it appears that there were only minor differences between patients and controls in terms of wage increases. The exception is lung cancer, where the disease apparently has a beneficial impact on wage development. It should be noted that, due to poor survival, very few lung cancer patients remain in the labour market after onset of disease, and those who do may not be typical.

When interpreting the results in Table 3, it should be noted that the figures only relate to the individuals who were still in the labour market. Those who left the labour market due to disease or death were excluded from these calculations. Hence, the population figures do not reflect the entire matched study population, but only those still in the labour market in 2000.

Table 4 summarises the productivity costs of an increase in particulate emissions at 10-microgram per m^3 at patient and societal level. Hence, it combines the findings of Tables 2 and 3 on the productivity costs of disease to the impact of particulate emissions on these diseases. In Table 4, the productivity costs of disease are multiplied by the elevated

TABLE 4: Total productivity costs per 100,000 at risk—aged 50–70 (2000-€).

	Hazard ratio of leaving the labour market R[1]	Relative risk of disease[2]	Annual wage (2000 €)[3]	Annual average productivity cost €[4]	Annual average wage loss 2000 €[5]	Productivity cost first year €[6]	Accumulated productivity cost over ten years €[7]
Coronary heart disease	1.129	1.175	29,913	675	70	507,148	4,455,856
Stroke	1.122	1.29	28,737	1,017	842	877,430	7,709,195
Lung cancer	1.355	1.14	27,154	1,350	−1,046	278,009	2,442,619
COPD	1.14	1.14	26,258	515	77	140,843	1,237,461

Sources:
[1] Attributable risk of leaving the labour market: hazard ratios as presented in Table 2.
[2] Relative risk of disease when exposed to increased particulate emission, according to sources [3, 4].
[3] Annual wage in 2000 for controls, as in Table 3.
[4] The annual average productivity cost per patient per year 2000, computed according to (ii) .
[5] The annual average wage loss in year 2000, according to (iii) .
[6] First-year productivity cost per 100,000 population aged 50–70, computed according to (iv) .
[7] Accumulated productivity cost per 100,000 population aged 50–70 over ten years. Computed as the findings of column 6, over a ten-year period, taking into account a declining labour market participation rate and a discount rate of 3 percent p.a.

risk of disease when exposed to increased particulate emissions. The resulting productivity costs from a 10-microgram increase in particulate emission are presented as the average per exposed person, per 100,000 population aged 50–70 years in the first year and per 100,000 population aged 50–70 years accumulated over ten years. The latter figure represents the net present value of one year's exposure. During the ten-year period, almost all patients have left the labour market. The results in the last two columns of Table 4 are computed according to (iv) and hence represent a saving that can be harvested when mitigation efforts succeed.

In the first year after disease incidence, the productivity cost of a 10-microgram per m^3 increase in particulate emission amounts to about 1.8 million EURO per 100,000 population in the age group 50–70. Assuming a linear effect, the accumulated impact of one year's incidence amounts to more than 9 million EURO over a ten-year period.

4. Discussion

We have found that pollution-related disease impacts on labour market affiliation, and therefore there is a societal gain from reducing air pollution. This finding points towards an important consequence of particulate emissions on labour market affiliation through health effects and hence indicates that a potential productivity gain may arise from successful mitigation of air pollution. To our knowledge, this topic has not been analysed by other authors.

We also looked at the wage development and compared patients suffering pollution-related disease and controls. We found no significant wage differences attributable to pollution-related disease.

The analysis was designed as a comparison of a group of exposed individuals with a group of controls. The control group was selected using a propensity score approach, aiming at achieving a comparable control group with characteristics similar to the exposed group. By selecting a control group that was as similar to the patient group as possible, we aimed to analyse the counterfactual: what would have happened if they had not become ill. One challenge of this exercise is the selection of the characteristics that comprise the propensity score: that is, determining which characteristics of patients and controls are important in the analysis of labour market affiliation and wages. In the analysis, we have used a variety of available socioeconomic variables in the composition of the propensity score.

Therefore, socioeconomic and demographic parameters that may impact on labour market behaviour should be captured by the matching procedure, at least to some extent. One of the disadvantages of the propensity score approach is that not all characteristics weigh the same in the score and more minor variations may not be captured. The variables that weigh the most in the propensity score are those contributing the most to explain disease occurrence. This weighing of variables is not possible when matching is conducted using individual variables, which was one of the reasons we did not adopt that approach. Another option of course would be regression analyses on the entire population including adjustment for relevant covariates. Such an approach could include application of instrumental variables [10], addressing potential unobservable individual effects. Though this may be part of explaining the relation between disease and labour market behaviour, we chose to focus on relative effects instead, in a trial-like setup. The similarity of wages before the incidence year indicates that matching was successful.

We have focused on a variety of characteristics in our matching procedure. These include age, gender, and length of education, but also socioeconomic status and comorbidity. Other variables may also be important in explaining the complex relation between pollution, health, and labour market behaviour. We suggest that the relation between labour market behaviour and health is as complex as reflected in our model, and perhaps even more so. While acknowledging this, we may tentatively conclude that a decrease in particulate emissions may be associated with reduced disease incidence and mortality which may have a positive impact on labour market affiliation and productivity.

The evidence of smoking as an important risk factor for disease dates several years back [11, 12]. Compared to smoking, particulate emissions only have marginal effect on disease development. This should be borne in mind, in particular when analysing diseases such as COPD and lung cancer, in which smoking is an important risk factor. If the studies that describe interactions between mortality and air pollution do not capture the effect of smoking as an effect modifier sufficiently, the impact of air pollution on health may be slightly overestimated. It is also possible that other risk factors interact with smoking and pollution exposure [13], causing some uncertainty in our findings. The actual magnitude of our results may thus be somewhat uncertain. Nevertheless, it remains clear that particulate emissions incur significant costs due to their health effects and that mitigation of emissions would be associated with a substantial saving to society.

5. Conclusion

We have illustrated how the potential impact of air pollution may influence social production by application of a matched study design that renders a study population similar to that of a trial. We found that there is a significant productivity cost related to the health effects of pollution. These results suggest that there may be a productivity gain associated with mitigation of particulate emissions.

Further economic research could incorporate our findings into a cost-benefit analysis of a given mitigation intervention. In addition, our findings could be supported by further epidemiological research into the association between air pollution and disease.

Acknowledgments

This study was supported by a grant from the Danish National Strategic Research Council (Grant no. 2104-06-0027). Earlier versions of the paper have been presented at meetings of Centre for Energy, Environment and Health and at the Nordic Health Economists meeting in Odense, August 2011.

References

[1] "Description of the CEEH integrated "Energy-environment-health-cost" modelling framework syste," 2010, http://ceeh.dk/CEEH_Reports/Report_1/index.html.

[2] CEEH scientific report no. 7a, "description of the CEEH health effect model," 2011, http://ceeh.dk/CEEH_Reports/Report_7a/index.html.

[3] K. A. Miller, D. S. Siscovick, L. Sheppard et al., "Long-term exposure to air pollution and incidence of cardiovascular events in women," *New England Journal of Medicine*, vol. 356, no. 5, pp. 447–458, 2007.

[4] C. A. Pope III, R. T. Burnett, M. J. Thun et al., "Lung cancer, cardiopulmonary mortality, and long-term exposure to fine particulate air pollution," *Journal of the American Medical Association*, vol. 287, no. 9, pp. 1132–1141, 2002.

[5] D. E. Abbey, M. D. Lebowitz, P. K. Mills, F. F. Petersen, W. L. Beeson, and R. J. Burchette, "Long-term ambient concentrations of particulates and oxidants and development of chronic disease in a cohort of nonsmoking california residents," *Inhalation Toxicology*, vol. 7, no. 1, pp. 19–34, 1995.

[6] C. A. Pope III, M. J. Thun, M. M. Namboodiri et al., "Particulate air pollution as a predictor of mortality in a prospective study of U.S. Adults," *American Journal of Respiratory and Critical Care Medicine*, vol. 151, no. 3 I, pp. 669–674, 1995.

[7] D. B. Rubin, "Estimating causal effects from large data sets using propensity scores," *Annals of Internal Medicine*, vol. 127, no. 8, pp. 757–763, 1997.

[8] P. R. Rosenbaum and D. B. Rubin, "The central role of the propensity score in observational studies for causal effects," *Biometrika*, vol. 70, no. 1, pp. 41–55, 1983.

[9] M. E. Charlson, P. Pompei, K. A. Ales, and C. R. MacKenzie, "A new method of classifying prognostic comorbidity in longitudinal studies: development and validation," *Journal of Chronic Diseases*, vol. 40, no. 5, pp. 373–383, 1987.

[10] J. A. Hausman and W. E. Taylor, "Panel data and unobservable individual effects," *Econometrica*, vol. 49, pp. 1377–1398, 1981.

[11] C. D. Jenkins, R. H. Rosenman, and S. J. Zyzanski, "Cigarette smoking. Its relationship to coronary heart disease and related risk factors in the Western Collaborative Group Study.," *Circulation*, vol. 38, no. 6, pp. 1140–1155, 1968.

[12] W. B. Kannel, W. P. Castelli, and P. M. McNamara, "Cigarette smoking and risk of coronary heart disease. Epidemiologic clues to pathogensis. The Framingham Study.," *National Cancer Institute monograph*, vol. 28, pp. 9–20, 1968.

[13] P. J. Villeneuve, M. S. Goldberg, R. T. Burnett, A. van Donkelaar, H. Chen, and R. V. Martin, "Associations between cigarette smoking, obesity, sociodemographic characteristics and remote-sensing-derived estimates of ambient $PM_{2.5}$: results from a canadian population-based survey," *Occup Environ Med*, vol. 68, no. 12, pp. 920–927, 2011.

6

"We Are Not Being Heard": Aboriginal Perspectives on Traditional Foods Access and Food Security

Bethany Elliott,[1] Deepthi Jayatilaka,[1] Contessa Brown,[2] Leslie Varley,[3] and Kitty K. Corbett[4]

[1] *Population and Public Health, Provincial Health Services Authority, Vancouver, Canada V6Z 2H3*
[2] *Heiltsuk Nation, Bella Bella, Canada V0T 1Z0*
[3] *Aboriginal Health, Provincial Health Services Authority, Vancouver, Canada V5Z 4C2*
[4] *Faculty of Health Science, Simon Fraser University, Burnaby, Canada V5A 1S6*

Correspondence should be addressed to Bethany Elliott, bethany.elliott@phsa.ca

Academic Editor: Habibul Ahsan

Aboriginal peoples are among the most food insecure groups in Canada, yet their perspectives and knowledge are often sidelined in mainstream food security debates. In order to create food security for all, Aboriginal perspectives must be included in food security research and discourse. This project demonstrates a process in which Aboriginal and non-Aboriginal partners engaged in a culturally appropriate and respectful collaboration, assessing the challenges and barriers to traditional foods access in the urban environment of Vancouver, BC, Canada. The findings highlight local, national, and international actions required to increase access to traditional foods as a means of achieving food security for all people. The paper underscores the interconnectedness of local and global food security issues and highlights challenges as well as solutions with potential to improve food security of both Aboriginal and non-Aboriginal peoples alike.

1. Introduction

According to the Food and Agriculture Organization of the United Nations, "Food security exists when all people, at all times, have physical, social, and economic access to sufficient, safe, and nutritious food that meets their dietary needs and food preferences for an active and healthy life" [1]. Although this definition is intended to be inclusive of the dietary needs and food preferences of "all people," concepts beyond the conventional food system, for example, traditional or country foods, are often overlooked in food security discussions. Two food systems—conventional and traditional—play on food security of indigenous peoples in Canada, referred to as Aboriginal peoples. (The term Aboriginal peoples, as defined by the Canadian Constitution Act, includes Indian—a term which is now commonly replaced by the more accepted term First Nations, Inuit, and Métis peoples). The conventional food system, with which most readers are familiar, prioritizes agribusiness products intended for global consumer markets (market foods). The traditional food system, according to Kuhnlein and Chan [2], "includes all of the food species that are available to a particular culture from local natural resources and the accepted patterns for their use within that culture" and incorporates the sociocultural meanings of these foods, their acquisition, processing, and use within a specific culture. Aboriginal people in Canada have relied on foods from this traditional system since time immemorial, but also access market foods through the conventional system. This unique perspective is often missed in mainstream food security discourse; therefore, we argue that integrating Aboriginal knowledge and perspectives in whole of society strategies is imperative in creating food security for all people.

To date, research on Aboriginal food security has focused on traditional foods within communities living on reserves (tracts of crown land, set apart for the use, and benefit of an Indian band [3]). However, with approximately 60% of the Aboriginal population in Canada now living off reserve [4] a better understanding of the importance of traditional foods in the urban context is crucial to ensuring Aboriginal food security. As a whole, Aboriginal peoples living both on and off reserve are among the most food insecure groups in Canada. In the province where this research project took place (British Columbia, Canada), 41% of Aboriginal households on reservations are food insecure [5]. A Canada-wide survey found that 33% of all off-reserve Aboriginal households are food insecure, compared with only 9% among the general population [6].

Both on and off reserves, Aboriginal food insecurity is correlated with many diet-related health concerns. The rate of diabetes among Aboriginal peoples in British Columbia (BC) is 40% higher than the rest of the population, and its incidence continues to rise [7]. The prevalence of heart disease in BC Aboriginal peoples is 25% higher than the general population [7]. In addition, in British Columbia, 54% of Aboriginal people identified themselves as either overweight (31.8%) or obese (22.6%) [7]. Food insecurity and inadequate nutrition play a central role in these chronic health conditions.

Evidence suggests that traditional foods are more nutritious than conventional diets consisting of market foods. Studies in Canada found that traditional foods contain higher amounts of nutrients and less fat, sodium, and carbohydrates (especially sucrose) than market foods [8–14]. The First Nations Food, Nutrition, and Environment Study examined BC Aboriginal traditional foods and found that dietary quality (i.e., nutrient and energy intake) was improved on days when Aboriginal peoples consumed traditional foods [5]. Due to the health benefits of traditional foods, researchers have warned of the dietary and health risks associated with the "nutrition transition"—a gradual westernization of Aboriginal diets to include more preprocessed market foods and drinks and less traditional foods [2, 5, 11, 15]. However, despite this transition, Aboriginal peoples continue to consume traditional foods [5, 16] and endeavour to pass down traditional knowledge of land and food systems to younger generations, increasing food security, and self-sufficiency within their communities [17].

In light of the importance of traditional foods to health and food security of Aboriginal peoples, and their increasing migration to urban settings, the Aboriginal Health and Food Security programs of the Provincial Health Services Authority (PHSA) undertook a collaborative research project to assess the challenges and solutions to accessing traditional Aboriginal foods in the urban context of Vancouver, BC. The research team had representation from the Aboriginal Health and Food Security programs of PHSA and included a graduate student from the University of Toronto, and a research consultant of Aboriginal heritage. The research team engaged both Aboriginal and non-Aboriginal partners and was guided by a project Advisory Committee consisting primarily of Aboriginal peoples living in Vancouver with knowledge of Aboriginal food security and/or traditional foods.

This paper describes (1) the collaborative research process, demonstrating how traditional knowledge and "ways of knowing" can be incorporated into food security research; and (2) the findings from this process, highlighting a whole of society approach to enhance access to traditional foods as a means to achieve food security for all peoples. This paper demonstrates the interconnectedness of local and global food security issues and highlights that the challenges and solutions presented have the potential to impact food security of both Aboriginal and non-Aboriginal peoples alike.

2. Methodology

2.1. Guiding Principles and Advisory Committee. To ensure that the research project was both meaningful to the Aboriginal community and respectful of their traditional knowledge, the project was guided by the OCAP principles developed by Canada's National Aboriginal Health Organization [18]. The principles are guidelines to help researchers conduct studies that are appropriate and beneficial for Aboriginal peoples and to ensure the ethical application of such research. The OCAP principles are *ownership* of cultural knowledge/data/information by the community or group; the right of Aboriginal peoples to seek *control* of all aspects of research and information management processes that impact them; the right of Aboriginal peoples to *access* information and data about themselves and their communities, and to manage access to their collective information; and the right of Aboriginal peoples to physically *possess* the data collected.

The OCAP principles are not a prescription for Aboriginal research, but serve as a guide that may be applied and interpreted by the Aboriginal community involved in the research process. The principles were brought to the project Advisory Committee for an open and direct conversation about how these principles should be applied. The Advisory Committee had no reservations about sharing their knowledge, preferring to build the research relationship on trust and communication rather than rules and regulations dictating knowledge transfer. Although the Advisory Committee interpreted the OCAP principles more loosely than some communities, this conversation was essential to ensure a common understanding and to reiterate the commitment to a respectful research process.

To ensure that the project was relevant, respectful, and important to urban Aboriginal peoples, the Advisory Committee was involved in every stage of the project—from developing the research question and methodology to the analysis, conclusions, and dissemination. The Advisory Committee met in person approximately once a month and offered feedback between meetings via telephone or email. At monthly meetings, the group always shared a healthy meal together, and whenever possible, traditional foods were served. Advisory Committee members were acknowledged with honoraria for their knowledge and time.

2.2. Sample and Recruitment. Intergenerational teaching/learning was an identified priority for the Advisory Committee and their associated community groups/organizations. To facilitate such learning, the project aimed to recruit 12 Aboriginal young people (youth) aged 19–30 years old and six community-identified Elders (or "Elders-in-Training" to participate in the study. (Elders-in-Training were Aboriginal peoples who were too young to be recognized as Elders, but were knowledgeable in traditional practices and active teachers in their communities.)

Two Advisory Committee members were particularly active in youth recruitment, registering interested participants through Aboriginal youth programs in Vancouver and presentations at community gatherings. The number of youth interested in participating exceeded study capacity; therefore, 15 youth were randomly selected to participate. The research team intentionally oversampled, anticipating that some youth may not attend. Youth who were not selected to participate were invited to stay involved by receiving project updates and final reports. For their participation, youth received a monetary honorarium consistent with other research projects and in keeping with the OCAP principles.

Through their personal and professional networks, the Advisory Committee identified respected Elders who were knowledgeable in traditional foods and practices. All six Elders contacted agreed to participate in the study and received an honorarium for their contribution of knowledge.

In total, fifteen youth and six Elders provided informed consent and participated in the study.

2.3. Research Design and Knowledge Generation. A common critique of traditional foods studies is the priority of western science over traditional knowledge and Aboriginal perspectives [19–23]. To avoid this pitfall, the research team and Advisory Committee prioritized culturally relevant practices and aimed to generate knowledge based on the lived experiences of urban Aboriginal peoples. A participatory research study drawing on narrative inquiry approaches was designed, and received ethics approval from the University of Toronto. Narrative inquiry is a qualitative research approach that incorporates participants' lived experiences through stories. Knowledge is co-constructed as participants tell their stories and the researcher listens, asks questions, and interprets what he/she hears [24]. In this study, narratives were employed to generate knowledge based in urban Aboriginal experiences. The narratives were created using the Story/Dialogue Method of gathering experiential knowledge developed by Labonte and Feather [25]. This method was selected due to its synchrony with the traditions, practices, and ways of knowing in many Aboriginal cultures.

The Story/Dialogue Method documents experiential knowledge through sharing of stories in a structured format. In small "Story Groups," participants are asked to share a story from their personal experience. The group then move through a series of questions, progressively reaching deeper levels of analysis of the story. Four categories of questions are discussed:

(1) *"What?"* questions clarify the details of the story;

(2) *"Why?"* questions seek an explanation for the events of the story;

(3) *"So What?"* questions synthesize what was learned from the story; and

(4) *"Now What?"* questions cause participants to consider future actions to improve the outcome of similar stories.

After participants move through all four levels of questions, they collectively create "Insight Cards" to capture the key discussion points for each set of questions. Each insight is written on a separate card, and participants work together to arrange the cards into categories or themes. The Story Groups then create a summary statement (a "Theory Note") for each grouping, followed by a comprehensive summary statement linking all the themes together (a "Composite Theory Note").

The Advisory Committee reviewed the Story/Dialogue Method and appreciated its resonance with storytelling—a deeply rooted cultural practice. However, the method was deemed too structured for an Aboriginal audience. Therefore, the method was adapted so participants were not responsible for the structured questioning and recording of comments and insights. Instead, trained facilitators were incorporated to gently guide the discussion to deeper levels of analysis. The facilitators also took over the majority of the note taking tasks, allowing participants to fully engage in the conversation. Although participants still created Insight Cards and organized the cards into categories, the term "Theory Note" was not used with participants, as it was deemed overly academic and potentially off-putting for a community setting. Due to time limitations of the day, the final summary ("Composite Theory Note") was omitted. Two non-Aboriginal and four Aboriginal peoples were recruited and trained in the adapted storytelling methodology.

The adapted Story/Dialogue Method proved to be effective in reaching the research aims of the project and incorporating traditional ways of knowing and generating knowledge. Other cultural traditions were also incorporated into the methodology—traditional foods were provided for lunch; Elders offered an opening welcome and closing prayer song; and talking circles were used to share introductions, personal stories, and feedback. The storytelling was held at the Aboriginal Friendship Centre in Vancouver, a well-known hub for Aboriginal peoples in the city.

2.4. Analysis. A major strength of the chosen methodology was the ability for participants to conduct the primary analysis of the themes emerging from their own stories and experiences. Participants collectively identified the key insights that they determined to be important to share with a wider audience. Each Story Group created Insight Cards. Some groups compiled their insight cards into one written summary, while other groups shared their summary orally. In an effort to incorporate culturally relevant approaches, facilitators readily accepted oral sharing of knowledge and took notes on what was shared.

Following the storytelling day, the research team conducted a secondary analysis by compiling the Insight Cards and written and oral summaries from all Story Groups into one cohesive story and three variations of a visual model. Participant quotes were taken directly from facilitator's notes and the Insight Cards developed by the story groups. The story and visual models were reviewed by the Advisory Committee to ensure that they were both accurate and culturally appropriate. After incorporating Advisory Committee feedback and selecting the most appropriate model, the

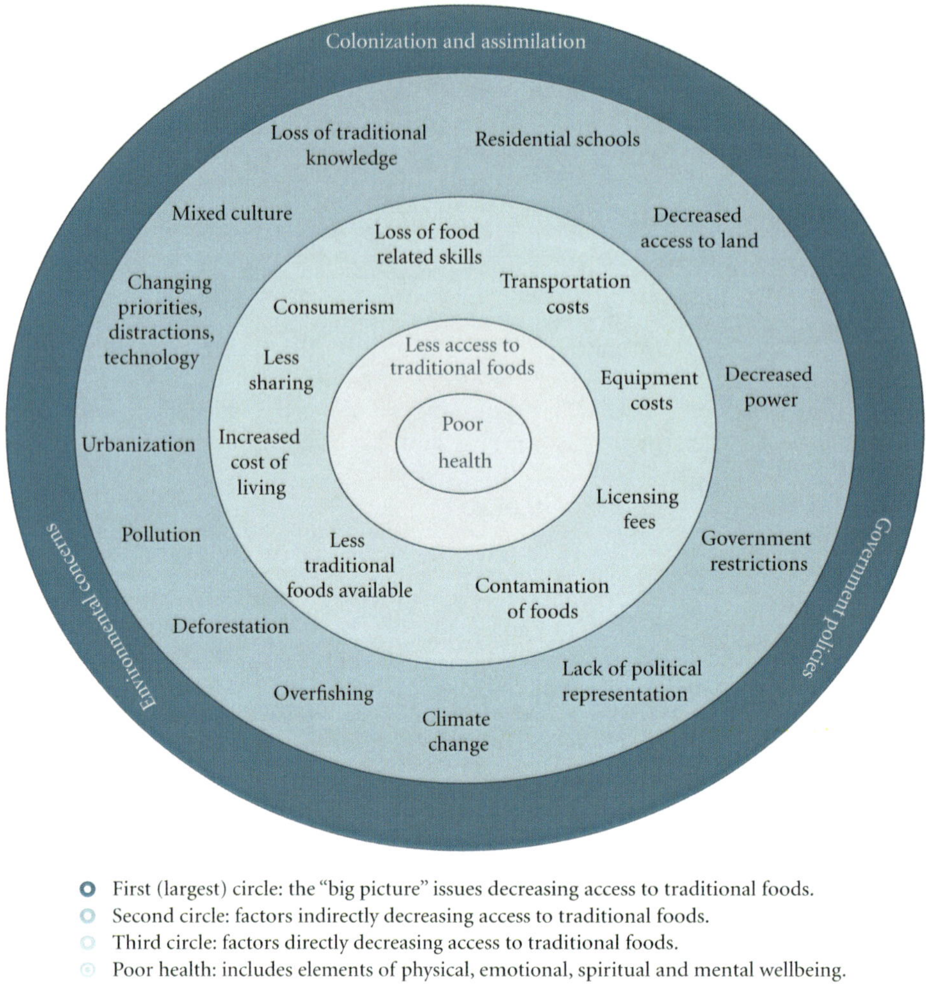

Figure 1: Factors that limit access to traditional foods in the city.

Committee and all participants were invited to a follow-up event held one month after the initial storytelling day. Participants offered feedback on the accuracy and clarity of the messages presented. This participatory approach to analysis allowed participants to "speak for themselves" and control how their stories and ideas were represented to a wider audience.

3. Results

Participant-identified challenges and solutions to accessing traditional foods in Vancouver are presented in Figures 1 and 2. As highlighted in the reviewed literature and echoed by our participants, access to traditional foods improves health. As such, both diagrams are centred on the health of Aboriginal peoples. Participants noted that the Aboriginal concept of health is holistic and includes physical, emotional, mental, and spiritual health—leading to overall wellbeing. Traditional foods, due to their connectivity with cultural practices and traditional knowledge, impact not only physical health, but also emotional, mental, and spiritual health.

3.1. Factors That Limit Access to Traditional Foods in the City. Just as consumption of traditional foods improves the diet and health of Aboriginal peoples, less access to traditional foods leads to a poorer diet and poorer health. The many factors that impede access to traditional foods are organized in concentric circles around "poor health" in Figure 1, with more direct influences placed closer to the centre. The circular representation, rather than a linear model, was purposely selected by the Advisory Committee because of the interrelated and overlapping nature of these factors over time.

Living in an urban centre brings unique challenges to accessing traditional foods. Participants stated that traditional foods are often shared through family networks, but due to distance or disconnection from their family and/or home community, they receive less traditional foods when they live in the city. Some participants suggested returning to the reserve "to learn and get traditional teachings," while one youth participant noted that her family chose to distance themselves from the community: "Mom did not like the negative things on the reserve, so that is why she kept me away from the reserve." Participants also noted that sharing

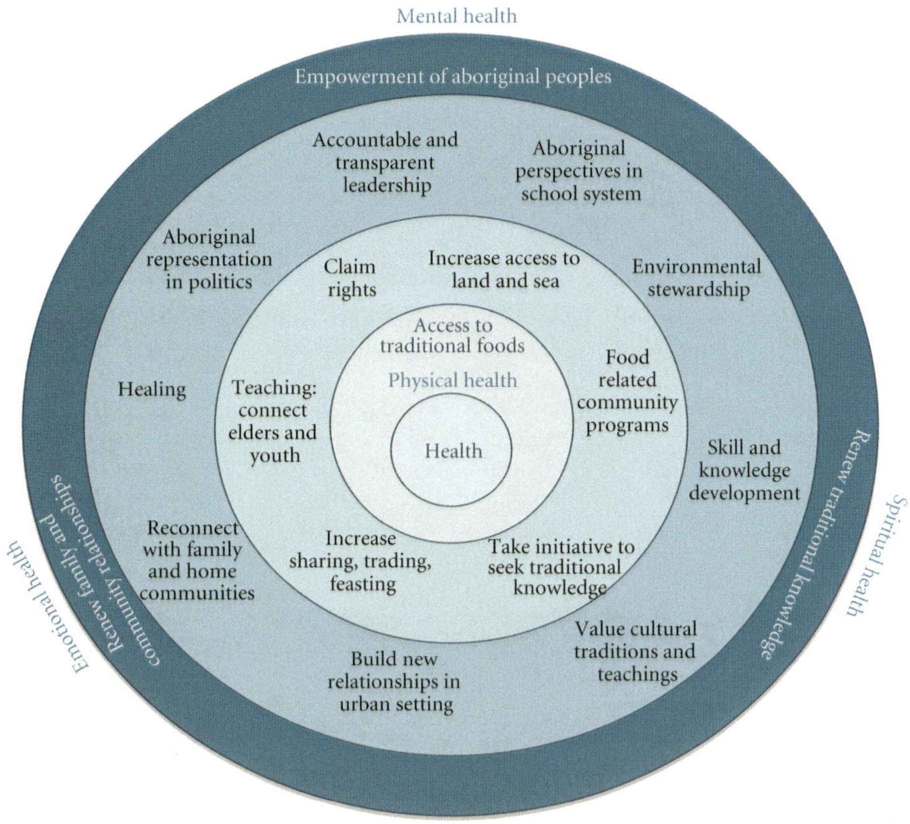

- First (largest) circle: the "high level" solutions to increasing access to traditional foods.
- Second circle: factors indirectly affecting access to traditional foods.
- Third circle: factors directly affecting access to traditional foods.
- Health includes:
  (i) physical health (healthy eating of traditional foods),
  (ii) emotional health (social support through relationships),
  (iii) spiritual health (increased cultural connectivity),
  (iv) mental health (increased sense of cultural identity, pride and vision).

FIGURE 2: Actions to increase access to traditional foods in the city.

of traditional foods has been affected by the increase in consumer mentality in the city, stating "Previously, it was very much about sharing. Now, everything is about money… We are measured only by how much we can buy." Youth raised in urban environments stated that they grew up in a "mixed culture" and struggled to maintain traditional ways of living, while attempting to succeed in a fast-paced urban environment: "We need to learn how to live our old ways and new ways together, and still be successful as Native Peoples." Youth said that in the city they have fewer opportunities to learn from Elders, and many stated they did not have the knowledge or skills to gather and prepare traditional foods.

While traditional knowledge continues to be preserved and shared in Aboriginal communities, participants stated that this knowledge is being lost over generations. Participants traced this gradual loss of traditional knowledge and skills back to residential schools, where, for generations, children were removed from their families and communities and forced to learn European ways of living, eating, and speaking. As one Elder shared, "It all comes back to residential schools, but we have the knowledge in our DNA. It's our duty to share it before it is extinct." As highlighted in the literature, assimilation practices initiated a "nutrition transition" among Aboriginal peoples by introducing them to less healthy non-traditional foods. One youth described the nutrition transition as the introduction to the "five white sins: flour, salt, sugar, alcohol, and lard." Participants underscored that colonization and forced assimilation have had a lasting impact on traditional knowledge and family dynamics, both of which impact access to traditional foods.

At a macrolevel, participants identified that government policies and the changing environment continue to impact access to traditional foods. For example, many participants stressed that "the Department of Fisheries and Oceans does not allow us to fish off our territory"—pointing to the reservation boundaries that contain Aboriginal peoples and limit access to fishing, hunting, and gathering grounds, particularly for those living off reserve. Discussions on government policies also highlighted licensing fees that make hunting and fishing too expensive for many Aboriginal peoples, impacting their ability to afford and share traditional foods: "Now we need licenses to collect everything from oysters to crab to kytons. It wasn't like this before. We could just go and collect what we wanted." Furthermore, continuing increases in transportation and equipment costs leave many families unable to afford the equipment or gas needed to hunt, fish, or gather foods. As one Elder stated, "Traditional foods should not be a privilege (for the wealthy), it should be available for all!" Lack of Aboriginal control over how land and waterways are being used, environmental pollutants that contaminate food and food sources, deforestation, climate change, and overfishing were all discussed as factors reducing the availability of traditional foods. Participants felt that not enough people were raising these issues with decision makers and noted the insufficient political representation of Aboriginal peoples in the Canadian government as a significant issue.

Overall, the challenges to accessing traditional foods discussed through storytelling match those identified in the literature reviewed, despite the fact that most of the previous Canadian studies focused on reserve or northern communities. However, participants highlighted the additional challenge of living in an urban setting. Costs of living are higher in the city; there is less opportunity for traditional teachings, and youth in particular stated that it is difficult to balance urban living with traditional values.

3.2. Solutions to Increase Access to Traditional Foods in the City. The solutions to increasing access to traditional foods are represented in Figure 2. Similar to Figure 1, health is at the centre. The more indirect, overarching solutions identified by participants—empowerment of Aboriginal peoples, renewal of traditional knowledge, and renewal of family and community relationships—are located in the outermost circle. These overarching solutions not only impact traditional foods access and physical health (nutrition), but also have positive effects on mental, emotional, and spiritual health. Participants emphasized this holistic view of health.

Overall, participants stressed the need to collectively heal from the past injustices of colonization and assimilation. As one participant highlighted, "We must learn from the past and forgive in order to be the best we can be." Renewal of family and community relationships was seen as important for connecting youth and Elders, facilitating the teaching of traditional knowledge to the younger generation, encouraging the sharing and trade of traditional foods, and celebrating together in cultural feasts. According to participants, "feasts are a fun and engaging way to bring family and community together" and they "provide an opportunity for young people to serve, associate with, and show respect for Elders." When urban Aboriginal peoples are far from their family or home community, participants stressed the importance of "building relationships with the surrounding Aboriginal communities and peoples who are native to the area" to facilitate teaching, sharing, and trading.

Elders underlined the importance of youth valuing traditional knowledge and investing time and energy into learning and gaining skills. As one Elder stressed: "Be there to experience and be shown. Physically do it!" Similarly, youth acknowledged the need to take initiative in seeking traditional knowledge from Aboriginal community programs/events, relatives, and Elders. As one Story Group expressed, youth should "communicate with Elders about traditional food, rather than expecting them to come to you." However, they recognized that this is not always easy: "Elders are role models and want to pass on their knowledge, but some youth do not have the opportunities or resources to learn from them." Participants also noted that traditional knowledge and practices are closely linked to environmental stewardship, stating that it could help protecting food sources from mismanagement, over-extraction, and pollution.

Participants saw the renewal of traditional knowledge as key to Aboriginal empowerment. Some Elders present had gone to residential schools, and through that system, "language, culture, and pride in traditions were lost." Youth wanted to see an appreciation of indigenous knowledge in both Aboriginal and non-Aboriginal communities, and an inclusion of Aboriginal perspectives, history, and culture in the school curriculum. For example, some youth said they had switched from the "regular" social studies class to the First Nations option and stressed the importance of Aboriginal and non-Aboriginal students learning "both sides of the story" in Canadian history.

Elders and youth emphasized the need for accountable and transparent leadership across the board, empowering Aboriginal peoples to claim their rights and access land and water systems. The need for Aboriginal voice in public policy making was highlighted, with participants firmly stating, "We are not being heard!" They saw political representation as vital to improving access to traditional foods—not only in urban settings, but for all Aboriginal peoples.

Solutions for increasing access to traditional foods are less common in academic literature. However, participants in the storytelling event were more excited by discussing potential solutions and actions than by reiterating challenges. By allowing participants to direct the conversation, the discussion naturally shifted to focus on positive actions that could be taken at local, regional, and national levels.

3.3. Summary of Findings. Figure 3 summarizes the main factors that impact access to traditional foods in Vancouver, as described by study participants. Challenges and solutions are brought together to demonstrate how all factors are interrelated and collectively impact access to traditional foods and holistic health. Participants identified a comprehensive range of influences, from local (e.g., interpersonal relationships), to regional (e.g., government policies), to global (e.g., environmental concerns).

Many of the challenges and solutions to accessing traditional foods articulated in the storytelling workshop

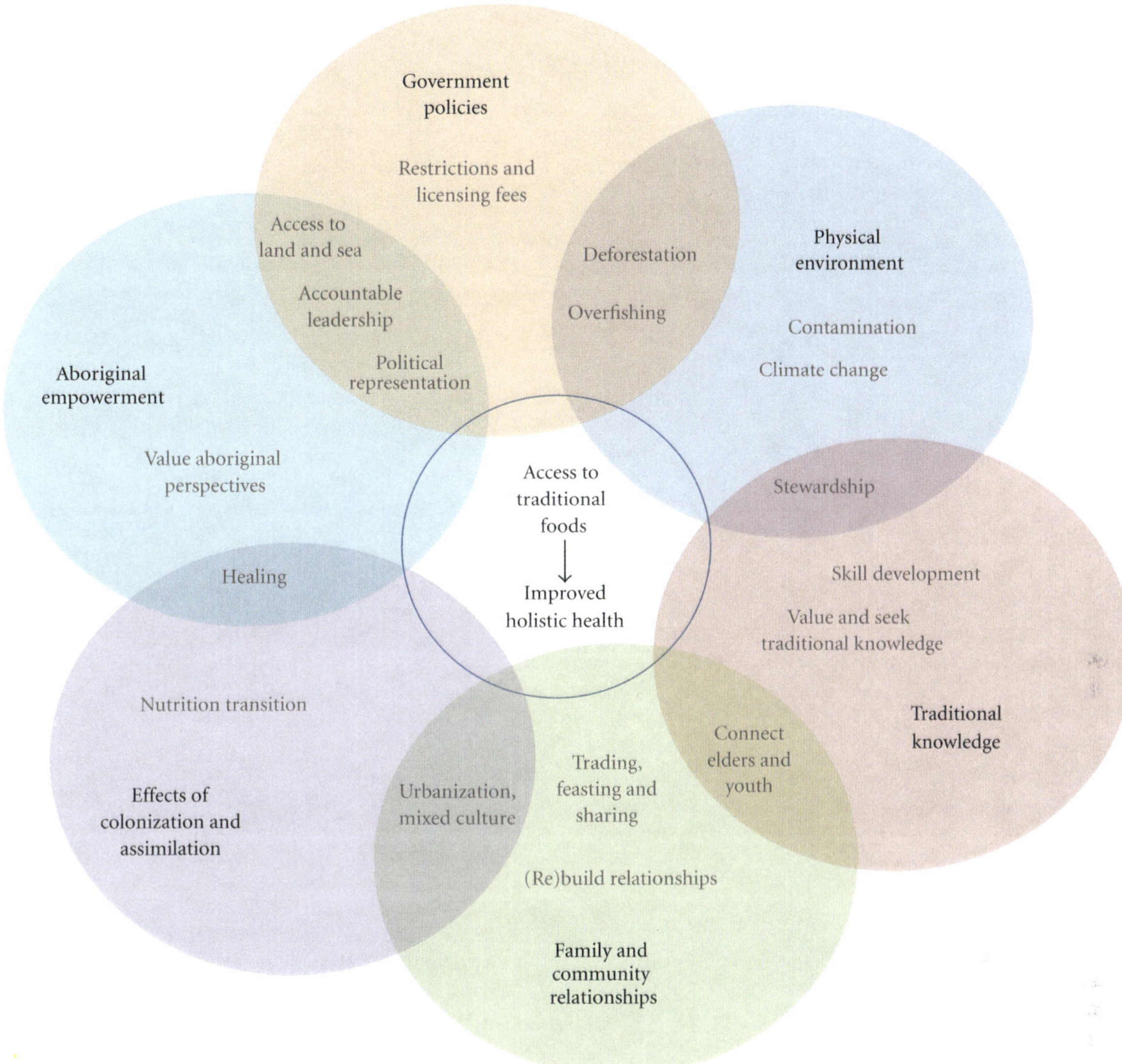

FIGURE 3: Summary of main factors that impact access to traditional foods in vancouver.

parallel challenges and solutions of food security more broadly. The influence of societal priorities and values, social support, environmental concerns, and government policy impact the food security of all people. Community and family connections play an important role in community and household food security among both Aboriginal and non-Aboriginal peoples, and traditional knowledge of Aboriginal groups offers valuable insight into the changes occurring in our environment and food sources. The comprehensive range of factors identified by the research participants can be applied beyond the Aboriginal context and provide insights for food security in a diversity of settings.

4. Conclusions

The value placed on traditional knowledge, taking time to build respectful relationships between Aboriginal and non-Aboriginal partners, and the incorporation of Aboriginal perspectives in the research design, implementation, and analysis were imperatives in the success of the project. The trusting and open relationship between Aboriginal and non-Aboriginal partners allowed for the incorporation of traditional knowledge and Aboriginal perspectives in all aspects of the research process. Incorporating traditional practices—such as gift giving, sharing circles, and storytelling—not only helped to strengthen relationships, but also strengthened the research findings. The adapted Story/Dialogue Method resonated with the cultures and traditions of research participants and enabled participants to determine the content of discussion and final reports. Where other research projects focused on challenges to accessing traditional foods, participants in the storytelling event preferred to talk about—and even plan to implement—solutions to increasing access in the city. The adapted Story/Dialogue Method not only gave participants ownership over the research content, but also fostered a renewed interest and excitement about traditional foods, resulting in grassroots actions by the participants. Many participants resolved to seek out traditional food and knowledge. One youth collected the contact information of an Elder in order to connect with her for teaching and learning opportunities. Collectively, the group started a Facebook page to promote local trading of traditional foods, brainstormed a television series to pitch to Aboriginal Peoples Television Network, and promoted local community gardens that provide traditional teachings. However, participants also recognized that many of the challenges and solutions discussed are beyond their control.

The knowledge generated from the project highlights the need for a whole of society response to increase and sustain access to traditional foods as a means to achieve Aboriginal food security. Participants highlighted a wide range of factors affecting their access to traditional food, from local to international influences. They clearly articulated that some factors lie within their immediate communities, such as family and community relationships, teaching and learning traditional knowledge, and strong local leadership. Other factors rest with the national and international community, such as government policies and regulations that impact traditional food sources, the physical environment, and impacts of climate change and contamination, and the "nutrition transition" from traditional to conventional diets. To fully appreciate the factors impacting access to traditional foods, it is important to look beyond the individual or their communities and incorporate the regional, national, and international factors at play.

Including Aboriginal knowledge and perspectives in food security research and discourse not only identifies unique challenges and solutions, but also highlights issues that are of relevance to all of society. In every society, food security is impacted by local factors such as social relationships and food skills and knowledge, and broader factors such as government policies, the physical environment, dependence on the conventional food system, and adequate voice and political representation of marginalized or vulnerable (i.e., food insecure) populations. The participants comprehensively articulated the interconnectedness of local and global factors impacting not only access to traditional foods, but also the food security of Aboriginal and non-Aboriginal peoples alike. In order to holistically address food security issues and achieve food security for all, Aboriginal peoples must be engaged as equal partners, with their knowledge and worldview prevailing in decisions within their own communities and also being solicited and incorporated into society-wide and global policies.

Acknowledgments

The authors would like to express their sincere thanks to the following individuals and groups for making this project successful: other members of the project's Advisory Committee—Kim van der Woerd, Alvin Dixon, Hilda Green, Lea Jensen, Jeri Sparrow, Samantha Tsuruda, Herb Varley; the youth and Elder participants; the recruited storytelling facilitators—Vina Brown, Kylee Swift; PHSA's Chronic Disease Prevention in Aboriginal Communities Steering Committee; the Urban Aboriginal Community Garden Kitchen Project; academic supervisors at the University of Toronto-Blake Poland, Suzanne Jackson, and Michael Goodstadt; and the Urban Aboriginal Friendship Centre.

References

[1] Food Agriculture Organization of the United Nations (FAO), *The State of Food Insecurity in the World 2001*, FAO, Rome, Italy, 2002.

[2] H. V. Kuhnlein and H. M. Chan, "Environment and contaminants in traditional food systems of northern indigenous peoples," *Annual Review of Nutrition*, vol. 20, pp. 595–626, 2000.

[3] Aboriginal Affairs and Northern Development Canada, *Terminology*, 2010, http://www.aadnc-aandc.gc.ca/eng/1100100014642.

[4] Statistics Canada, *Census 2006: Aboriginal Peoples in Canada in 2006*, 2010, http://www12.statcan.ca/census-recensement/2006/as-sa/97-558/p16-eng.cfm.

[5] L. Chan, O. Receveur, D. Sharp, H. Schwartz, A. Ing, and C. Tikhonov, *First Nations Food, Nutrition and Environment Study (FNFNES): Results from British Columbia (2008/2009)*, University of Northern British Columbia, Prince George, Canada, 2011.

[6] Health Canada, *Canadian Community Health Survey, Cycle 2.2, Nutrition (2004). Income-Related Household Food Security in Canada*, Minister of Health, Office of Nutrition Policy and Promotion, Health Products and Food Branch, Health Canada, Ottawa, Canada, 2006.

[7] Province of British Columbia, Provincial Health Officer Aboriginal 2009 Report, 2009 http://www.hls.gov.bc.ca/pho/pdf/abohlth11-var7.pdf.

[8] S. M. Downs, A. Arnold, D. Marshall, L. J. McCargar, K. D. Raine, and N. D. Willows, "Associations among the food environment, diet quality and weight status in Cree children in Québec," *Public Health Nutrition*, vol. 12, no. 9, pp. 1504–1511, 2009.

[9] G. M. Egeland, P. Berti, R. Soueida, L. T. Arbour, O. Receveur, and H. V. Kuhnlein, "Age differences in vitamin A intake among Canadian Inuit," *Canadian Journal of Public Health*, vol. 95, no. 6, pp. 465–469, 2004.

[10] N. Simoneau and O. Receveur, "Attributes of vitamin A- and calcium-rich food items consumed in K'asho Got'ine, Northwest Territories, Canada," *Journal of Nutrition Education and Behavior*, vol. 32, no. 2, pp. 84–93, 2000.

[11] O. Receveur, M. Boulay, and H. V. Kuhnlein, "Decreasing traditional food use affects diet quality for adult Dene/Metis in 16 communities of the Canadian Northwest Territories," *Journal of Nutrition*, vol. 127, no. 11, pp. 2179–2186, 1997.

[12] H. V. Kuhnlein, R. Soueida, and O. Receveur, "Dietary nutrient profiles of Canadian Baffin Island Inuit differ by food source, season, and age," *Journal of the American Dietetic Association*, vol. 96, no. 2, pp. 155–162, 1996.

[13] E. E. Wein, "Foods and nutrients in reported diets versus perceived ideal diets of Yukon Indian people," *Journal of Nutrition Education and Behavior*, vol. 28, no. 4, pp. 202–208, 1996.

[14] E. E. Wein, J. H. Sabry, and F. T. Evers, "Nutrient intakes of native Canadians near Wood Buffalo National Park," *Nutrition Research*, vol. 11, no. 1, pp. 5–13, 1991.

[15] S. Damman, W. B. Eide, and H. V. Kuhnlein, "Indigenous peoples' nutrition transition in a right to food perspective," *Food Policy*, vol. 33, no. 2, pp. 135–155, 2008.

[16] M. Batal, K. Gray-Donald, H. V. Kuhnlein, and O. Receveur, "Estimation of traditional food intake in indigenous communities in Denendeh and the Yukon," *International Journal of Circumpolar Health*, vol. 64, no. 1, pp. 46–54, 2005.

[17] D. Morrison, Final Activity Report. *B.C. Food Systems Network: Working Group on Indigenous Food Sovereignty*, 2008, http://www.indigenousfoodsystems.org/content/bc-food-systems-network-working-group-indigenous-food-sovereignty-final-report.

[18] First Nations Centre, *OCAP: Ownership, Control, Access and Possession. Sanctioned By the First Nations Information Governance Committee, Assembly of First Nations*, National Aboriginal Health Organization, Ottawa, Canada, 2007.

[19] P. Tobin, M. French, and N. Hanlon, "Appropriate engagement and nutrition education on reserve: lessons learned from the Takla First Nation in Northern BC," *Journal of Aboriginal Health*, vol. 6, no. 1, pp. 49–57, 2010.

[20] E. Power, *Food Security for First Nations and Inuit in Canada: Background Paper*, First Nations and Inuit Health Branch, Health Canada, 2007.

[21] L. Simpson, "Toxic contamination undermining Indigenous food systems and Indigenous sovereignty," *Pimatiziwin*, vol. 1, no. 2, pp. 130–134, 2003.

[22] L. T. Smith, *Decolonizing Methodologies: Research and Indigenous Peoples*, Zed Books, New York, NY, USA, 1999.

[23] J. D. O'Neil, B. Elias, and A. Yassi, "Poisoned food: cultural resistance to the contaminants discourse in Nunavik," *Arctic Anthropology*, vol. 34, no. 1, pp. 29–40, 1997.

[24] M. Savin-Baden and L. Van Niekerk, "Narrative inquiry: theory and practice," *Journal of Geography in Higher Education*, vol. 31, no. 3, pp. 459–472, 2007.

[25] R. Labonte and J. Feather, *Handbook on Using Stories in Health Promotion Practice*, Health Canada, 1996.

7

An Alternative Approach to Water Regulations for Public Health Protection at Bathing Beaches

Amir M. Abdelzaher,[1,2] Helena M. Solo-Gabriele,[1,2] Matthew C. Phillips,[1,2] Samir M. Elmir,[1,3] and Lora E. Fleming[1,4,5]

[1] *NSF NIEHS Oceans and Human Health Center, University of Miami, Miami, FL 33149, USA*
[2] *Department of Civil, Architectural, and Environmental Engineering, University of Miami, Coral Gables, FL 33146-0630, USA*
[3] *Miami-Dade County Health Department, Miami, FL 33056, USA*
[4] *Department of Epidemiology & Public Health and Marine Biology & Fisheries, University of Miami, Miami, FL 33136, USA*
[5] *European Centre for Environment and Human Health, University of Exeter Medical School, Truro, Cornwall TR1 3HD, UK*

Correspondence should be addressed to Helena M. Solo-Gabriele; hmsolo@miami.edu

Academic Editor: Boo Kwa

New approaches should be considered as the US Environmental Protection Agency (EPA) moves rapidly to develop new beach monitoring guidelines by the end of 2012, as these guidelines serve as the basis by which states and territories with coasts along the oceans and Great Lakes can then develop and implement monitoring programs for recreational waters. We describe and illustrate one possible approach to beach regulation termed as the "Comprehensive Toolbox within an Approval Process (CTBAP)." The CTBAP consists of three components. The first is a "toolbox" consisting of an inventory of guidelines on monitoring targets, a series of measurement techniques, and guidance to improve water quality through source identification and prevention methods. The second two components are principles of implementation. These include first, "flexibility" to encourage and develop an individualized beach management plan tailored to local conditions and second, "consistency" of this management plan to ensure a consistent national level of public health protection. The results of this approach are illustrated through a case study at a well-studied South Florida recreational marine beach. This case study explores different monitoring targets based on two different health endpoints (skin versus gastrointestinal illness) and recommends a beach regulation program for the study beach that focuses predominately on source prevention.

1. Introduction

There is a growing health concern related to swimming in contaminated waters. Globally, each year, there are in excess of an estimated 120 million cases of gastrointestinal disease and in excess of an estimated 50 million cases of more severe respiratory diseases associated with swimming and bathing in wastewater-polluted coastal waters [1]. Since the 1950s, epidemiologic studies have been designed to evaluate the relationship between swimming in point source-impacted beaches and health risks (i.e., gastrointestinal disease, respiratory, eye, nose, and throat illnesses); they have concluded that symptoms for all these illnesses were increased in swimmers compared to nonswimmers [2, 3]. Outbreak reports from the CDC also confirm that illnesses in the USA are occurring from swimming in contaminated waters [4]. The excess illnesses associated with coastal water pollution can also result in substantial economic burdens. A study in Orange County, CA, estimated 3.3 million US dollars per year in excess illness costs for Newport and Huntington Beaches associated with bathing in marine waters [5].

Swimming-related illness is predominately associated with exposure to microbial pathogens, which may enter the water through point sources such as sewage outfalls. However, recent studies have demonstrated that swimming-related illnesses can occur at nonpoint source beaches [6, 7] and even possibly from beach sand contact [8–10]. These developments highlight the ongoing challenge to beach managers and public health professionals in monitoring the beach environment and protecting the health of its users [11, 12]. To address this challenge, we provide background information about existing regulations; describe a possible alternative approach given the existing regulations; and then apply this alternative approach to a well-studied South Florida recreational marine beach to illustrate one possible outcome of the alternate approach.

1.1. Current US Regulation. At the US federal level, jurisdiction over recreational waters is provided through the Clean Water Act (CWA). The CWA provides the US EPA with jurisdiction over two approaches for the control of water quality. First, it provides jurisdiction to regulate discharges of pollutants into the waters of the United States. Specifically, the CWA regulates discharges that represent point sources of pollution, that is, industrial, municipal, and other discharges via conveyances such as pipes or man-made ditches. Second, the CWA provides the authority to set point-of-use standards for surface waters. Waterbodies must not exceed contaminant levels beyond allowable values as determined by their "designated use" (swimming, bathing, surfing, water skiing, etc.). In most situations, the authority to issue discharge permits and to set designated use standards is delegated by the EPA to the states, thereby providing the states with the full authority to implement, that is, monitoring compliance, permitting, and enforcement.

The Beaches Environmental Assessment and Coastal Health (BEACH) Act of 2000, an amendment to the CWA, sets forth beach water quality guidelines for 30 eligible states and territories with coasts along the oceans and Great Lakes. These guidelines include limits for *Enterococcus* in marine waters and for both *Enterococcus* and *E. coli* in freshwater. A single-maximum value, as well as a monthly geometric mean, is recommended by the Act [13]. While all 30 states affected by the BEACH Act follow these guidelines, many states employ unique additional sets of parameters to assess the safety of recreational waters (Table 1) [14]. In the U.S water monitoring includes measures at approximately 3,000 beaches for fecal indicator bacteria, resulting in 18,500 closures or advisory days in 2009 issued for recreational beaches [14] (Figure 1).

Seventeen of the 30 states under the BEACH Act preemptively close at least some of their beaches after significant rainfall. Twenty-eight states vary sampling based on season and sampling more often during the summer months. Twenty-two states vary the frequency of sampling based on usage and sample more often at beaches with higher human usage. Twenty-five states base the location of their sampling on usage or proximity to a possible source of contamination. Two states (Massachusetts and Hawaii) test waters for pharmaceutical chemicals that would be discharged with human sewage. Seven states have predictive models in effect for some of their beaches; many of which have proven to be more effective than the culture-based monitoring techniques [15]. Four states bordering the Gulf of Mexico close beaches after hurricanes. Texas monitors for *V. vulnificus* in addition to *Enterococcus* and Hawaii adds *C. perfringens* to their microbial testing. New York and Rhode Island utilize sanitary surveys in their monitoring efforts, taking into consideration environmental parameters (such as tidal stage, wild life, and seaweed). New Hampshire has an internet-based system in place where advisories are posted based on self-reported illnesses acquired from swimming at certain beaches [14]. Florida monitors its coastal beaches on a weekly basis year round using *Enterococcus* as the fecal microbe indicator. Florida applies the 2004 EPA's Recreational water Quality Criteria (RWQC) for a single sample and geometric mean to issue beach advisories [16].

Table 1: Number of states applying various beach monitoring techniques [14].

Regulatory practice	Number of states
Sampling location	
Ankle	2
Knee	15
Waist	13
Frequency of sampling based on	
Usage	22
Season	28
Location of sampling based on Usage or point source	25
States allowed to issue advisories	30
States allowed to issue closures	17
Presumptive rainfall standards	17
Predictive models used	5
Unique microbial indicators used	2
Chemical indicators used	2

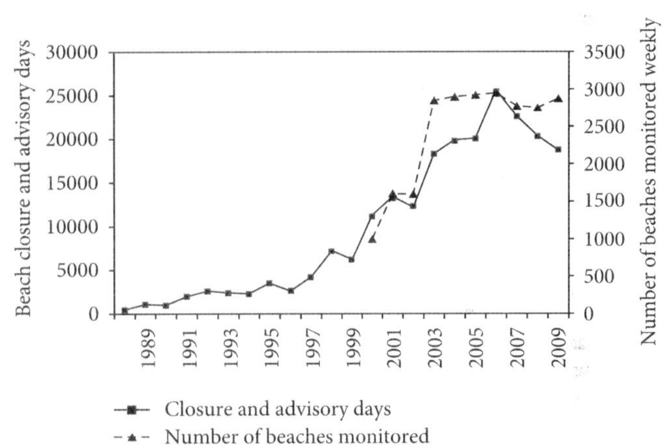

Figure 1: Number of beaches monitored and days of closures and advisories in the US [11, 14].

1.2. International Regulations. International regulations include those of the World Health Organization (WHO) and the European Union (EU) [17, 18]. The WHO approach differs from the US traditional monitoring guidelines in that

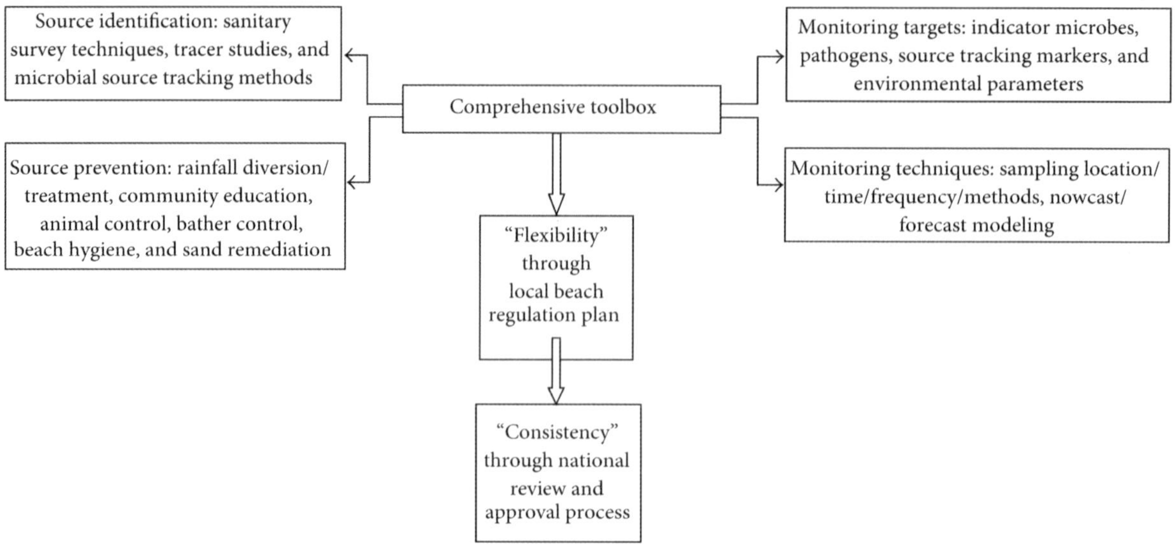

Figure 2: Comprehensive Toolbox within an Approval Process (CTBAP) Approach. This approach is based upon three steps which include: an inventory through the comprehensive toolbox (CTB) and two implementation principles to ensure "flexibility" and "consistency". The inventory (a.k.a. comprehensive toolbox, CTB) consists of the methods and tools to address recreational water quality and include guidance for source identification and prevention along with guidance for monitoring targets and techniques. The principles of implementation are "flexibility" which is to be incorporated into the local beach regulation plan and "consistency" through a national review panel charged with assuring a consistent level of public health protection."

the susceptibility of the beach to fecal pollution (i.e., the likelihood of various fecal sources from reaching the water) is taken into account when determining the monitoring criteria [17]. Beaches without a known point source of human fecal pollution are allowed higher levels of fecal indicator microbes than ones which do.

The EU [18] regulates the sampling program (frequency of sampling, location of sampling, and time of sampling), including algae and/or their toxins as indicators of human health risk [19] and, most importantly, the requirement of "beach water profiles" for all beaches in the EU. The beach water profile is a critical addition to the regulation since it requires beaches to be assessed for physical, geographical, and hydrological conditions as well as potential pollution sources. These profiles are to be updated every 2 to 4 years depending on their history (i.e., whether determined to be excellent, good, sufficient, or poor) [18].

2. Methods, Alternative Approach to Current Beach Regulations

The proposed method is based upon an alternative approach which takes into consideration existing beach regulations. It is clear that the US regulations focus on contaminant discharges and monitoring for fecal microbe indicator levels, whereas international regulations rely more heavily on the allowable water quality levels, which for the WHO include an expectation of flexibility based upon susceptibility of the beach.

Specifically, we propose the establishment of an effective criterion which we call the "Comprehensive Toolbox within an Approval Process, (CTBAP)" (Figure 2). The CTBAP is based upon three steps which include an inventory and two implementation principles. The inventory (a.k.a. comprehensive toolbox, CTB) consists of the methods and tools to address recreational water quality. These include guidance for source identification and prevention, along with guidance for monitoring targets and techniques. The two principles of implementation are "flexibility" which is to be incorporated into the local beach regulation plan and "consistency" to provide a consistent level of public health protection at the national level. A consistent national level of health protection implies that the monitoring targets provide the same level of risk, regardless of geographic location. So instead of setting the allowable indicator bacteria level at one consistent value, which is currently practiced through the US regulations, health risks would be set at a consistent level. The underlying theory behind this approach is to allow and expect for state, county, or even beach-specific flexibility, with a national approval mechanism for a nationally comparable level of human health protection. The methods and techniques in the alternative approaches would then be incorporated into the CTB.

This national CTB with initial organization at the federal level would create a resource which local teams (consisting of managers and scientists as well as other parties with expertise in the specific local conditions) may use to strategize the local beach management plan that would work best for them. A national CTB, in addition to providing options for monitoring targets and techniques, should also include guidance concerning sampling time, location, frequency, and method; predictive modeling (forecast and nowcast); information on how to communicate beach conditions to beach goers; sanitary survey methods; source tracking/tracer study methods; health risk study techniques to include quantitative microbial risk assessments, epidemiologic studies, self-reporting systems; pollution prevention methods via infrastructure, community education, animal control, and so forth. This CTB will need to be updated continuously by the national regulatory agency to keep up with the knowledge gained from new advances in the field of recreational water quality monitoring and pollution prevention.

Specifically to provide "flexibility" to state and local beach regulators, we recommend (1) an allowable range of targets based upon the susceptibility of the beach to fecal pollution as in the WHO approach and (2) an allowance for additional measures and controls as in the EU approach. We believe the concept of flexibility can also go further to include allowances for multiple lines of evidence to establish an overall safety level. For example, currently in recreational water quality monitoring, some states include multiple measures, but typically these measures are independent; if the threshold for either measure is exceeded, then an advisory is issued. Another component of the "flexibility" paradigm would be to allow for a safety assessment based upon integrated lines of evidence. An integrated line of evidence is consistent with the approach used for air quality standards. For example, for air quality standards, multiple constituents are measured, and collectively they are integrated to develop a "hazard" index, that is, Air Quality Index (AQI) [20]. A similar approach can be included as an option in the CTBAP process for developing standards for recreational bathing, where multiple lines of evidence can be used to collectively evaluate the probability of illness. These multiple lines of evidence can include measures of indicator microbes, results from modeling, weather conditions, measures of additional microbes (including possibly pathogens), and other factors.

The second principle, that of "consistency," establishes a consistent health protection level across the country. One concern in providing too much flexibility to the states is that health protection will not be equal across the nation. The solution for this may be a national and diverse team of experts under a national agency (such as the US EPA) which could regularly review the proposed beach regulation plans of the individual states. Given the specificity of the beach, the current state of the science, and experiences as well as beach regulation plans of other beaches, this panel will either approve or recommend certain modifications to the beach regulation plan. This will allow for the development of a site-specific plan that is acceptable and comparable to other beach regulation plans. Therefore, the baseline used is not a single microbiological criterion, which may give a false sense of equal protection (since recommended indicators perform differently at different beaches and under different conditions), but a single team of expert reviewers who would assess health risk.

In order to implement such an approach, beach regulators should be given a reasonable amount of time to develop their beach regulation plans after the release of the CTB by the EPA. Until then, the traditional criteria may remain in effect. As the number of approved plans increases, a matrix may develop similar to that proposed by Boehm et al. 2009 [11]. The matrix as recommended by these authors would be based on certain factors (such as climate conditions and pollution sources) as well as any other factor that is deemed important by the state and/or local regulatory agency. Although this direction of beach regulation is recommended for the upcoming years and decades as science advances rapidly, such an approach will also be more difficult to apply than the traditional approach of beach regulation and requires initially a larger burden on both the local beach regulators and the EPA. Therefore, the actual implementation of such an approach will depend on when such an approach becomes feasible at the local and national levels.

3. Results, Outcomes from Applying the Recommended Approach

To illustrate some of the aspects of the recommended approach, a well-studied nonpoint source beach is used as a case study. Assuming the existence of a comprehensive toolbox as proposed above from which guidance may be derived, along with the local conditions known about this beach, a beach regulation plan may be developed. What follows is a discussion of the different aspects that may be included in such a beach regulation plan which would then be submitted to the national regulatory panel for review and approval. Given that the case study beach is well studied, the data from the actual beach may be used in order to guide the development of the proper monitoring techniques/targets and source identification/prevention approaches to be included in the beach regulation plan. Regulators for beaches not well studied may need to couple knowledge of their beach with any available studies from similar beaches (similar in terms of pollution sources, geographic region, beach use, resources, etc.) in order to develop their site-specific beach regulation plan.

3.1. Beach Water Profile. The case study beach is located on Virginia Key within Miami-Dade County, Florida, USA, geographically classified as "subtropical" with an average ambient temperature of 24.8°C. This beach is the only beach in the county that allows pets [21]. Given the fact that admission is free and that the beach is located in a central location accessible by many of the county's residents, the beach can become overcrowded especially on weekends and holidays, during hours when the beach is open (between dawn and dusk) [22].

Extensive evaluation of the vicinity of the study beach did not find contributions from point sources of pollution to this beach (such as sewage outfalls, failing lift stations, and cross connections of sewage with storm drains), or less obvious nonpoint sources (such as septic tanks) [23]. This beach is usually in compliance with regulatory monitoring criteria but periodically (i.e., 0.9 times per year averaged from 2002 to 2012) has been placed under a beach advisory due to microbial water quality violations (Florida Healthy Beaches Program Database).

At the study beach, indicator microbe levels vary significantly both spatially (location) and temporally (time)

TABLE 2: Possible sampling strategies for the study site. The choice of sampling time and place depends upon which source (shoreline or offshore) is considered to be more strongly associated with human health.

	Target background levels for study site	
	Highest background Enterococci levels	Lowest background Enterococci levels
Primary source of Enterococci that would be measured	Microbes from shoreline	Microbes from offshore sources not from shoreline sand
Sampling strategy	During morning, near peak high tide, or after rainfall and as close as possible to the shoreline.	During noon and afternoon, after peak low tide, avoiding rain events, and sampling offshore.

[24–26], as is frequently observed at other beaches [27–30]. Enterococci, the current microbial target recommended for marine waters and used by regulators at the study beach, varied based on the location of sampling, with higher levels observed near the shoreline and lower levels observed offshore. These spatial differences are hypothesized to be due to Enterococci release from the intertidal sand zone where microbes are believed to regrow and persist [31–33]. Temporal variability is driven at the site by a combination of tidal, rainfall, and solar radiation effects [31, 34, 35].

Given the extensive beach-specific data, it becomes clear that any monitoring target (i.e., such as Enterococci) should include a monitoring technique that considers both spatial and temporal variability for the study beach (Table 2). If Enterococci from the shoreline sand are considered to be related to human health, the monitoring technique should be designed so that this Enterococci signal would be the most obvious. This would mean sampling at locations and times where microbial concentrations are expected to be most elevated and during times that people may be exposed to those waters (i.e., during the morning, after peak hightide or rainfall events, and as close as possible to the shoreline). However, if a relationship between Enterococci and human health at this study beach is believed to be driven by offshore sources of Enterococci, such as inadvertent sewage spills, regulators may consider developing sampling strategies that target these sources. This would entail sampling at locations and times where microbial concentrations from sand sources are expected to be least (i.e., during noon and afternoon, after peak low tide, avoiding sampling after rain events, and sampling offshore possibly at waist deep waters) (Table 2). In this case, elevated Enterococci levels would indicate a new offshore and potentially hazardous pollution source. Currently samples are collected in waist deep water which is consistent with a focus on identifying offshore sewage impacts and avoiding the high background levels associated with the nonpoint sources that originate from the intertidal zone.

3.2. Monitoring Targets and Disease Endpoints. Monitoring targets can include microbial, chemical, hydrologic, or another indicator of a health risk, whereas disease endpoints can include gastrointestinal, skin, respiratory, eye, and ear illnesses. The most common disease endpoint evaluated traditionally for recreational swimming is gastrointestinal illness (GI). A common method to compare potential monitoring targets to disease end-points is through epidemiologic studies. This is accomplished through identifying the associations between human health outcomes and monitoring targets. In the vast majority of beaches in the USA, an epidemiologic study specifically for that beach is not available, and therefore epidemiologic studies at similar beaches or other methodologies such as quantitative microbial risk assessment (QMRA) [36] may be used to assist in identifying appropriate monitoring targets.

At the study beach, a randomized control epidemiology study with comprehensive water microbial and environmental monitoring was completed [6, 34, 37]. During the epidemiology study, an increased risk of self-reported skin, respiratory, and gastrointestinal illnesses were associated with recreational bathing [6]. Statistically significant associations were observed between (a) skin disease and Enterococci levels determined by membrane filtration, (b) skin disease and to 24-hour antecedent rainfall, and (c) respiratory illness and the inverse of water temperature [37]. Neither environmental conditions nor microbes evaluated in this study were found to statistically relate to self-reported gastrointestinal illness. However, the results of the study did indicate a possible pattern between gastrointestinal illness and both F^- coliphage and *Giardia* spp., both being detected on 4 of the 15 total study days (Table 3) [34], and both were detected on 3 of the 5 days characterized by the highest excess gastrointestinal illness (see the number represented by asterisk (*) in Table 3). Given the principle of "flexibility", these targets, F^- coliphage and *Giardia* spp., should be thus considered as additions to the CTB that is used to assess water quality at this site.

With respect to disease end-points, we implement the concept of flexibility through the consideration of multiple health endpoints [34] (Table 2), which is based on measured health endpoints from more than one type of illness (e.g., gastrointestinal, skin, and respiratory). With this methodology, regulators are potentially guarding against a wider range of health impacts that may result from bathing, and hence from other pollution sources besides human sewage containing enteric pathogens. However, the multiple health endpoints, when applied to the data available for the study beach, were driven by the increased report of skin illnesses given their predominance relative to other illnesses. Therefore, for the case study beach, the multiple health endpoints approach may be considered where one microbial target would be used to assess risks from skin illnesses and another target would be used to assess gastrointestinal illness.

TABLE 3: Criteria of development based on GI illness health risk values based on microbial targets measured at study site during the beaches epidemiologic study [34].

	Sampling day	1	2	3	4	5	6	7	8	9	10	11	12	13	14	15
Microbe measure	Enterococci by MF (CFU/100 mL)	<2	15*	4*	15	13	99	109*	<2	3	29*	50	13	<2*	14	<2
	F^- coliphage (PFU/100 mL)	<0.3	**1***	**17***	<0.3	<0.3	<0.3	<0.3*	<0.3	<0.3	<0.3*	<0.3	**0.3**	**0.3***	<0.3	<0.3
	Giardia (cysts/100 L)	**1.1**	<0.5*	<0.5*	<0.5	<0.5	<0.5	**2.1***	<0.5	<0.5	**2.3***	<0.5	<0.5	**1.5***	<0.5	1
Excess illness (%)	GI	0.0	9.7*	4.8*	0.1	2.2	2.4	5.8*	0.2	0.5	4.2*	1.9	−0.1	4.1*	0.0	−4.9
	Skin	10.3	3.0*	4.8*	−2.3	4.2	8.6	8.3*	7.7	2.8	15.6*	11.5	5.1	5.9*	0.0	−1.1
	Respiratory	0.5	0.0*	5.1*	−4.7	0.0	0.0	5.9*	7.3	2.2	2.0*	2.0	0.0	−2.0*	0.0	0.0
	Cumulative	10.8	12.7*	14.6*	−6.8	6.3	10.9	20.0*	15.1	5.6	21.8*	15.4	5.1	8.0*	0.0	−6.0

*Corresponds to days with highest gastrointestinal illness.

3.3. Source Identification and Prevention. Although monitoring is an important aspect of beach regulation, source identification followed by source prevention is the key to establishing the safety of the beach environment in a long-term sustainable manner. This focus is also consistent with the jurisdiction of the EPA through the CWA to minimize contaminant discharges. However, the beach profiled for the study site did not identify point sources of pollution. Instead, several nonpoint sources were identified including rainfall runoff [31], bather shedding [38, 39], dog feces [21], and sand diffusion [40, 41]. Such observations are not only observed at the study beach but also at many other beach sites throughout the USA and beyond [11, 15, 42]. All of these sources come in contact with the beach sand and/or are directly released from the beach sand. Furthermore, analysis of the beach sand at the site has identified potential pathogenic microbes including protozoa, helminthes, fungi, and the bacteria, *S. aureus* [43, 44].

The focus should be thus on remediation of sand sources through multiple means, such as controlling runoff [45] and solid waste control [46], limiting the number of pets, birds [47], and minimizing human shedding through the provision of showers [43].

To address the need to remediate nonpoint diffuse sources of contamination, various source identification techniques [48] need to be available to beach regulators in the CTB in order for them to include these techniques in their beach regulation plan. Sanitary survey approaches, tracer study techniques, and microbial source tracking methodologies need to be simplified and made more accessible to regulators through inclusion in the CTB. Once sources are identified, through the guidance of the CTB, beach regulators can conduct various source prevention techniques as part of their beach regulation plan.

4. Discussion and Conclusions

The complexity of the beach system, especially that of beaches not dominated by a point source of pollution [34], implies that more novel and comprehensive approaches will be needed in order to more effectively protect the health of bathers, while at the same time limiting overconservatism which may lead to unnecessary beach closures and economic loss [5]. The CTBAP proposes the development of a comprehensive toolbox which provides an inventory of potential monitoring targets, measurement techniques, and guidance for source identification and prevention. The implementation would be based upon principles of "flexibility" where states are encouraged to identify their own targets as they develop beach management plans and "consistency" which includes an assessment of the plans at the national level to ensure a consistent level of human health protection.

To that end, the specific recommendations for the study beach reviewed here focus on controlling discharges and providing more flexibility for the allowable levels at the point-of-use. The study beach's main pollution source as described above is the sand which serves as a reservoir for indicator and pathogenic microbes inoculated into the sand by anthropogenic- and animal-related sources. Therefore, the continued monitoring of the sand and remediation as needed are recommended to prevent the sand from becoming a source of microbes that constantly contaminates the water via environmental conditions such as tidal action and rainfall. This is in addition to the source prevention techniques mentioned earlier (i.e., runoff diversion and treatment and bather and dog source remediation and prevention) to preemptively limit sand and water pollution.

Within the confines of the current US regulations, it is understood that the EPA has limited authority, including limitations to regulating water only (as opposed to regulating beach sands). Within this limitation and given the need to control pollution sources, it is recommended that states, as part of their implementation plans, consider the inclusion of sand measures as part of their monitoring program. Ideally beach management plans should include a focus on maintaining sand quality as a means of improving water quality. Ideally the CTB, established at the federal level, would acknowledge sand as a potential source and ideally the CTB would also provide guidance for measuring, modeling, and remediating microbes from sand sources.

With respect to allowable levels at the point-of-use, no relationship was found at the study site between fecal indicator bacteria and gastrointestinal illness. Indicator levels at the site are strongly dictated by environmental conditions which may not be related to the pathogens of concern and hence the lack of health relation. However, given the potential association with skin illness, Enterococci should still remain in this beach's monitoring criterion. Therefore, the recommended criteria should include Enterococci, with the understanding that an elevation in values may indicate a potential skin illness risk as opposed to a gastrointestinal illness-related health risk. This should then be taken into account by regulators in determining whether or not to place beach advisories based on this indicator alone. If such advisories are placed, it is recommended that the risk communication strategy take into account the potential disease outcome (e.g., recommending freshwater showers after using the beach).

Enterococci would also be beneficial to evaluate potential sewage contamination from offshore sources; as such the sampling protocol should include sampling, as explained earlier, where levels would be expected to be low based on sampling time and location (i.e., sampling in waistdeep water during noon or afternoon). High levels in these situations should be taken seriously as they may indicate the influence of other offshore fecal sources of pollution (e.g., from moored boats) besides the expected dominant source of sand diffusion.

A study is also recommended for this beach to determine whether the addition of F^- coliphage and *Giardia* spp. may serve as indicators of gastrointestinal-related illness given the prior limited epidemiologic results, and hence their addition to the monitoring program. This may be accomplished through an approach other than traditional epidemiology studies such as quantitative microbial risk assessments. If further studies warrant their use, F^- coliphage may be added as a monitoring target along with Enterococci, while *Giardia* spp. may be used as a confirmatory target for the presence of gastrointestinal health risk. The proposed beach regulation plan for point-of-use monitoring would be similar to the existing sampling plan for this beach except with a different understanding of how to use Enterococci and interpret its levels, an emphasis on source prevention (e.g., minimize dog fecal contamination, runoff management, solid waste management, etc.), and potential supplementary monitoring (F^- coliphage and *Giardia* spp.) to assist in predicting gastrointestinal illness.

Implementation of the "Comprehensive toolbox within an Approval Process," for this particular study site would greatly benefit from guidance with respect to minimizing impacts from sand sources, would benefit from guidance in assessing measures of F^- coliphage and *Giardia* spp., would benefit from guidelines for sample collection and processing, and would benefit from guidelines for assessing nontraditional disease end-points such as skin ailments. These components can be added to the CTB once approved through the federal level review board thereby ensuring a comparable national protection level through this panel.

The authors acknowledge that development of a CTBAP would require a considerable amount of additional resources. Evaluation of state proposals and incorporating the approved methods into a federally maintained CTB requires validation of alternative approaches on a continuous basis, along with consensus building and considerable engagement with the states and beach managers. Implementation of the CTBAP would thus require a considerable investment in time and resources by both federal and state governments, an investment that could payoff in the long-term through improvements in water quality and ultimately public health. As implied by Dwight et al., [5], excess illness costs associated with recreational swimming are on the order of many of millions of dollars per year for two California beaches alone. Considering all of the beaches nationally, the payoff could be substantial for investments aimed at improving methods for monitoring and improving water quality at recreational beach sites.

Acknowledgments

This study was funded in part by the National Science Foundation (NSF) and the National Institute of Environmental Health Sciences (NIEHS) Oceans and Human Health Center at the University of Miami Rosenstiel School (NSF 0CE0432368/0911373) and (NIEHS P50 ES12736); an NSF REU in Oceans and Human Health; and ESF and ERDF Convergence funding to the European Centre for Environment and Human Health (University of Exeter).

References

[1] H. Shuval, "Estimating the global burden of thalassogenic diseases: human infectious diseases caused by wastewater pollution of the marine environment," *Journal of Water and Health*, vol. 1, no. 2, pp. 53–64, 2003.

[2] T. J. Wade, N. Pai, J. N. S. Eisenberg, and J. M. Colford Jr., "Do U.S. Environmental Protection Agency water quality guidelines for recreational waters prevent gastrointestinal illness? A systematic review and meta-analysis," *Environmental Health Perspectives*, vol. 111, no. 8, pp. 1102–1109, 2003.

[3] A. Prüss, "Review of epidemiological studies on health effects from exposure to recreational water," *International Journal of Epidemiology*, vol. 27, no. 1, pp. 1–9, 1998.

[4] S. H. Lee, D. A. Levy, G. F. Craun, M. J. Beach, and R. L. Calderon, "Surveillance for waterborne-disease outbreaks—United States. 1999–2000," *Morbidity and Mortality Weekly Report*, vol. 51, no. 8, pp. 1–47, 2002.

[5] R. H. Dwight, L. M. Fernandez, D. B. Baker, J. C. Semenza, and B. H. Olson, "Estimating the economic burden from illnesses associated with recreational coastal water pollution—a case study in Orange County, California," *Journal of Environmental Management*, vol. 76, no. 2, pp. 95–103, 2005.

[6] J. M. Fleisher, L. E. Fleming, H. M. Solo-Gabriele et al., "The BEACHES Study: health effects and exposures from non-point source microbial contaminants in subtropical recreational marine waters," *International Journal of Epidemiology*, vol. 39, no. 5, pp. 1291–1298.

[7] J. M. Colford Jr., T. J. Wade, K. C. Schiff et al., "Water quality indicators and the risk of illness at non-point source beaches in Mission Bay, California," *Epidemiology*, vol. 18, pp. 27–35, 2007.

[8] C. D. Heaney, E. Sams, S. Wing et al., "Contact with beach sand among beachgoers and risk of illness," *American Journal of Epidemiology*, vol. 170, no. 2, pp. 164–172, 2009.

[9] C. D. Heaney, E. Sams, A. P. Dufour et al., "Fecal indicators in sand, sand contact, and risk of enteric illness among beachgoers," *Epidemiology*, vol. 23, no. 1, pp. 95–106, 2012.

[10] T. Shibata and H. M. Solo-Gabriele, "Quantitative microbial risk assessment of human illness from exposure to marine beach sand," *Environmental Science & Technology*, vol. 46, no. 5, pp. 2799–2805, 2012.

[11] A. B. Boehm, N. J. Ashbolt, J. M. Colford et al., "A sea change ahead for recreational water quality criteria," *Journal of Water and Health*, vol. 7, no. 1, pp. 9–20, 2009.

[12] United States Environmental Protection Agency (U.S. EPA), "Report of the expert's scientific workshop on critical research needs for the development of new or revised recreational water quality criteria," EPA-823-R-07-006, Office of Water, Washington, DC, USA, 2007.

[13] United States Environmental Protection Agency (U.S. EPA), "Ambient water quality criteria for bacteria," EPA A440/5-84-002.U.S. EPA, Washington, DC, USA, 1986.

[14] National Resource Defense Council (NRDC), *Testing the Waters. A Guide to Water Quality at Vacation Beaches*, New York, NY, USA, 2010.

[15] D. S. Francy, E. E. Bertke, and R. A. Darner, "Testing and refining the Ohio Nowcast at Two Lake Erie Beaches. U. S. Geological survey," Open-File Report 2009-1066, 2008.

[16] United States Environmental Protection Agency (U.S. EPA), "Water Quality Standards for Coastal and Great Lakes Recreation Waters Rule (BEACH Act)," 69 FR 67217, 2004.

[17] World Health Organization (WHO), *Guidelines for Safe Recreational Water Environments. Vol. 1: Coastal and Fresh Waters*, WHO, Geneva, Switzerland, 2003.

[18] European Union (EU), "Directive 2006/7/EC of the European Parliament and of the Council of 15 February 2006 concerning the management of bathing water quality and repealing directive 76/160/EEC," *Official Journal of the European Union*, vol. 64, pp. 37–51, 2006.

[19] L. E. Fleming, B. Kirkpatrick, L. C. Backer et al., "Review of Florida red tide and human health effects," *Harmful Algae*, vol. 10, no. 2, pp. 224–233, 2011.

[20] United States Environmental Protection Agency (U.S. EPA), "AQI: A guide to air quality and your health," EPA-456/F-09-00. Research Triangle Park, Office of Air Quality Planning and Standards, North Carolina, NC, USA, 2009.

[21] M. E. Wright, H. M. Solo Gabriele, S. Elmir, and L. E. Fleming, "Microbial load from animal feces at a recreational beach," *Marine Pollution Bulletin*, vol. 58, no. 11, pp. 1649–1656, 2009.

[22] J. D. Wang, H. M. Solo-Gabriele, A. M. Abdelzaher, and L. E. Fleming, "Estimation of enterococci input from bathers and animals on a recreational beach using camera images," *Marine Pollution Bulletin*, vol. 60, no. 8, pp. 1270–1278, 2010.

[23] T. Shibata, H. M. Solo-Gabriele, L. E. Fleming, and S. Elmir, "Monitoring marine recreational water quality using multiple microbial indicators in an urban tropical environment," *Water Research*, vol. 38, no. 13, pp. 3119–3131, 2004.

[24] A. A. Enns, L. J. Vogel, A. M. Abdelzaher et al., "Spatial and temporal variation in indicator microbe sampling is influential in beach management decisions," *Water Research*, vol. 46, no. 7, pp. 2237–2246, 2012.

[25] A. Piggot, J. Klaus, S. Johnson, M. C. Phillips, and H. M. Solo-Gabriele, "Enterococci levels are related to sediment biofilms at recreational beaches in South Florida," *Applied and Environmental Microbiology*, vol. 78, no. 17, pp. 5973–5982, 2012.

[26] Z. Feng, A. Reniers, B. K. Haus, and H. M. Solo-Gabriele, "Modeling sediment-related enterococci loadingrelease, transport and inactivation at an embayed non-point source beach," *Water Resources Research*, 2012.

[27] M. B. Nevers and R. L. Whitman, "Policies and practices of beach monitoring in the Great Lakes, USA: a critical review," *Journal of Environmental Monitoring*, vol. 12, no. 3, pp. 581–590, 2010.

[28] A. B. Boehm, S. B. Grant, J. H. Kim et al., "Decadal and shorter period variability of surf zone water quality at Huntington Beach, California," *Environmental Science and Technology*, vol. 36, no. 18, pp. 3885–3892, 2002.

[29] M. C. Phillips, H. M. Solo-Gabriele, A. M. Piggot, J. S. Klaus, and Y. Zhang, "Relationships between sand and water quality at recreational beaches," *Water Research*, vol. 45, no. 20, pp. 6763–6769, 2011.

[30] Z. Ge, R. L. Whitman, M. B. Nevers, and M. S. Phanikumar, "Wave-induced mass transport affects daily *Escherichia coli* fluctuations in nearshore water," *Environmental Science & Technology*, vol. 46, no. 4, pp. 2204–2211, 2012.

[31] M. E. Wright, A. M. Abdelzaher, H. M. Solo-Gabriele, S. Elmir, and L. E. Fleming, "The inter-tidal zone is the pathway of input of enterococci to a subtropical recreational marine beach," *Water Science and Technology*, vol. 63, no. 3, pp. 542–549, 2011.

[32] T. D. Bonilla, K. Nowosielski, M. Cuvelier et al., "Prevalence and distribution of fecal indicator organisms in South Florida beach sand and preliminary assessment of health effects associated with beach sand exposure," *Marine Pollution Bulletin*, vol. 54, no. 9, pp. 1472–1482, 2007.

[33] E. W. Alm, J. Burke, and A. Spain, "Fecal indicator bacteria are abundant in wet sand at freshwater beaches," *Water Research*, vol. 37, no. 16, pp. 3978–3982, 2003.

[34] A. M. Abdelzaher, M. E. Wright, C. Ortega et al., "Daily measures of microbes and human health at a non-point source marine beach," *Journal of Water and Health*, no. 93, pp. 443–457, 2011.

[35] T. Shibata, H. M. Solo-Gabriele, C. D. Sinigalliano et al., "Evaluation of conventional and alternative monitoring methods for a recreational marine beach with non-point source of fecal contamination," *Environmental Science & Technology*, vol. 44, no. 21, pp. 8175–8181, 2010.

[36] C. Haas, J. Rose, and C. Gerba, *Quantitative Microbial Risk Assessment*, John Wiley & Sons, New York, NY, USA, 1999.

[37] C. D. Sinigalliano, J. M. Fleisher, M. L. Gidley et al., "Traditional and molecular analyses for fecal indicator bacteria in non-point source subtropical recreational marine waters," *Water Research*, vol. 44, no. 13, pp. 3763–3772, 2010.

[38] S. M. Elmir, M. E. Wright, A. Abdelzaher et al., "Quantitative evaluation of bacteria released by bathers in a marine water," *Water Research*, vol. 41, no. 1, pp. 3–10, 2007.

[39] S. M. Elmir, T. Shibata, H. M. Solo-Gabriele et al., "Quantitative evaluation of enterococci and Bacteroidales released by adults and toddlers in marine water," *Water Research*, vol. 43, no. 18, pp. 4610–4616, 2009.

[40] X. Zhu, J. D. Wang, H. M. Solo-Gabriele, L. E. Fleming, and S. Elmir, "A microbial water quality model for recreational marine beaches," *Water Research*, vol. 45, pp. 2985–2995, 2011.

[41] M. C. Phillips, H. M. Solo-Gabriele, A. J. H. M. Reniers, J. D. Wang, R. T. Kiger, and N. Abdel-Mottaleb, "Pore water transport of enterococci out of beach sediments," *Marine Pollution Bulletin*, vol. 62, no. 11, pp. 2293–2298, 2011.

[42] B. D. Badgley, B. S. Nayak, and V. J. Harwood, "The importance of sediment and submerged aquatic vegetation as potential habitats for persistent strains of enterococci in a subtropical watershed," *Water Research*, vol. 44, no. 20, pp. 5857–5866, 2010.

[43] L. R. Plano, A. C. Garza, T. Shibata et al., "Shedding of *Staphylococcus aureus* and methicillin-resistant *Staphylococcus aureus* from adult and pediatric bathers in marine waters," *BMC Microbiology*, vol. 11, article 5, 2011.

[44] A. H. Shah, A. M. Abdelzaher, M. Phillips et al., "Indicator microbes correlate with pathogenic bacteria, yeast, and helminthes in sand at a subtropical recreational beach site," *Journal of Applied Microbiology*, vol. 110, no. 6, pp. 1571–1583, 2011.

[45] A. Griesbach, "California's clean beach initiative: is it working?" in *Proceedings of the National Beach Conference*, p. 56, Miami, Fla, USA, March 2011.

[46] R. J. Hernandez, Y. Hernandez, and N. Jimenez, "Recolonization of enterococci in shore line sand after full scale beach renovation," in *Proceedings of the National Beach Conference*, p. 373, Miami, Fla, USA, March 2011.

[47] R. R. Converse, J. L. Kinzelman, E. A. Sams et al., "Dramatic improvements in beach water quality following gull removal," *Environmental Science and Technology*, vol. 46, no. 18, pp. 10206–10213, 2012.

[48] Wisconsin Department of Natural Resources (WDNR), Wisconsin's Nonpoint Source Program Management Plan, FFY 2011–2015, 2011, http://dnr.wi.gov/topic/Nonpoint/documents/NPSProgramMgmtPlan6282011.pdf.

8

The Distributional Characteristics of Heavy Metal in Jiangsu Province Shoal Sea

Yu Wenjin[1,2] and Zou Xinqing[3]

[1] *Key Laboratory of Meteorological Disaster of Ministry of Education, Nanjing University of Information & Technology, Nanjing 210044, China*
[2] *Hohai University, Key Laboratory of Coastal Disaster, Nanjing 210093, China*
[3] *Ministry of Education Key Laboratory for Coast and Islands Development, Nanjing University, Nanjing 210093, China*

Correspondence should be addressed to Yu Wenjin; yuwenjin2003@tom.com

Academic Editor: David O. Carpenter

After the analysis of surface samples and core samples collected in Xinyanggang tidal land, the contents of Pb, Cu, Zn, and Cr were obtained and analyzed in this paper. The heavy metal accumulation rule and pollution status were studied by Index of geo-accumulation, latent ecological risk index method, and elements accumulation index method. The research suggests that (1) the contents of heavy metal Pb, Cu, Zn, and Cr in Xinyanggang tidal land have the same change trend, and such trend remains unchanged after the data were normalized, while the fluctuation range becomes smaller. (2) After analyzing the heavy metal content in the surface samples, it was revealed that the contents of heavy metals are getting lower from high tidal zone to low tidal zone, but the ranges of the change were different. Cu, Ni, and Zn emerge obvious decline from supratidal zone to subtidal zone, while the changes of Cr and Pb are not obvious. (3) Pb and Cr contents in Xinyanggang tidal land present accumulative character, as Pb in Xinyanggang is 3 times as much as the local background value, whose EF reaches 3.774. (4) RI value in Xinyanggang is 23.552, which indicates that though Xinyanggang tidal land has some heavy metal pollution and accumulation, there are no ecosystem risks, and the whole Xinyanggang core area environment quality is relatively good.

1. Introduction

As a special coastal wetland, tidal wetland is a complicated multiple-functional ecosystem with unique ecovalue and resource potential. In tidal zone, heavy metals cannot be purified through water self-purification; they normally sink into sediments after deposition and accumulation in tidal land through complicated physical, chemical, and biological process. Xu carried out researches on the spatial distributions of heavy metals and their dynamic accumulating characteristics in Shanghai coastal tidal land [1] which indicate that, in large scale, the spatial distribution pattern of the heavy metal Cu, Zn, Cr, and Pb in tidal flat sediments was not directly affected by coastal pollution discharges, rather they were closely related to sediment dynamics; while in small scale, the content of heavy metals in the tidal land near the drain was closely related to the drain. Bi Ch [2] studied different variation patterns of the existing form of heavy metal Cu, Zn, Cr, and Pb in different seasons, different locations in tidal land near the Bailonggang drain, and the shape, content, and distribution in the root sediments, finding that the contents of heavy metals in the tidal land near the Bailonggang drain were all obviously above the background value in the Shanghai tidal flat and that the sewage input had some impact on the existing form of heavy metals in sediments.

Northern-Jiangsu tidal wetland, which is a typical muddy tidal flat wetland, has the greatest area, the maximum ecosystem types, and the most complicated erosion-accumulation changes in China, even in the world. It was formed by the sediments from the ancient Yellow River Delta and Changjiang River Delta, which were washed by wave collisions and tides in the Yellow Sea and the East China Sea. With the length of 444 km, Jiangsu coastal wetland has the area of 5,100 km^2. Within this area, there are abundant river and marsh developed. The ecosystem in the core area of

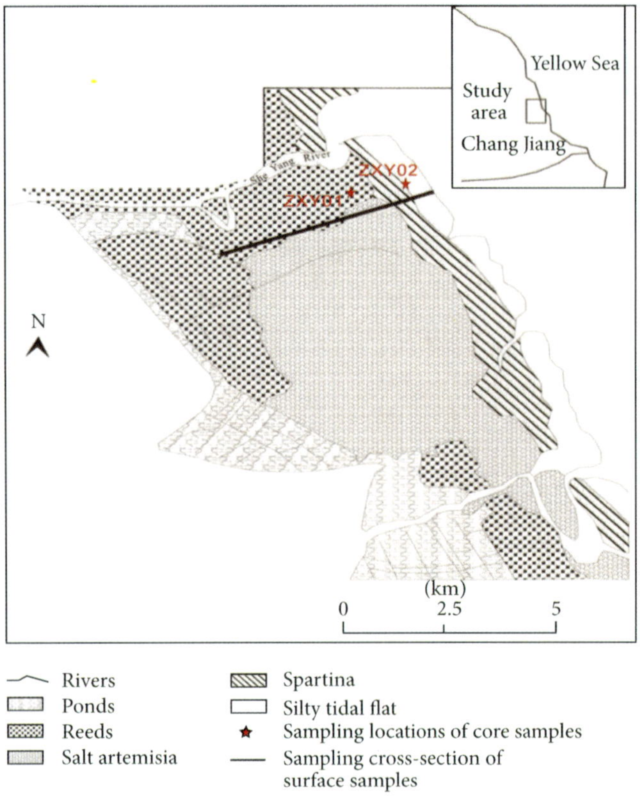

FIGURE 1: Map of sampling locations.

Yancheng Reserve remains in natural status, with limited human impacts. Therefore through analysis of tidal flat surface samples and core samples in the core area of the Reserve and the contents of heavy metal Cu, Zn, Cr, and Pb in different geomorphologies and different vegetation conditions and upon verifying between indicators, the following works had been done, that the distribution pattern of the above indicators was discussed, the biogeochemical process in different vegetations and sediments was analyzed, and the roles of different tidal flat geomorphologies and their vegetations in the enrichment of the heavy metals in the whole tidal wetland were compared.

2. Materials and Methods

2.1. The Collection of Samples and Disposal. Between August 17 and 19 2005, two cores (SY01, SY02) were collected in the core area of Yancheng red-crown crane National Natural Reserve (Xinyanggang in Sheyang County); surface samples were collected every 20 m along the cross-section from the west to the east, 220 samples in all, the sampling locations refer to Figure 1. Two cores were collected using 70 mm inner diameter and 75 mm outer diameter PVC pipes which directly access into the ground. It was pointed by the hand GPS, precision 10 m. After sealing at field, we brought them to the lab, took out the samples, dissected, took photos, and described the lithologic characters and deposition configurations. We conserved one-half of the dissected core samples and the other half was divided every 2 cm, 72 parts in total, using freeze-drying machine ALPHA-1-4 produced by the German Martin Christ Company to hypothermia lyophilize samples. For the computation method of water content and volume, refer to Ren M E, 1983. The grain size of the samples was analyzed using the Laser Particle Size Analyzer Mastersizer 2000 produced by Britain, accomplished in the Ministry of Education Key Laboratory For Coast and Islands Development, Nanjing University. The grain size parameters computation used the Moment method.

We took 260 lyophilized samples (including all the surface samples, core samples choosing 0–50 cm, and 50–100 cm every other sample), removed plant debris and stones, ground and passed then through 100 mesh sieve, preserved then in plastic bottles, and then kept then in dryer in order to determine the content of heavy metals. The heavy metal tests were carried out in ICP-MS Heavy Metal Analysis Room of the State Key Laboratory for Mineral Deposits Research, Nanjing University. The process is as follows: weigh 0.5 g sample accurately, then resolve it using HNO_3-HCL-$HCLO_4$ acid in the triangular flask, slake it in the 2040 programmable slacker, and determine the volume, and determine the content of Cu, Zn, Pb, Ni, Fe, Cr, Fe, Li, Al, and other heavy metals in soil using ICP-MS.

The instruments used are the following: Orient MDS-9000 Microwave Slaking System (Xi'an Aoruite Technology Development Corporation); HP4500series300 Plasma Mass Spectrometer (Hewlett-Packard); Ultra-pure Water NG (MLLi-Q) manufactured by American MLLipore Company. All containers were soaked overnight using 20% hydrogen nitrate and rinsed with water three times.

2.2. Data Handling and Methods. The map of sampling locations and a part of figures and tables were made using Mapinfo 7.0 and Coreldraw 10; most figures and data statistical analysis were accomplished using excel 2000 and Origin 6.0, and part of the data was handled and statistically analyzed with SPSS10. and with SPSS10. The correlation analysis between heavy metals and the correlation analysis between heavy metals and grain size were also carried out.

2.3. The Heavy Metal Pollution Evaluation Method

2.3.1. Index of Geoaccumulation. In order to evaluate the enrichment conditions and pollution conditions of heavy metals in the core area, the Index of geoaccumulation, I_{geo}, presented by German scientist, Muller, was adopted [3], which was used to quantitatively analyze heavy metal pollution in fluids. Its equation can be seen as follows:

$$I_{geo} = \log_2\left(\frac{C_n}{AB_n}\right). \tag{1}$$

In the above equation, C_n is the content of the n element in the sediment, B_n is the geochemical background value of the bedrock, and A is the constant for modifying the fluctuation of the background value caused by lithogenous movement, usually 1.5. According to this method, the heavy metal pollution in the sediments was divided into 7 degrees, as can be seen in Table 1.

TABLE 1: Index of geoaccumulation and pollution ratings.

Degree	0	1	2	3	4	5	6
I_{geo}	<0	[0, 1]	[1, 2]	[2, 3]	[3, 4]	[4, 5]	[5, 6]
Pollution degree	No pollution	Light pollution	Partial pollution	Middle pollution	Heavier pollution	Heavy pollution	Serious pollution

TABLE 2: Grade standard of E_f^i and RI.

Pollution coefficient E_r^i	Pollution index RI	Pollution level
<40	<150	Light ecological risk
40–79	150–299	Middle ecological risk
80–159	300–600	Strong ecological risk
160–320	>600	Very strong ecological risk
>320		Extremely strong ecological risk

2.3.2. Heavy Metal Latent Ecological Risk Assessing Method. In this paper, the Latent ecological index method put forward by the Sweden scientist Hakanson was adopted [4], which is a method for assessing heavy metals in soils or in the sediments from the perspective of sedimentation based on the nature and the environmental behavior characteristics of heavy metal. This method not only considers the heavy metal content in soils, but also links the ecological effects of heavy metals, environmental effects, and toxicological effects together and adopts the comparable, equivalent attribute Index classification method for evaluation. Potential ecological index correlates to the individual pollution coefficient, heavy metal toxicity coefficient, and potential ecological risk individual coefficient; its equation can be seen as follows:

$$\mathrm{RI} = \sum E_r^i,$$
$$E_r^i = T_r^t \times C_f^i, \qquad (2)$$
$$C_f^i = \frac{C_0^i}{C_n^i}.$$

In the above equations, E_r^i is the potential ecological risk individual coefficient, and T_r^i is the heavy metal toxicity; its corresponding coefficient adopts heavy metal toxicity standardized coefficient developed by Hakanson as evaluation basis; the heavy metal toxicity level priority is Pb = Cu > Zn, and the toxicity coefficient is Hg: 40, Cd: 30, As: 10, Pb: 5, Cu: 5,Cr: 2, Zn: 1. C_f^i is the individual pollution coefficient, C_n^i is the reference value, and C_0^f the measured value of the surface heavy metal in soil. The heavy metal individual pollution coefficient can refer to Aloupi and Angelidis [5], and the heavy metal pollution ecological risk coefficient and the ecological risk index can be seen in Table 2.

2.3.3. Sediment Enrichment Factor Method of Heavy Metals. Using the K_{SEF}, sediment enrichment factor method to evaluate the degree of the heavy metal pollution is developed by Kemp [6], and its equation is

$$K_{\mathrm{SEF}} = \frac{(S_E/S_{\mathrm{Al}} - a_E/a_{\mathrm{Al}})}{(a_E/a_{\mathrm{Al}})}. \qquad (3)$$

In the above equation, K_{SEF} is the heavy metal enrichment factor in sediments, S_E is the content of heavy metals in sediments, S_{Al} is the Al content in sediments, a_E is the heavy metal content in uncontaminated sediments, and a_{Al} is content of Al in the uncontaminated sediments. Al was chosen to be the reference element due to its inertness in its migration. In Xingyanggang Al could be replaced by Li. In sediments the greater K_{SEF} is, the heavier the heavy metal pollution can be. If $K_{\mathrm{SEF}} > 0$, it means that there is heavy metal enrichment, and the enrichment level can be signified by its value. Using K_{SEF} method for heavy metal geochemical correction in sediments not only can remove the impact of particle size, but also can avoid impact of the secondary nature of sediments on the measured values. In order to reflect the enrichment of the heavy metals, the enrichment factor equation was introduced as following:

$$EF = \frac{M_0/\mathrm{Li}_0}{M_B/\mathrm{Li}_B}. \qquad (4)$$

In the above equation, M_0 relates to heavy metals content in the tidal flat surface, M_B is the background value of the heavy metal, and EF means enrichment factor. Li_0 means the content of Li in the tidal flat sediments, and Li_B means the background value of Li. The enrichment factor classification standard can be shown in Table 3.

3. Results and Discussions

3.1. The Vertical Variation Pattern of Heavy Metals. After the study on the particle size and the vertical variation pattern of the heavy metals of the core ZXY01, ZXY02, it could be found that (1) the tendency of heavy metal Zn, Pb, and Cu in ZXY01 was basically the same; on the whole it decreased fluctuatingly from the surface to the downward, at −15 cm, −30 cm, and −55 cm, it formed the peak value, while at −25 cm, −55 cm it formed the valley value; (Pb was noticeably increasing only bellow −60 cm, different from the other two metals); the peak and valley values of them were in good coordination. The contents of Fe, Ca, and Mn were fluctuatingly increasing; at −25 cm and −55 cm it formed the peak value, so they were synchronous (refer to Figure 3). Ni, Cr, and Mg had no obvious increasing tendency; they fluctuated in a certain scope but formed peak value at −25 cm and −55 cm all the same. (2) After using Li as the standard normalized

TABLE 3: Enrichment degree of heavy metals.

EF	<0.25	0.25~0.5	0.5~0.75	0.75~1.5	1.5~2	2~4	>4
Enrichment degree	Extremely depletion	Strong depletion	Weak depletion	Proximity enrichment	Weak enrichment	Strong enrichment	Extremely enrichment

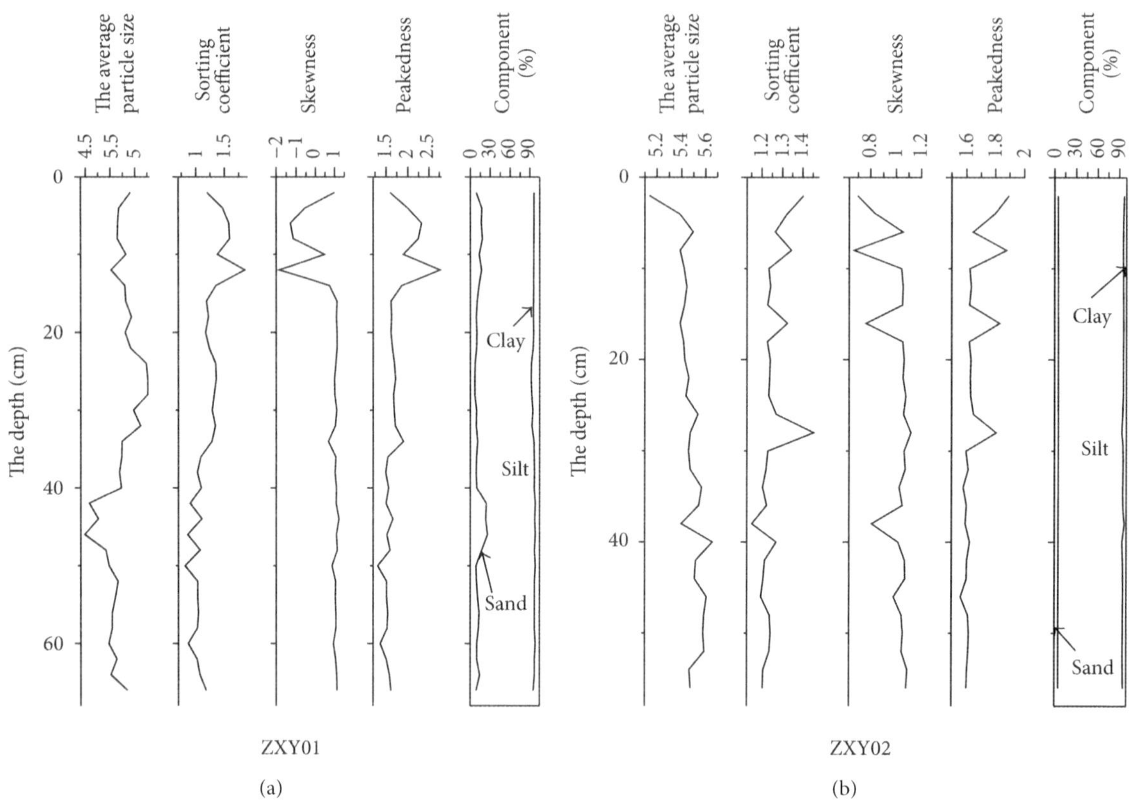

FIGURE 2: Grain size character diagram of cores ZXY01 and ZXY02 in the Xinyanggang tidal flat.

element, the fluctuation range of normalized heavy metals was all significantly narrower than that of the heavy metal content, with the former peaks and troughs lagging behind the latter. The basic fluctuation trend did not change, while the trend of Pb/Li opposed to that of Pb content. Obviously, Pb displayed different distribution characteristics from that of other elements. Except that the content of heavy metals Zn, Pb of ZXY02 fluctuated with depth in a certain range, the remaining heavy metals shown in Figure 3 increased with the depth. After being normalized, the fluctuation scope of heavy metals significantly narrowed, and the fluctuation trends of the elements were similar to that of the contents of heavy metals with the exception of Pb. (3) Compared with ZXY01, the normalized value of ZXY02 was relatively more stable. In these two cores, normalized Pb displayed different characteristics from the other elements, indicating that the sources of Pb and other elements were different, and some Pb pollution might also exist in the core.

When comparing grain size of ZXY01 with ZXY02, the content of clay and sand of ZXY01 was more than that of ZXY02, and the change from top to bottom was greater. The silt content of ZXY02 was higher than that of the other, while the content of clay and sand from the top to the bottom was relatively stable (Figure 2). Compared with the most heavy metal deposition pattern in North Jiangsu, the heavy metal deposition was mainly controlled by clay content and material source in the sediment and was positively correlated with clay content. This was the reason why the content of Cu and Zn of ZXY02 was less than that of ZXY01 and the changes were more stable (Figure 3). Only the Pb content change had unique accumulating law, and it could be deduced that human activity contributed a great deal to the accumulation of Pb in this area.

3.2. The Horizontal Distribution Pattern of Heavy Metals. The heavy metal content distribution characteristics of the horizontal section show the decrement trend from high tide zone to low tide zone, but the decrement speed varied. As observed the content of Cu, Ni, and Zn declined more notably from the upsurge to the low ebb, while Cr, Pb had no obvious decreasing trend, showing that the content of Cr, Pb in tidal flat sediments was not significantly affected by water dynamic. Particularly Pb gas deposits accounted for larger proportion. Seeing from fluctuation amplitude, Zn, Pb had larger fluctuation amplitude, respectively, 79.19~63.92 (μg/g) and 71.54~58.7 (μg/g), and the other elements had

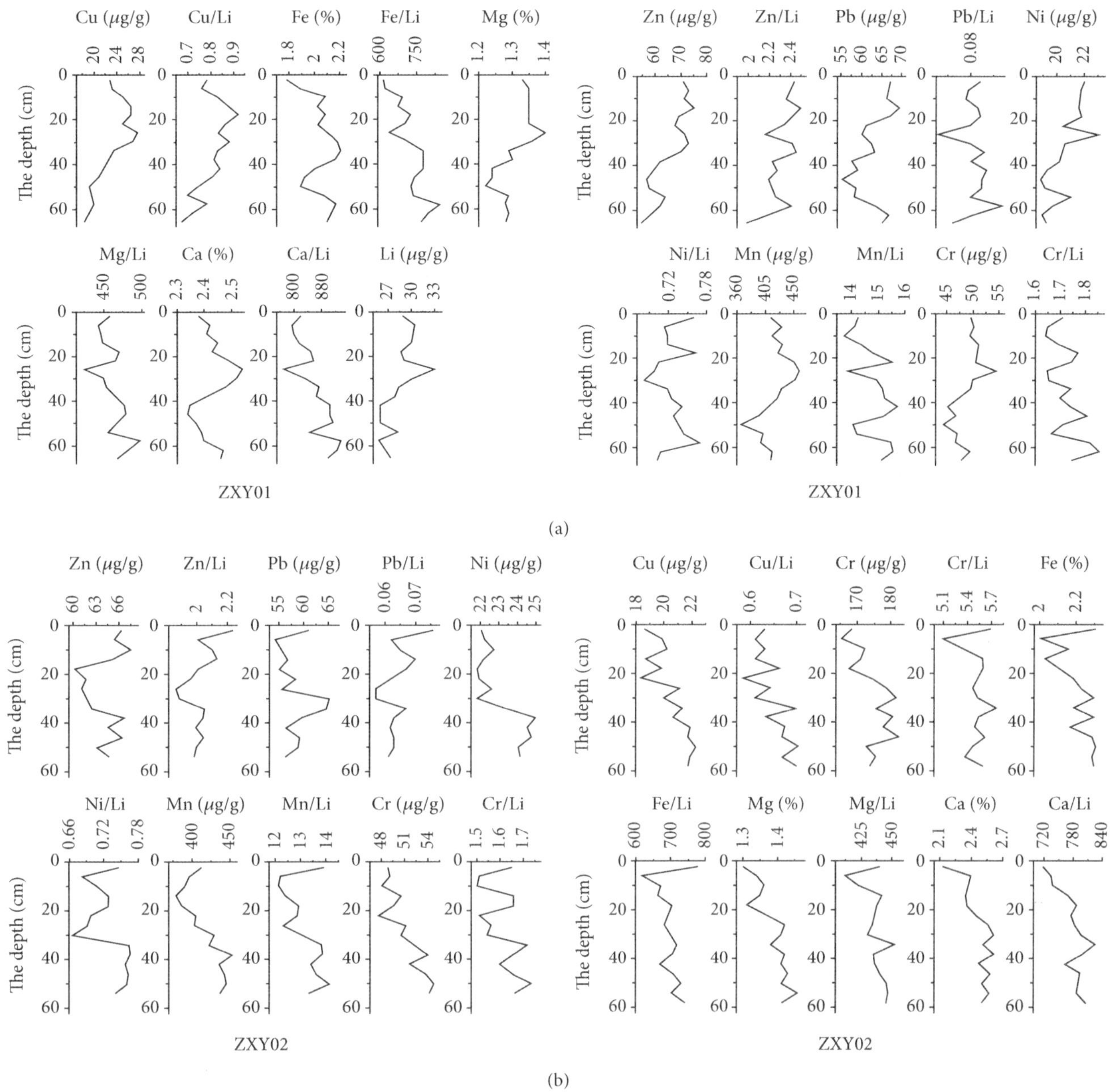

Figure 3: Metal content change map of Xinyanggang pillars ZXY01 and ZXY01.

smaller fluctuation amplitude, copper: 29.98~24.07 (μg/g), Ni: 25.08~19.52 (μg/g), and Cr: 58.31~48.79 (μg/g). As can be seen from Table 4, the content change scope of surface heavy metals of Xingyanggang core area was smaller than that of Sheyang County in comparison, so it could be seen that overall protective effect was better in the core area.

4. Heavy Metal Pollution Evaluation

4.1. The Present Heavy Metal Pollution Analysis. After analyzing 220 surface samples, in general, the content of the chemical elements of Xingyanggang tidal wetlands in the surface sediments was in the following order: Mn>Pb>Zn>V>Cr>Cu>Li>Ni. In this paper, representative elements Cu, Pb, Zn, and Cr were used to evaluate tidal flat heavy metal pollution as indicators, which could indicate the human activity impacts on the tidal flats. Many researchers use the average value of shale presented by Turekian and Wedepohl [7] or the average crustal abundance value presented by Taylor [8] as a reference background value. However, in different regions due to different sediment sources, background values should be chosen which had comparable mineral compositions with contaminated sediments and had unpolluted sediment elements value, namely, from the deepest core sites with the absence of bioturbation, so the trace elements prior to the industrialization activities were estimated to be background values [5] Xingyanggang region was a traditional agricultural area, the core area protected well, and no large-scale development conducted, basically in pristine natural state. Throughout

TABLE 4: Heavy metal content of surface samples in Xingyanggang tidal flat.

Elements	Surface samples of Sheyang County		Surface samples in Xingyanggang tidal flat	
	Mean value	Variation scope	Mean value	Variation scope
Zn	72.2	79.19~63.92	68.95	73.14~64.02
Pb	65.76	71.54~58.7	65.83	71.88~56.01
Co	14.28	15.37~12.99	14.27	15.53~13.09
Ni	22.96	25.08~19.52	22.52	23.85~21.3
Mn	481	506.6~449.7	443.98	477.1~397.8
Cr	53.6	58.31~48.79	52.83	56.28~48.42
Cu	27.77	29.98~24.07	20.84	22.87~18.14
Li	32.8	36.39~28.87	31.49	33.78~30.05

TABLE 5: Heavy metal content and background values in Xinyanggang tidal land.

Area	Pb (μg/g)	Zn (μg/g)	Cu (μg/g)	Cr (μg/g)	Li
Background value in Xinyanggang tidal flat	21.05	88.5	21.35	46.8	38
Mean value in Xinyanggang tidal flat	65.83	68.95	20.84	52.83	31.49
Maximum value in Xinyanggang tidal flat	71.88	73.14	22.87	56.28	33.78
Minimum value in Xinyanggang tidal flat	56	64.02	18.14	48.42	30.05
Background value in north shore tidal flat of Changjiang estuary	22.1	112	27.7	33.6	—
Background value in eastern China tidal flat	20	65	15	60	38
Marine survey value in Jiangsu tidal flat heavy metal survey in 1986	25	80	30	45.7	
Marine baseline survey value of Dafeng County in 1997	28.06	—	—		
I_{geo}	1.06	−0.954	−0.62	−0.409	−0.857
Pollution degree	Heavier pollution	No pollution	No pollution	No pollution	No pollution
K_{SEF}	2.774	−0.06	0.192	0.362	
EF	3.774	0.94	1.178	1.362	
Enrichment degree	Strong enrichment	Proximity enrichment	Proximity enrichment	Proximity enrichment	

Sheyang County industrialization just started in the mid-1980s. Considering that the Xingyanggang tidal flat material sources come from the Old Yellow River sediments, the Yangtze River sediments, and Jiangsu radial sand ridges, in this paper, the soil reference value adopted the heavy metal Pb, Cu, Zu, and Cr average background value of Yangtze River estuary northern shore tidal flat and eastern China tidal flat as the value [9] (see Table 5). For classification standards of heavy metal individual pollution coefficient, one can refer to (Editor-in-chief by Nanjing Institute of Soil, CAS, 1978).

The research reveals that contents of elements Pb, Cr in Xinyanggang intertidal sediments are different from those in Yangtze River mouth sediments, Yellow River Mouth sediments, China shallow sea sediments, and Jiangsu soil and showed difference of enrichment level (Table 4). According to China's marine sediment quality standard, Pb exceeded sediment standard value of the bottom (50 μg/g). Cu, Cr, and Pb in Xinyanggang tidal flat were all beyond the background values, in which Pb is the worst, with the EF value reaching 3.774, which was three times higher than the background values of China east coast. Meanwhile Pb enrichment degree in Xinyanggang tidal flat reaches the strong enrichment scope (Table 5). In conclusion, Pb pollution is significant. K_{SEF} values of Cu, Cr, and Pb are greater than zero and had a certain degree of enrichment. Pb is more significant, corresponding to its EF value. From EF and K_{SEF} value, Zn had no enrichment, Pb had significant enrichment, and Cr, Cu had slight enrichment. Cu's EF value reaches 1.173, exceeding China east coast background value but less than that of north bank of Yangtze River estuary. EF value of Cr reaches 1.326, lower than the background value of China east coast but higher than that of north bank of Yangtze River estuary. In other words, the enrichment degrees of Cu and Cr are close to the background values, with no significant pollution deposition occured. Because of the industry developed in this region, Pb's pollution is significant.

From I_{geo} value, Xinyanggang Pb pollution reaches partial pollution degree, while Zn, Cr, Cu, and Li are not polluting, corresponding to the former research results in the preamble.

4.2. The Vertical Change of Heavy Metal Pollution. According to ^{210}Pb dating method, the average sedimentary rate of Xinyanggang tidal flat was 2.85/a, so that heavy metal pollution change process in the last 25 years can be obtained from the study of core samples (Figure 4). It is showed by ZXY01

TABLE 6: Estimation result of the ecological damage of heavy metals from Xinyanggang tidal flat.

	Tide beach	In the tidal flat	The ebb shoal
C^i_{Pb}	3.127	3.055	3.190
C^i_{Cu}	2.108	1.842	1.198
C^i_{Zn}	1.339	2.069	1.006
E^i_{Pb}	15.635	22.7775	20.950
E^i_{Cu}	15.540	11.210	5.990
E^i_{Zn}	6.439	6.052	2.017
RI	23.552	36.0835	27.946
The evaluation results	Slight ecological risk	Slight ecological risk	Slight ecological risk

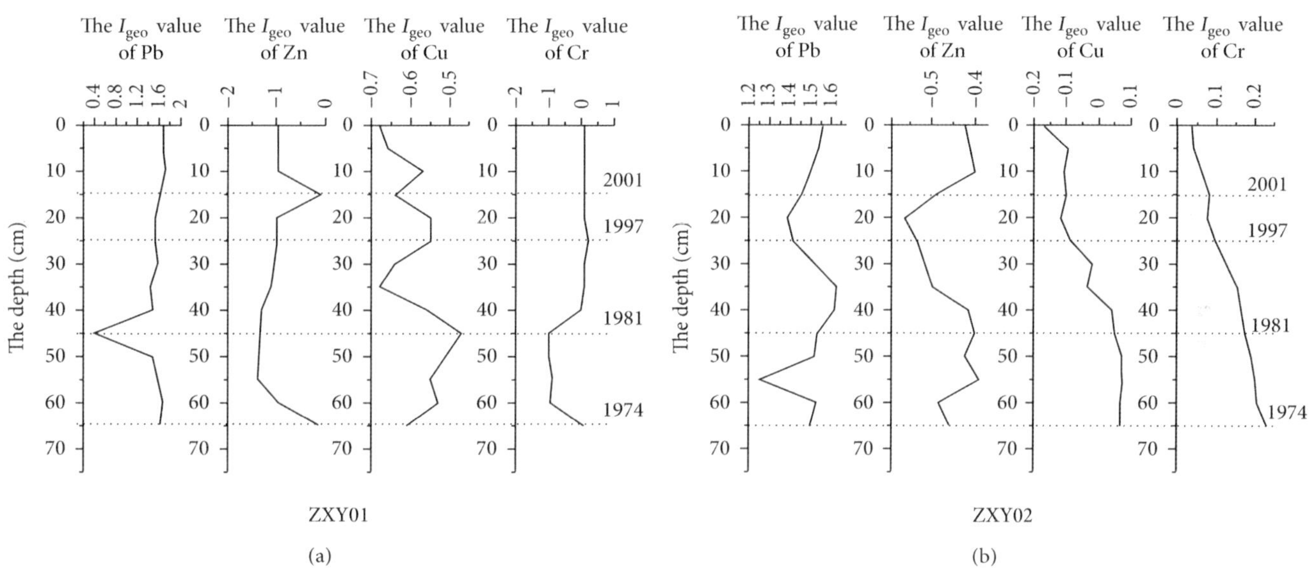

FIGURE 4: Vertical change process of heavy metal pollution in Xingyanggang tidal flat.

and ZXY02 that since 2001, I_{geo} value of Pb in Xinyanggang is above 1, indicating middle plus level pollution. From 1974 to 1981, Pb pollution was on the downward trend, which was because lead content in fuel was controlled by law. From 1981 to 1997, Pb pollution fluctuated in the low level; after 1997, Pb pollution was on an upward trend, which was related to the development of Sheyang chemical and metallurgical industries, and so forth [10]. Thus, it was proposed that a buffer zone should be set up between the core area and the development zone to better protect the core area environment. The research showed that no significant Cu, Zn pollution occurred in the tidal flat of Xinyanggang core zone, and Cu, Zn pollution was on the downward trend. Although there was minor contamination of Cr (–1–0.2), it was only a lighter extent and on a downward trend. This showed that since the nature Reserve establishment in the core area in recent years, good effects have achieved.

4.3. The Potential Ecological Harm Analysis of Heavy Metals. Upon study, it was found that there were a certain enrichment and pollution of heavy metal Pb, Cr in Xinyanggang core area. In order to find out the heavy metal impact in the core area on the national protection animal, the red-crowned crane, and on the ecological environment pollution, the potential ecological index method was adopted which was presented by Swedish scientist Hakanson, which is a method for assessing heavy metals in soils or in the sediments from the perspective of sedimentation based on the heavy metal nature and its environmental behavior characteristics. This method not only considers the content of heavy metals in soil, but also links the ecological effects of heavy metals, environmental effects and toxicological effects together. The results showed that (see Table 6) Pb, Zn, Cu, and Cr had no ecological pollution, Pb had the highest indexes, and its E^i_r and C^i_f reached 15.635 and 3.127, both in the minor scope of ecological harm. The indicators' order from high to low was Pb, Cr, Cu, and Zn, all in a safe area, and ecological pollution hazards had not appeared yet. RI value was 23.552, far less than light ecological hazard upper limit 150, indicating that although there were some heavy metal enrichment and pollution in the core area, yet no ecological hazards had been produced, and overall environment quality in Xinyanggang core area was excellent.

5. Conclusions

Through research it could be found that (1) the contents of heavy metal Pb, Cu, Zn, and Cr in Xinyanggang tidal land have the same change trend, and the fluctuation range becomes greater from deep part to surface. After using Li as the standard normalized element, the fluctuation ranges of all heavy metal normalized elements were significantly narrower than that of the heavy metals' content, with the former peaks and troughs lagging behind the latter. The main fluctuation trend keeps unchanged. The change trend of Pb/Li was counter to that of Pb content. (2) From the heavy metal content distribution characteristics of the horizontal section, we can find that they all displayed the decreasing trend from high tide to low tide, but the decreasing speed varied. The contents of Cu, Ni, and Zn declined more notably from the upsurge to the low ebb, while Cr, Pb had no obvious decreasing trend. (3) Cr and Pb in Xinyanggang tidal flat showed different enrichment degree, in which Pb exceeded the standard most, with EF value reaching 3.774, three times as much as the background values of China east coast. Its enrichment degree in Xinyanggang tidal flat reaches the strong enrichment scope, so Pb pollution is significant. (4) Xinyanggang RI value is 23.552, far less than light ecological hazard upper limit 150, indicating that although there are some heavy metal enrichment and pollution in the core area, no ecological hazard has been produced yet, and overall environment quality in Xinyanggang core area was excellent.

Acknowledgments

This study was jointly supported by the National Basic Research Program of China (973 Program) (no. 2012CB955903), Public Welfare (Project no. 201005006-01), and the MOST major special project of science and technology (2013CB956500).

References

[1] Z. L. Chen, S. Y. Xu, L. Liu et al., "The space distributes and Backlog of heavy metal in Shanghai the strand shore tide pool deposition," *Acta Geographica Sinica*, vol. 6, pp. 641–650, 2000 (Chinese).

[2] J. Bi Ch, *The Research on the Heavy Metals Timespace Distributes the Regulation and Its Living Creature Usefulness on the Plant Root Fasten in Tidal Land*, Eastern China Normal University, Shanghai, China, 2001.

[3] G. Muller, "Index of Geo-accumulation in sediment of the Rhine Rive," *GEO Journal*, vol. 2, no. 3, pp. 108–118, 1969.

[4] L. Hakanson, "An ecological risk index for aquatic pollution control. A sedimentological approach," *Water Research*, vol. 14, no. 8, pp. 975–1001, 1980.

[5] M. Aloupi and M. O. Angelidis, "Geochemistry of natural and anthropogenic metals in the coastal sediments of the island of Lesvos, Aegean Sea," *Environmental Pollution*, vol. 113, no. 2, pp. 211–219, 2001.

[6] C. Izquierdo, J. Usero, and I. Gracia, "Speciation of heavy metals in sediments from salt marshes on the Southern Atlantic coast of Spain," *Marine Pollution Bulletin*, vol. 34, no. 2, pp. 123–128, 1997.

[7] K. K. Turekian and K. H. Wedepohl, "Distribution of the elements in some major units of the earth crust," *Geological Society of America Bulletin*, vol. 72, no. 2, pp. 175–191, 1961.

[8] S. R. Taylor, "Abundance of chemical elements in the continental crust: a new table," *Geochimica et Cosmochimica Acta*, vol. 28, no. 8, pp. 1273–1285, 1964.

[9] J. Li and C. J. Zhang, *Environmental Bank-Number Book*, Chinese Environment publish, 1988.

[10] W. J. Yu, X. Q. Zou, and D. K. Zhu, "The study on sedimentation rate and the character about heavy metal of tidal flat in northern Jiangsu province," *Marine Geology & Quaternary Geology*, vol. 2, pp. 25–31, 2007.

Exploring the Next Frontier for Tobacco Control: Nondaily Smoking among New York City Adults

Rachel Sacks, Micaela H. Coady, Ijeoma G. Mbamalu, Michael Johns, and Susan M. Kansagra

Bureau of Chronic Disease Prevention and Tobacco Control, New York City Department of Health and Mental Hygiene, CN-18, Queens, NY 11101, USA

Correspondence should be addressed to Rachel Sacks, rachel.sacks.mph@gmail.com

Academic Editor: Joanna Cohen

Objective. Among current smokers, the proportion of Nondaily smokers is increasing. A better understanding of the characteristics and smoking behaviors of Nondaily smokers is needed. *Methods.* We analyzed data from the New York City (NYC) Community Health Survey to explore Nondaily smoking among NYC adults. Univariate analyses assessed changes in Nondaily smoking over time (2002–2010) and identified unique characteristics of Nondaily smokers; multivariable logistic regression analysis identified correlates of Nondaily smoking in 2010. *Results.* The proportion of smokers who engage in Nondaily smoking significantly increased between 2002 and 2010, from 31% to 36% ($P = 0.05$). A larger proportion of Nondaily smokers in 2010 were low income and made tax-avoidant cigarette purchases compared to 2002. Smoking behaviors significantly associated with Nondaily smoking in 2010 included smoking more than one hour after waking (AOR = 8.8, 95% CI (5.38–14.27)); buying "loosies" (AOR = 3.5, 95% CI (1.72–7.08)); attempting to quit (AOR = 2.3, 95% CI (1.36–3.96)). *Conclusion.* Nondaily smokers have changed over time and have characteristics distinct from daily smokers. Tobacco control efforts should be targeted towards "ready to quit" Nondaily smokers.

1. Introduction

Nondaily smoking, also referred to as intermittent or occasional smoking, represents a new challenge for tobacco research and control, both nationally and in New York City (NYC). Expanding smoke-free environments and higher cigarette taxes have been associated with declines in daily smoking nationwide and on a state-by-state basis [1–4]. However, alongside this downward trend in daily smoking, Nondaily smoking has risen. Between 2002 and 2010, the proportion of Nondaily smokers within the US adult smoker population rose [5, 6].

A better understanding of the Nondaily smoking population is needed in order to inform the development of educational efforts and cessation interventions that address this shift in the smoking population [7–10]. Previous studies have characterized Nondaily smoking as either an indicator of a tobacco initiation period common among college students and young adults [11, 12], a transition stage among daily smokers that precedes cessation [13–15], or a stable, long-term smoking behavior [1, 13]. Due to their high rates of quit attempts [8, 16], Nondaily smokers are also seen as a "ready to quit" subgroup of smokers that could benefit from cessation advice [7, 17]. Yet tobacco control programs and healthcare providers may be overlooking these smokers, either because Nondaily smokers do not self-identify as "smokers" [1, 2, 13], do not perceive themselves at risk for the negative health consequences of smoking [1, 7, 17], or may be ineligible for cessation programs that provide pharmacotherapy [18].

Communicating the dangers of smoking to Nondaily smokers is further complicated by the existence of subgroups within this population. Previous studies have described Nondaily smokers as younger, predominantly female, better educated, and wealthier than daily smokers [14, 19]. Research has also found greater representation of racial/ethnic minorities among Nondaily smokers as compared to daily smokers [7, 17, 20], and particularly high levels of Nondaily smoking among Hispanics [21]. However, these broad demographic categories may not provide sufficient information to inform targeted cessation interventions for Nondaily smokers, especially considering the diversity of smoking behaviors seen in this population [1, 7]. The so-called social smokers who smoke primarily in social situations have been the subject of exploratory research that has identified associations between smoking and binge drinking, especially among college students [11, 22, 23]. By contrast, former daily smokers who have reduced their smoking in response to tax increases or smoke-free air laws represent a different subgroup of the Nondaily smoking population that may be older and more sensitive to tobacco control policies than social smokers [24–26].

NYC provides an ideal environment in which to examine a diverse population of smokers to both assess Nondaily smoking over time and more closely examine the demographic and smoking characteristics of Nondaily smokers. In 2002, NYC launched a comprehensive tobacco control plan that included (1) taxation, including four cigarette tax increases since 2002; (2) legislation, which rendered workplaces smoke-free, including restaurants and bars; (3) expansion of treatment options for smokers via provision of nicotine replacement therapy for daily smokers; (4) intensive antitobacco education via various media channels. After implementing this plan, the prevalence of adult smoking in NYC dropped significantly from 22% in 2002 to 16% in 2009 [27].

Using a population-based survey of NYC adults, our objectives were threefold: (1) to assess whether the proportion and characteristics of Nondaily smokers have changed between 2002 and 2010; using the 2010 data only, (2) to compare the demographic characteristics, and smoking behaviors of different types of smokers (Nondaily, light daily and heavy daily); (3) to explore characteristics associated with Nondaily smoking.

2. Materials and Methods

2.1. Data Collection and Sample. Nondaily smoking data were collected using the NYC Community Health Survey (CHS), a population-based, random-digit-dialed telephone survey of approximately 10,000 NYC adults, aged 18 or older. The NYC DOHMH has conducted the CHS annually since 2002. The survey is available in multiple languages, including Spanish, Russian, and Chinese. All interviews were conducted by trained interviewers.

In 2002, eligible households were contacted using landlines only. A total of 9,674 interviews were conducted, representing a 36% response rate and a 69% cooperation rate among contacted households [28]. In 2010, landlines and cell phone numbers were used to contact potential respondents, resulting in 8,665 interviews. Response and cooperation rates of 34% and 88% for landline users and 46% and 96% for cell phone users were achieved among those contacted.

2.2. Instrument. The NYC CHS instrument was adapted from the Centers for Disease Control's Behavioral Risk Factor Surveillance System (BRFSS) [29]. The tobacco module includes questions related to current smoking, secondhand smoke exposure, responses to increases in taxation of tobacco products, and smoking cessation.

Current smoking was defined as presently smoking on all or some days and having smoked at least 100 cigarettes in a lifetime; "Nondaily" smoking was defined as smoking on some days. Daily smokers were classified as "heavy" or "light" depending on the number of cigarettes smoked per day (CPD). Heavy smoking was defined as 11 or more CPD; light smoking as 10 or less CPD. Respondents who reported smoking 11 or more CPD on some days were classified as heavy smokers (19 cases in 2002 and 4 cases in 2010).

Missing CPD data was imputed (40 cases in 2002, 69 cases in 2010) using mean replacement. In 2002, the mean number of cigarettes per day was calculated using only everyday smokers. In 2010, respondents were first asked how many cigarettes they smoked on the days they smoked and then asked how many days per month they smoked. When the number of cigarettes smoked was available but number of days smoked was missing, the days smoked were replaced with the mean of days smoked for all Nondaily smokers. If both the number of cigarettes smoked and days smoked were missing, then values were imputed based on the mean for Nondaily smokers.

A quit attempt was defined as intentional cessation for at least 24 hours in the past year [30]. Binge drinking was defined as having more than five drinks (males) or more than four drinks (females) on a single occasion within the last 30 days [31].

The survey was modified between 2002 and 2010. Questions about the location of cigarette purchases produced a large number of missing responses. The instrument was subsequently modified to include specific modes of tax-avoidant purchase (internet/mail, another person/street in NYC, in New York State (NYS) outside NYC, other state, Indian reservation, outside USA, duty free).

The household measure of income has also changed. In 2002, respondents were asked to provide their yearly household income. For 2010, respondents' poverty level was measured based on federal poverty level (FPL) thresholds (<200% FPL, 200–<400% FPL, ≥400% FPL), annual income thresholds used to estimate the number of people in poverty nationwide. To enable comparisons between 2002 and 2010, a new poverty variable for 2002 was created and estimated from the income variable. The estimation incorporated observations with partial information on income and corrects for observations with insufficient information to assign an income category.

The 2010 survey also included items to measure how many days per week and month cigarettes were smoked to more accurately measure CPD. To assess a key dimension of nicotine dependency, the 2010 survey asked "how soon after waking up do you smoke your first cigarette?"

Because the CHS uses a complex sampling design, analyses require the use of a stratifying variable and a weighting variable. The stratifying variable has 34 strata that represent neighborhoods derived from the United Hospital Fund (UHF) classification system [32]. An additional stratum was added in 2010 to represent the cell phone only sample. The weighting variable adjusts for probability of selection and poststratification. Poststratification is accomplished by weighting each record up to the population of the neighborhood (as defined by UHF), while taking into account the respondent's age, gender, and race. Starting in 2009, responses were also weighted to account for the distribution of the adult population comprising three telephone usage categories (landline only, landline and cell, cell only) using data from the 2008 New York City Housing and Vacancy Survey.

For each survey year, cases were required to have nonmissing values for at least three or more of the following variables in order to meet BRFSS guidelines for completeness: age, Hispanic status, race/ethnicity, marital status, education, employment, and phone (do you have more than one telephone in your household?). From the base sample of complete interviews in 2002 ($N = 9,674$) and in 2010 ($N = 8,665$), our final analytic sample included 2,113 smokers in 2002 and 1,141 smokers in 2010.

2.3. Statistical Analysis. Changes in the number and proportion of Nondaily, light, and heavy smokers were assessed by comparing 2002 and 2010 data. Additionally, to compare characteristics and behaviors that were associated with being a Nondaily smoker, proportions were calculated for each variable of interest using the 2002 and 2010 datasets. Variables included were selected based on *a priori* knowledge of characteristics and behaviors associated with Nondaily smoking [1, 7, 14, 24]: age, race/ethnicity, gender, borough of residence, education level, and income; we also examined quit attempts, healthcare professional advice regarding cessation, having a smoke-free home policy, time to first cigarette after waking, source of last cigarette purchased (carton, pack, or loose single), and location of last cigarette purchase. Source and location of last cigarette were used to assess smokers' purchasing patterns for evidence of tax-avoidant purchases. Chi-square tests were used to identify significant variation between 2002 and 2010 among the stratifying variables. Significant chi-squares were followed up with pairwise comparisons between 2002 and 2010 prevalence estimates using t tests. A multivariable analysis was used to test the significance of changes in characteristics of the Nondaily smoker population between 2002 and 2010. Variables found to be significant in bivariate analysis ($P < 0.05$) were included in the multivariable model.

Next, using 2010 data, we compared demographic and smoking-related characteristics of Nondaily smokers to those of light smokers and heavy smokers, separately, in order to identify significant differences in these populations. Chi-square tests were used to identify significant variation between groups; significant chi-square tests were followed up with pairwise comparisons using t-tests. All differences were considered significant at $P < 0.05$.

A multivariable logistic regression model was used to identify characteristics associated with Nondaily smoking in 2010. The dependent variable was a dichotomous indicator of Nondaily (coded as 1) versus daily smoking (coded as 0). Independent variables found to be significant in bivariate analysis ($P < 0.05$) were considered candidates in the multivariable model. Potential confounding variables were also included in the model based on *a priori* knowledge of characteristics and behaviors associated with Nondaily smoking [1, 7, 12, 14].

To assess effect modification, we also included interaction terms derived from previous research. Several studies suggest that the relationship between Nondaily smoking and education may be modified by sex, and the association between Nondaily smoking and binge drinking may be modified by race [11, 17, 23]. Thus, we included terms for these interactions in the model. An interaction term between tax-avoidant purchasing behavior and smoking rules in the home was also included to help explain the relationship between Nondaily smoking and home smoking rules, which has been found in previous research [7]. The final model included three interaction terms: sex x education level; racial/ethnicity X binge drinking; and having a smoke-free home policy X tax-avoidant purchasing behavior. Significant effects were retained in the final model. Model fit was assessed using the likelihood ratio test. Adjusted odds ratios (AORs) and corresponding 95% confidence intervals (CIs) and P values were derived from the final models.

All analyses were conducted using the survey procedures in SAS v.9.1 (SAS Institute Inc., Cary, NC) and SAS-callable SUDAAN v.10 (Research Triangle Institute, Research Triangle Park, NC) to account for the complex survey design, incorporate the survey weights and age standardize estimates. In the descriptive analyses, all estimates were standardized to the US 2000 standard population using four age strata (18–24; 25–44; 45–64; 65+). All analyses (descriptive and multivariable) were weighted to the NYC adult population.

3. Results

3.1. Changes in Nondaily Smoking over Time. Between 2002 and 2010, NYC saw a 35% overall decline in adult smoking prevalence in NYC, from 22% to 14% (data not shown). Since 2002, the number of heavy smokers in NYC has declined by more than half, from an estimated 490,000 in 2002 (representing 8% of the adult population) to about 226,000 in 2010 (representing 4% of the adult population) (Figure 1). The number of Nondaily smokers declined by about one-quarter from an estimated 410,000 in 2002 (representing 7% of the adult population) to about 311,000 in 2010 (representing 5% of the adult population). The decrease in the number of light smokers was similar to that of Nondaily smokers. In 2002 and 2010, the majority of current smokers was either Nondaily or light smokers (62% and 73%, resp.).

In 2002, about one-third (31%) of adult smokers in NYC reported smoking only on some days (Table 1); that percentage significantly increased to 36% in 2010 ($P = 0.050$). Across both years (2002 and 2010), Nondaily smokers were most likely to be between 25 and 44 years old (range of 52-53% across years), white (41% in both years), and have at least some college education (55–61%). The majority of participants reported making a quit attempt in the last

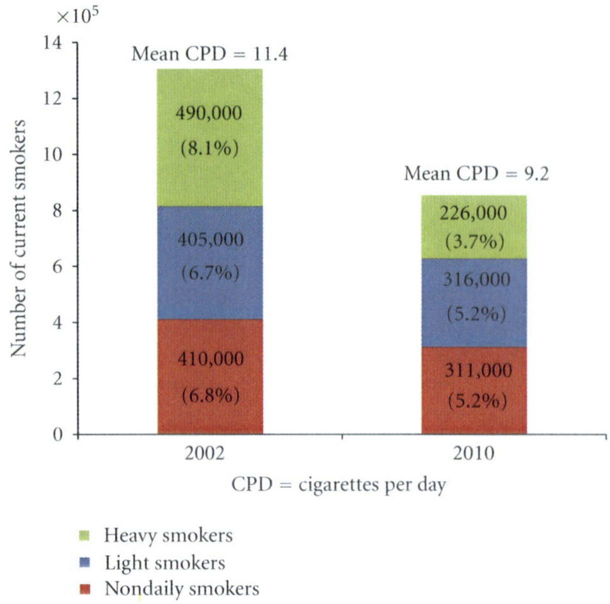

FIGURE 1: *Types of smokers, 2002 versus 2010.* Source: Community Health Survey 2002, 2010. Data are age-standardized to the US 2000 Standard Population. Estimated number and proportions are among the total NYC population aged 18 years and older.

12 months (range of 73-74% across years) and 27–29% engaged in binge drinking. Nondaily smokers were more likely to make tax-avoidant purchases in 2010 (29%) than in 2002 (12%).

Two demographic characteristics of Nondaily smokers differed across years (Table 1). While the proportion of Nondaily smokers living in the borough of Manhattan declined from 29% in 2002 to 16% in 2010 ($P < 0.001$), the proportion that resides in Queens increased (23% in 2002 versus 32% in 2010, $P = 0.022$). Finally, the proportion of Nondaily smokers in the lowest income category increased from 2002 to 2010 (33% versus 46%, $P = 0.004$), while the proportion in the middle income category declined (34% versus 22%, $P = 0.004$). The proportion of Nondaily smokers who did not allow smoking in the home increased (41% versus 52%, $P = 0.001$).

Multivariable logistic regression analyses designed to test if the changes in these characteristics were significant between 2002 and 2010 showed that only the decrease in residents in Manhattan remained significant after controlling for demographic characteristics and smoking behaviors (AOR = 0.3, 95% CI (0.10, 0.89); data not shown). Thus, there were fewer Nondaily smokers in Manhattan in 2010 than in 2002.

3.2. Characteristics Associated with Nondaily Smoking in 2010. Several significant differences in demographic and smoking characteristics were found between Nondaily, and light or heavy smokers in 2010 (Table 2). Whites were less likely to be Nondaily smokers than heavy smokers (41% versus 54%, $P < 0.05$), while blacks were more likely to be Nondaily smokers than heavy smokers (25% versus 10%, $P < 0.05$). Males were also more likely to be Nondaily smokers than heavy smokers (51% versus 66%, $P = 0.029$). The highest rate of quit attempts was among Nondaily smokers, while the percent of smokers advised to quit by a healthcare professional was lowest among Nondaily smokers in comparison to light and heavy smokers (44% versus 60% and 65%; $Ps < 0.01$). Compared to heavy smokers, more Nondaily smokers reported having rules about smoking in the home (52% versus 27%, $P < 0.001$). Most Nondaily smokers (79%) reported smoking their first cigarette of the day more than one hour after waking, in comparison to light smokers (41%) and heavy smokers (15%), $P < 0.001$. Significantly fewer Nondaily smokers smoked their last cigarette from a carton, as compared to heavy smokers (8% versus 35%, $P < 0.001$), and from a pack, as compared to light smokers (66% versus 77%, $P < 0.001$).

3.3. Correlates of Nondaily Smoking. The results of the multivariable model are reported in Table 3. In the adjusted model, Nondaily smokers were more likely to smoke their first cigarette of the day more than one hour after waking (AOR = 8.8, 95% CI (5.38–14.27)). Other variables associated with being a Nondaily smoker included buying single loose cigarettes (AOR = 3.5, 95% CI (1.72–7.08)), and making a quit attempt in the last year (AOR = 2.3, 95% CI (1.36–3.96)). Our results further suggest that the relationship between Nondaily smoking and having rules limiting smoking in the home varies as a function of cigarette purchasing behavior (AOR = 6.57, 95% CI (1.96–22.01)). Among smokers who try to avoid NYC cigarette taxes, Nondaily smoking was more common among those with rules limiting smoking in the home (AOR = 3.51, 95% CI (2.76–4.47)) but not for non-tax-avoidant smokers (AOR = 0.54, 95% CI (0.20–1.41)). Similarly, race moderated the relationship between binge drinking and Nondaily smoking (OR = 4.62, 95% CI (1.59–13.48)). The odds of being a Nondaily smoker was higher for racial/ethnic minorities who engage in binge drinking (AOR = 2.06, 95% CI (1.61–2.64)) but this did not hold for whites (AOR = 0.45, 95% CI (0.20–1.01)). There was also evidence that sex moderated the relationship between Nondaily smoking and educational attainment (OR = 2.49, 95% CI (0.91–6.82), $P = .08$). Males with at least some college education had more than twice the odds of being a Nondaily smoker (AOR = 2.6, 95% CI (1.23–5.43)), while the odds of being a Nondaily smoker among females did not vary by education (AOR = 1.03, 95% CI (0.80–1.35)). Income was collinear with education and excluded from the model.

4. Discussion

4.1. Key Results and Main Conclusions. Nondaily smokers now account for more than one-third of all adult smokers in NYC, and this proportion is much higher than the proportion seen nationally [6]. We noted a significantly higher proportion of Nondaily smokers were Queens residents in 2010 than in 2002, and rates of Nondaily smoking rose faster among New Yorkers in the lowest income

TABLE 1: Characteristics of Nondaily adult smokers aged 18 years and older, by select demographics—New York City Community Health Survey 2002 versus 2010.

	2002		2010		Chi-square test
	%	95% CI (LCI, UCI)	%	95% CI (LCI, UCI)	*P* value
Nondaily smokers overall	30.6	(28.1, 33.3)	35.6	(31.5, 40.0)	0.049
Age group					
18–24	17.4	(13.8, 21.7)	14.6	(9.5, 22.0)	
25–44	53.3	(48.4, 58.2)	52.0	(44.8, 59.1)	
45–64	23.6	(19.8, 27.9)	26.8	(21.4, 32.9)	0.723
65+	5.7	(4.0, 8.0)	6.6	(4.5, 9.6)	
Race/Ethnicity					
White non-Hispanic	40.7	(35.8, 45.9)	41.3	(34.6, 48.4)	
Black non-Hispanic	24.5	(20.4, 29.2)	25.0	(20.0, 30.8)	
Hispanic	24.3	(20.5, 28.6)	27.2	(21.5, 33.6)	0.516
Other non-Hispanic	10.4	(7.4, 14.4)	6.6	(3.8, 11.1)	
Male	49.0	(44.0, 54.1)	50.6	(43.8, 57.3)	0.955
Borough of residence					
Bronx	16.4	(12.9, 20.6)	16.7	(12.3, 22.2)	
Brooklyn	26.6	(22.5, 31.2)	30.2	(24.7, 36.5)	
Manhattan	28.7	(24.3, 33.5)	15.6*	(11.3, 21.1)	0.005
Queens	23.0	(18.6, 28.0)	32.4*	(26.2, 39.2)	
Staten Island	5.4	(3.8, 7.5)	5.1^	(2.7, 9.4)	
HS Graduate or Less (among adults aged 25+)	45.1	(40.0, 50.3)	39.2	(32.8, 46.0)	0.348
Income From All Sources (% federal poverty level)					
<200 FPL	33.4	(28.2, 39.0)	46.4*	(39.4, 53.5)	
200–<400 FPL	33.7	(28.4, 39.3)	21.6*	(16.2, 28.4)	0.016
≥400 FPL	33.0	(28.1, 38.3)	32.0	(25.5, 39.2)	
Smoking Cessation (past 12 months)					
Tried to quit smoking	73.9	(69.1, 78.3)	73.4	(67.1, 79.0)	0.776
Received provider advice to quit smoking	43.9	(38.9, 48.9)	43.5	(37.1, 50.1)	0.566
Smoking is not allowed in the home	40.9	(35.8, 46.2)	52.3	(46.0, 58.6)	0.001
Last cigarette purchased from tax-avoidant location	12.1	(9.1, 16.0)	29.3	(22.7, 36.8)	<.001
Binge drinking (last 30 days)	27.2	(23.1, 31.7)	28.7	(23.0, 35.1)	0.774

*Significant difference between 2002 and 2010, $P < .05$; indicated on variables with more than two levels.
^Estimate's Relative Standard Error (a measure of estimate precision) is greater than 30% or the sample size is too small, making the estimate potentially unreliable.
n/c: not calculated because one or more estimates is unreliable.
We present only one category for dichotomous variables to eliminate redundancy in the table.

category during that period. Together these trends suggest an increase in Nondaily smoking among lower-income New Yorkers—a departure from earlier studies that have associated Nondaily smoking with higher income and education levels [19, 24, 33]. Alongside these demographic shifts, there was an increase in purchasing behaviors associated with tax avoidance between 2002 and 2010. Price increases on cigarettes resulting from higher taxes seem the most plausible explanation for this shift. Within the context of NYC's tobacco control efforts, this trend suggests that low-income and price-sensitive smokers may be consuming fewer cigarettes in response to higher prices.

Binge drinking has been explored in previous studies, particularly as it relates to college students and social smoking [9, 11, 12, 23]. The small sample size of 18–24-year olds in our study prevents us from detecting and exploring trends among this age group. However, we documented that nearly one-third of Nondaily smokers have engaged in binge drinking and found that Nondaily smokers were more likely to be racial/ethnic minorities in comparison to heavy smokers.

Our results suggest that Nondaily smokers may be a "ready to quit" population that is less nicotine dependent than other groups of smokers [1, 7, 26]. Compared to light and heavy smokers, Nondaily smokers were more likely to have tried to quit smoking and to wait longer to smoke their first cigarette, suggesting a lower level of nicotine dependency [34]. Nondaily smokers were also more likely to purchase

Table 2: Characteristics of Nondaily, light and heavy smokers, current adult smokers aged 18 years and over—New York City Community Health Survey, 2010.

	Nondaily smoker %	Light smoker %	Heavy smoker %	P value
Overall	35.6	37.0	27.4*	0.009
Mean cigarettes per day (SE)	1.8 (0.1)	7.1 (0.2)*	23.4 (1.0)*	<.001
Age group				
18–24	14.6	16.4	5.0^	0.061
25–44	52.0	45.4	47.5	
45–64	26.8	30.5	36.3	
65+	6.6	7.7	11.2	
Race/Ethnicity				
White non-Hispanic	41.3	31.3*	54.0*	<.001
Black non-Hispanic	25.0	23.0	10.4*	
Hispanic	27.2	36.8	24.0	
Other non-Hispanic	6.6	9.0	11.6	
Male	50.6	47.1	66.4*	0.029
Borough of residence				
Bronx	16.7	18.5	15.5	0.428
Brooklyn	30.2	27.6	29.6	
Manhattan	15.6	22.7	19.3	
Queens	32.4	27.3	28.3	
Staten Island	5.1^	3.9	7.2	
HS graduate or less (among adults aged 25+)	39.2	44.3	48.5	0.020
Income (% federal poverty level)				
<200 FPL	46.4	53.6	49.4	0.207
200–<400 FPL	21.6	16.8	13.5*	
≥400 FPL	32.0	29.7	37.1	
Smoking Cessation (past 12 months)				
Tried to quit smoking	73.4	51.4*	54.8*	0.001
Received provider advice to quit	43.5	59.6*	64.8*	<.001
Smoking is not allowed in the home	52.3	44.2	27.1*	<.001
Time to first cigarette				
Within 60 minutes	21.5	59.0*	85.5*	<.001
More than 1 hour	78.5	41.0	14.5	
Source of last cigarette				
Carton	7.8	10.4	35.4*	<.001
Pack	66.1	76.6*	60.2	
Single/loosie/bummed/roll own	26.1	13.0*	4.4^	
Last cigarette purchased from tax-avoidant location	70.7	85.3*	60.8	<.001
Binge Drinking (last 30 days)	28.7	24.9	38.0	0.503

* Significantly different from Nondaily smokers, $P < .05$. See Section 2 for descriptions and definitions of smoker types.
^ Estimate's Relative Standard Error (a measure of estimate precision) is greater than 30% or the sample size is too small, making the estimate potentially unreliable.
We present only one category for dichotomous variables to eliminate redundancy in the table.

single loose cigarettes, and those who banned smoking in the home appear to comprise a price-sensitive subsgroup. Healthcare providers appear to be overlooking this group; however, Nondaily smokers were less likely to be advised to quit smoking by a healthcare professional.

Many researchers have noted that Nondaily smoking may increase as a result of expanding tobacco control legislation and cigarette price increases [2, 4, 35, 36]. The Chaiton and Cohen hypothesis regarding the "softening" of the smoking population may be a useful framework for

TABLE 3: Multivariable logistic analyses predicting Nondaily smoking versus daily smoking among current smokers, aged 18 years and over—New York City, 2010.

	Main effects model		Interaction effects model	
	Adjusted odds ratio	(95% CI) LCI, UCI	Adjusted Odds Ratio	(95% CI) LCI, UCI
Age Group				
18–44	0.83	(0.49, 1.40)	0.87	(0.51, 1.50)
45+	Ref.		Ref.	
Borough of Residence				
Brooklyn	1.10	(0.55, 2.22)	1.06	(0.52, 2.19)
Manhattan	0.66	(0.30, 1.48)	0.63	(0.27, 1.47)
Queens	1.03	(0.48, 2.22)	1.00	(0.45,2.20)
Staten Island	1.17	(0.42, 3.23)	1.02	(0.32, 3.20)
Bronx	Ref.		Ref.	
Time to first cigarette of the day				
More than 1 hour after waking up	8.32*	(2.05, 13.70)	8.76*	(5.38, 14.27)
Within 60 minutes of waking up	Ref.		Ref.	
Last cigarette purchased				
Carton	0.39*	(0.17, 0.91)	0.41*	(0.19, 0.90)
Single/loosie/bummed/rolled-your-own	3.61*	(1.79, 7.28)	3.49*	(1.72, 7.08)
Pack	Ref.		Ref.	
Cessation attempts in the past year				
Tried to quit smoking	2.15*	(1.28, 3.60)	2.32*	(1.36, 3.96)
Did not try to quit smoking	Ref.		Ref.	
Sex				
Male	0.87	(0.53, 1.40)	0.51	(0.22, 1.16)
Female	Ref.		Ref.	
Race/ethnicity				
All other races	1.11	(0.64, 1.91)	0.66	(0.3, 1.24)
White	Ref.		Ref.	
Rules about smoking in home				
Smoking is not allowed	1.10	(0.68, 1.79)	0.74	(0.43, 1.28)
Smoking is allowed in some or all areas	Ref.		Ref.	
Education (among adults aged 18+)				
Some college or more	1.75*	(1.06, 2.91)	1.03	(0.80, 1.35)
High school grad or less	Ref.		Ref.	
Last cigarette purchased				
Outside NYC/tax-avoidant	1.51	(0.80, 2.84)	0.54	(0.20, 1.41)
In New York City/nontax-avoidant	Ref.		Ref.	
Binge drinker				
Yes	1.06	(0.60, 1.88)	0.45*	(0.20, 1.01)
No	Ref.		Ref.	
Smoking not allowed in the home X tax-avoidant	—	—	6.57*	(1.96, 22.01)
All other race X binge drinker	—	—	4.62*	(1.59, 13.48)
Sex X some college or more education	—	—	2.49†	(0.91, 6.82)

† $P < .10$, * $P < .05$.

interpreting our findings in this regard [37]. Although more research is needed to measure nicotine addiction among Nondaily smokers in NYC, our results are consistent with the "softening" hypothesis. We saw a shift among the smoking population away from heavy daily smoking toward Nondaily smoking; we noted that low-income New Yorkers comprised a larger proportion of the Nondaily smoking population in 2010 as compared to 2002; we saw that Nondaily smokers were more likely than daily smokers to purchase single cigarettes than a pack. These factors point to the possibility that NYC's smoking population may be reducing their cigarette consumption in response to NYC's comprehensive tobacco control plan and transitioning toward becoming persistent Nondaily smokers.

4.2. Limitations. The NYC CHS is a population-based survey of smokers that relies upon self-reported data. Its cross-sectional design limits our ability to draw causal inferences. However, the surveys were large, conducted in multiple languages, and weighted to ensure they are representative of the NYC population; respondent opinions correlate well with both observed declines in smoking and predictions from the literature [5, 6]. In our analyses, a small number of smokers who reported smoking on some days only were classified as heavy smokers due to their high levels of consumption (23 cases total between 2002 and 2010). However, results from an exploratory analysis in which the 23 cases were classified as Nondaily smokers did not differ from the results presented here; thus, this classification did not impact our results. Finally, the change in the CPD imputation method between 2002 and 2010 could have contributed to decreases in mean CPD between 2002 and 2010.

4.3. Future Directions. New York has a greater percentage of Nondaily smokers than the US as a whole—a trend also seen in California, another jurisdiction with a strong tobacco control program [38]. This shift in smoking trends indicates that as tobacco control efforts spread around the nation, the phenomenon of Nondaily smoking may increase. Accordingly, new cessation policies and educational messaging may need to be tailored to this growing subpopulation of Nondaily smokers. NYC now has the highest cigarette excise taxes in the nation and comprehensive smoke-free air laws that prohibit smoking in bars, restaurants, and other public spaces. These distinctive environmental aspects may render our findings unique to NYC. Further research is needed to assess whether other jurisdictions with less comprehensive tobacco control policies are experiencing similar trends.

In bivariate analysis, we found that among Nondaily smokers a higher proportion were Queens residents in 2010 compared to 2002. Queens is home to many recent immigrants; 48% of the population is foreign-born, compared to 22% of the NYC population as a whole [39]. Because previous research has documented that Nondaily smoking is common among this group, particularly among Hispanic immigrants [21, 40], increasing rates of Nondaily smoking in Queens could reflect recent immigration in that borough. It should be noted that the changes in Queens were not significant in the full multivariable model, suggesting the decline was confounded by another predictor. However, our data do not allow us to identify immigration trends. Further research will be needed to explore this hypothesis in more detail.

Our findings also identified low levels of cessation advice by healthcare providers in this population, indicating that new questions may be necessary to screen effectively for Nondaily smoking in this setting. The question "are you a smoker?" may not resonate with Nondaily smokers; it may be more effective to ask if a patient smokes cigarettes every day, some days, or not at all. New Joint Commission guidelines, scheduled to take effect in 2012, encourage a similar approach, stipulating that healthcare providers screen patients for tobacco use in the past 30 days to assess and document their patients' smoking status [41]. Providers should adopt these new guidelines to better identify and treat Nondaily smokers.

Because Nondaily smokers may perceive themselves at lower risk for adverse health effects [40], and in view of findings here and in other studies that healthcare providers may not be routinely advising Nondaily smokers to quit [7], more research is needed on how to effectively assess and convey the health risks of Nondaily smoking. Furthermore, because common cessation aids may not be indicated for Nondaily smokers, incorporating assessments of nicotine dependency would be instrumental to future studies.

Many of the studies that have sought to categorize different subgroups of Nondaily smokers have often relied on qualitative studies that have been limited to specific populations, such as college students [16, 24–26]. Clear definitions of subgroups that account for both the smoking characteristics and behaviors documented in these smaller studies as well as broader trends seen in population-based studies [7, 40] would allow for better tailoring of antitobacco efforts toward the needs of Nondaily smokers. Price-sensitive smokers may be one such group; however, identifying the psychosocial characteristics of price-sensitive smokers could allow for better targeting of antitobacco interventions to their needs. Additional studies focusing on social smoking, particularly among young people, and on the prevalence of Nondaily smoking among recent immigrants to NYC would assist in the development of more effective interventions.

Acknowledgments

This work was supported in part by the New York City Department of Health and Mental Hygiene and by a cooperative agreement from CDC's Communities Putting Prevention to Work Program 3U58DP002419-01S1. The findings and conclusions in this paper are those of the authors and do not necessarily represent the views of the US Department of Health and Human Services or the Centers for Disease Control and Prevention.

References

[1] R. E. Schane, S. A. Glantz, and P. M. Ling, "Nondaily and social smoking: an increasingly prevalent pattern," *Archives of Internal Medicine*, vol. 169, no. 19, pp. 1742–1744, 2009.

[2] S. Shiffman, "Light and intermittent smokers: background and perspective," *Nicotine & Tobacco Research*, vol. 11, no. 2, pp. 122–125, 2009.

[3] D. M. Burns, J. M. Major, C. M. Anderson, and J. W. Vaughn, "Changes in cross-sectional measures, numbers of cigarettes smoked per day, and time to first cigarette—California and national data," in *Smoking and Tobacco Control Monograph 15: Those Who Continue to Smoke*, National Cancer Institute, Bethesda, Md, USA, 2003.

[4] R. Luoto, A. Uutela, and P. Puska, "Occasional smoking increases total and cardiovascular mortality among men," *Nicotine & Tobacco Research*, vol. 2, no. 2, pp. 133–139, 2000.

[5] Centers for Disease Control and Prevention, "Cigarette smoking among adults—United States, 2002," *Morbidity and Mortality Weekly Report*, vol. 53, no. 20, pp. 427–431, 2004.

[6] Centers for Disease Control and Prevention, "Vital signs: current cigarette smoking among adults aged ≥18 years—United States, 2005–2010," *Morbidity and Mortality Weekly Report*, vol. 60, pp. 1207–1212, 2011.

[7] E. K. Tong, M. K. Ong, E. Vittinghoff, and E. J. Pérez-Stable, "Nondaily smokers should be asked and advised to quit," *American Journal of Preventive Medicine*, vol. 30, no. 1, pp. 23–30, 2006.

[8] H. A. Tindle and S. Shiffman, "Smoking cessation behavior among intermittent smokers versus daily smokers," *American Journal of Public Health*, vol. 101, no. 7, pp. e1–e3, 2011.

[9] L. J. Rutten, E. M. Augustson, K. A. Doran, R. P. Moser, and B. W. Hesse, "Health information seeking and media exposure among smokers: a comparison of light and intermittent tobacco users with heavy users," *Nicotine & Tobacco Research*, vol. 11, no. 2, pp. 190–196, 2009.

[10] D. E. Levy, L. Biener, and N. Rigotti, "The natural history of light smokers: a population-based cohort study," *Nicotine & Tobacco Research*, vol. 11, no. 2, pp. 156–163, 2009.

[11] C. J. Berg, K. A. Lust, J. R. Sanem et al., "Smoker self-identification versus recent smoking among college students," *American Journal of Preventive Medicine*, vol. 36, no. 4, pp. 333–336, 2009.

[12] A. H. Levinson, S. Campo, J. Gascoigne, O. Jolly, A. Zakharyan, and Z. V. Tran, "Smoking, but not smokers: identity among college students who smoke cigarettes," *Nicotine & Tobacco Research*, vol. 9, no. 8, pp. 845–852, 2007.

[13] R. E. Schane, P. M. Ling, and S. A. Glantz, "Health effects of light and intermittent smoking: a review," *Circulation*, vol. 121, no. 13, pp. 1518–1522, 2010.

[14] K. M. Hassmiller, K. E. Warner, D. Mendez, D. T. Levy, and E. Romano, "Nondaily smokers: who are they?" *American Journal of Public Health*, vol. 93, no. 8, pp. 1321–1327, 2003.

[15] D. Hennrikus, R. Jeffery, and H. Lando, "Occasional smoking in a Minnesota working population," *American Journal of Public Health*, vol. 86, no. 9, pp. 1260–1266, 1996.

[16] S. H. Zhu, J. Sun, S. Hawkins, and S. Cummins, "A population study of low-rate smokers: quitting history and instability over time," *Health Psychology*, vol. 22, no. 3, pp. 245–252, 2003.

[17] D. R. Trinidad, E. J. Pérez-stable, S. L. Emery, M. M. White, R. A. Grana, and K. S. Messer, "Intermittent and light daily smoking across racial/ethnic groups in the United States," *Nicotine & Tobacco Research*, vol. 11, no. 2, pp. 203–210, 2009.

[18] 2008 PHS Guideline Update Panel, Liaisons, and Staff, "Treating tobacco use and dependence: 2008 update—U.S. public health service clinical practice guideline executive summary," *Respiratory Care*, vol. 53, no. 9, pp. 1217–1222, 2008.

[19] P. M. Wortley, C. G. Husten, A. Trosclair, J. Chrismon, and L. L. Pederson, "Nondaily smokers: a descriptive analysis," *Nicotine & Tobacco Research*, vol. 5, no. 5, pp. 755–759, 2003.

[20] P. Fagan and N. Rigotti, "Light and intermittent smoking: the road less traveled," *Nicotine & Tobacco Research*, vol. 11, no. 2, pp. 107–110, 2009.

[21] L. R. Reitzel, T. J. Costello, C. A. Mazas et al., "Low-level smoking among Spanish-speaking Latino smokers: relationships with demographics, tobacco dependence, withdrawal, and cessation," *Nicotine & Tobacco Research*, vol. 11, no. 2, pp. 178–184, 2009.

[22] H. R. White, B. C. Bray, C. B. Fleming, and R. F. Catalano, "Transitions into and out of light and intermittent smoking during emerging adulthood," *Nicotine & Tobacco Research*, vol. 11, no. 2, pp. 211–219, 2009.

[23] E. L. Harrison, R. A. Desai, and S. A. McKee, "Nondaily smoking and alcohol use, hazardous drinking, and alcohol diagnoses among young adults: findings from the NESARC," *Alcoholism*, vol. 32, no. 12, pp. 2081–2087, 2008.

[24] N. J. Evans, E. Gilpin, J. P. Pierce et al., "Occasional smoking among adults: evidence from the California Tobacco Survey," *Tobacco Control*, vol. 1, pp. 169–175, 1992.

[25] S. Shiffman, T. R. Kirchner, S. G. Ferguson, and D. M. Scharf, "Patterns of intermittent smoking: an analysis using ecological momentary assessment," *Addictive Behaviors*, vol. 34, no. 6-7, pp. 514–519, 2009.

[26] Q. B. Nguyen and S. Zhu, "Intermittent smokers who used to smoke daily: a preliminary study on smoking situations," *Nicotine & Tobacco Research*, vol. 11, no. 2, pp. 164–170, 2009.

[27] New York City Department of Health and Mental Hygiene, "Health department announces an eight-year decline in smoking-related deaths in New York City as smoking remains at an all-time low," October 2010, http://www.nyc.gov/html/doh/html/pr2010/pr050-10.shtml.

[28] New York City Department of Health and Mental Hygiene, "Community health survey: methodology," November 2010, http://www.nyc.gov/html/doh/html/survey/chs-methods.shtml.

[29] Centers for Disease Control and Prevention (CDC), *Behavioral Risk Factor Surveillance System Survey Questionnaire*, U.S. Department of Health and Human Services, Centers for Disease Control and Prevention, Atlanta, Ga, USA, 2001, http://www.cdc.gov/brfss/questionnaires/pdf-ques/2001brfss.pdf.

[30] E. A. Gilpin, J. P. Pierce, and A. J. Farkas, "Duration of smoking abstinence and success in quitting," *Journal of the National Cancer Institute*, vol. 89, no. 8, pp. 572–576, 1997.

[31] New York City Department of Health and Mental Hygiene, "Who's still smoking? Cigarette use among adults in New York City," *Vital Signs*, vol. 6, no. 2, 2007.

[32] New York City Department of Health and Mental Hygiene, "*New York City United Hospital Fund (UHF) Neighborhoods and Zip Codes*," 2006, http://www.nyc.gov/html/doh/downloads/pdf/survey/uhf_map_100604.pdf.

[33] C. G. Husten, "How should we define light or intermittent smoking? Does it matter?" *Nicotine & Tobacco Research*, vol. 11, no. 2, pp. 111–121, 2009.

[34] M. E. Mooney, E. O. Johnson, N. Breslau, L. J. Bierut, and D. K. Hatsukami, "Cigarette smoking reduction and changes in nicotine dependence," *Nicotine & Tobacco Research*, vol. 13, no. 6, pp. 426–430, 2011.

[35] T. Korhonen, U. Broms, E. Levälahti, M. Koskenvuo, and J. Kaprio, "Characteristics and health consequences of intermittent smoking: long-term follow-up among Finnish adult twins," *Nicotine & Tobacco Research*, vol. 11, no. 2, pp. 148–155, 2009.

[36] J. P. Pierce, M. M. White, and K. Messer, "Changing age-specific patterns of cigarette consumption in the United States, 1992–2002: association with smoke-free homes and state-level tobacco control activity," *Nicotine & Tobacco Research*, vol. 11, no. 2, pp. 171–177, 2009.

[37] M. O. Chaiton, J. E. Cohen, and J. Frank, "Population health and the hardcore smoker: Geoffrey Rose revisited," *Journal of Public Health Policy*, vol. 29, no. 3, pp. 307–318, 2008.

[38] California Department of Public Health, California Tobacco Program, *California Tobacco Control Update 2009: 20 Years of Tobacco Control in California*, Sacramento, Calif, USA, 2009.

[39] US Census Bureau, "State and County Quickfacts," 2010, http://quickfacts.census.gov/qfd/states/36/36081.html.

[40] L. K. Ackerson and K. Viswanath, "Communication inequalities, social determinants, and intermittent smoking in the 2003 Health Information National Trends Survey," *Preventing Chronic Disease*, vol. 6, no. 2, p. A40, 2009.

[41] Joint Commission, 2011, http://www.jointcommission.org/specifications_manual_for_national_hospital_inpatient_quality_measures.

10

A Systematic Review of Physical Activity Interventions in Hispanic Adults

Melinda J. Ickes[1] and Manoj Sharma[2, 3]

[1] Department of Kinesiology and Health Promotion, University of Kentucky, 111 Seaton Building, Lexington, KY 40506, USA
[2] Department of Health Promotion & Education, University of Cincinnati, Teachers College 527 C, P.O. Box 210068, Cincinnati, OH 45221, USA
[3] Department of Public Health, University of Cincinnati, Teachers College 527 C, P.O. Box 210068, Cincinnati, OH 45221, USA

Correspondence should be addressed to Melinda J. Ickes, melinda.ickes@uky.edu

Academic Editor: Edward Trapido

Healthy People 2020 aims to achieve health equity, eliminate disparities, and improve the health of all groups. Regular physical activity (PA) improves overall health and fitness and has the capability to reduce risk for chronic diseases. Identifying barriers which relate to the Hispanic population is important when designing PA interventions. Therefore, the purpose was to review existing PA interventions targeting Hispanic adults published between 1988 and 2011. This paper was limited to interventions which included more than 35% Hispanic adults ($n = 20$). Most of the interventions were community based ($n = 16$), although clinical, family-based, and faith-based settings were also represented. Interventions incorporated theory ($n = 16$), with social cognitive theory and transtheoretical model being used most frequently. Social support was integral, building on the assumption that it is a strong motivator of PA. Each of the interventions reported success related to PA, social support, and/or BMI. Lessons learned should be incorporated into future interventions.

1. Introduction

In the United States, Hispanic Americans are the largest ethnic group after non-Hispanic whites. Hispanics or Latinos are persons of Cuba, Mexico, Puerto Rico, South or Central-America, or other Spanish culture or origin, regardless of race [1]. Between 2000 and 2007, this Latino population grew nearly 30%, currently representing 15.75% (48.4 million) of the U.S. population [2]. Projections estimate that by the year 2050, there will be 132.8 million Hispanic individuals, comprising over 30% of the USA. population [2]. The rapid increase in the Hispanic population throughout the USA. requires an understanding of Hispanic culture, health care needs, and methods to approaching health promotion [3].

One of the overarching goals of Healthy People 2020 is to achieve health equity, eliminate disparities, and improve the health of all groups [4]. In order for this to occur, it is necessary to look at the underlying factors which contribute to such disparities. Unfortunately, within the Hispanic subgroup of the USA. population, health disparities are prevalent. It is known that obesity is a significant public health concern across the USA. In fact, 68% of the adult population was classified as overweight (BMI > 25 or higher), and 33.8% classified as obese (BMI > 30 or higher) in 2007-2008 [5]. Yet, rates of overweight and obesity are significantly higher among Latinos/Mexican Americans. In 2009, Hispanic Americans were 1.2 times as likely to be obese than non-Hispanic whites [6]. In Latino women, in particular, rates have increased at alarming rates, with 73% were considered overweight or obese, compared to 61.6% of the general female population [1].

Consequences related to overweight and obesity have been cited time and time again and have been associated with an increased risk of coronary heart disease, type 2 diabetes, certain types of cancer, hypertension, dyslipidemia, stroke, liver disease, gallbladder disease, sleep apnea, respiratory problems, and osteoarthritis [7]. Unfortunately disparities related to some of these chronic diseases in Latino communities are very prevalent. Coronary heart disease is the leading cause of death in Latinos, much like the general population;

however, the death rates are higher than the national average [8, 9]. In Hispanic women, coronary heart disease mortality was 40% greater than non-Hispanic whites [10]. Rates of diabetes are 2 to 3 times greater compared to non-Hispanic whites [11]. Compared to non-Hispanic whites, Hispanics in the USA. are more likely to die from diabetes (41%), stroke (18%), and chronic liver disease (62%) [6]. Implications regarding the high incidence of morbidity and mortality among the Hispanic population lend to the importance of addressing such disparities.

Regular physical activity has benefits to improve overall health and fitness and the capability to reduce risk for many of the above-mentioned chronic diseases. According to the *2008 Physical Activity Guidelines for Americans*, physical activity is anything that gets your body moving. For adults, it is recommended that both aerobic and muscle-strengthening activities be included each week: 150 minutes of moderate-intensity aerobic activity and muscle-strengthening activities on two or more days a week that work all major muscle groups [12].

Unfortunately, the proportion of the USA. population that is participating in physical activity is dismal in comparison to the known benefits. In 2008, 32.6% of the population reported no leisure-time physical activity, and only 18.2% of adults met the physical activity guidelines for Americans [4]. *Healthy People 2020* has indicated lack of physical activity as a priority area for our nation, including objectives to reduce the proportion of adults who engage in no leisure-time physical activity and to increase those adults who are meeting the recommended levels of physical activity [4].

In the Latino population, physical inactivity appears to be more prevalent when comparing among Hispanics (37%), blacks (33%) and whites (22%) [6]. According to Neighbors et al. [13], although all Hispanic groups were less active than were non-Hispanic white individuals; much variability was seen across the subgroups: Cuban and Dominican participants were the least active (19.8% met recommendation), whereas Mexican American participants were the most active (31.9% met recommendation). In terms of gender, women were less active than were men across all subgroups. Among Hispanic women, 74% report that they do not participate in leisure-time physical activity, and this seems to decline with age [14]. There are many factors which inhibit individuals from participating in regular physical activity.

According to *Healthy People 2020*, some of the factors negatively associated with adult physical activity include advancing age, low income, lack of time, lack of motivation, overweight or obesity, and perception of poor health [4]. With the changing demographics of the USA. population, it is necessary to look at specific factors which relate to the growing Hispanic population. According to Crespo and colleagues, greater acculturation tends to be associated with increased physical activity among this segment of the population [14]. Research has indicated that Mexican Americans grasp the perceived benefits of physical activity, yet this does not translate to greater likelihood of participation [15].

Barriers to physical activity which have been reported by Latinos are varied, but common themes relate to time constraints and environmental access. Juarbe and colleagues questioned their Hispanic participants and found they perceived little or no time for social interactions (including physical activity) outside home and family because of their multiple role responsibilities [15]. Environmental variable significantly correlated with physical activity including perceived neighborhood safety and perceived access to facilities that enabled physical activities to occur [16].

Focusing on factors which contribute to the initiation of physical activity is necessary to truly impact this behavior among Hispanics. Key motivators for physical activity include a desire to be healthy for the family and the anticipated physical and psychological benefits [11]. Since activity preferences may vary among different cultures, culturally focused strategies have been advocated. Dancing, walking, gardening, and family-oriented activities are preferred in the Hispanic population [11, 17].

Support networks, or the extent to which a person is connected to others, are considered predictive of health behaviors. Within the Latino population, social support is described as having a friend who is supportive [18], knowing people who exercise or seeing people exercise [19], or being involved in a group exercise activity [20]. Reportedly, means of social support increase the likelihood of participation in physical activity [11, 17]. Self-efficacy, an individual's beliefs regarding their capacities to perform in a certain manner or produce certain results in their lives [21], has also been identified as a factor which contributes to the initiation and/or maintenance of physical activity among Hispanics [22, 23]. Considering the lack of physical activity among Hispanic Americans, and the associated barriers, the Institute of Medicine (IOM) has expressed an urgent need to initiate interventions which influence obesity-related behaviors among diverse ethnic groups [24].

2. Purpose

The goal of this systematic paper is to summarize the existing evidence related to physical activity interventions with the goal of obesity prevention in Hispanic adults, published between January 1988 and April 2011, in order to determine the benefits and limitations of specified strategies.

3. Methods

3.1. Study Abstraction. An extensive literature search was conducted independently by two researchers to collect studies for inclusion in this paper to increase the likelihood that all pertinent articles were retrieved. Searches were performed using the databases Academic Search Complete, CINAHL, ERIC, Health Source: Nursing/Academic Edition, MEDLINE, Scopus, SPORT Discus, and WOK Web of Science Citation Index Expanded. Various combinations of the following keywords were used including "Hispanic" or "Latino"; "adults"; "physical activity" or "exercise." Limits of scholarly journals (peer reviewed) were set. Additional articles were identified by searching each included article reference section as well as those included in two related review articles: one focused on interventions in Hispanic women and girls and covered articles until 2007 [25] and another focused on Hispanic children and adults and covered articles until 2006 [26]. Any discrepancies were discussed until both authors agreed.

3.2. Inclusion/Exclusion Criteria. Inclusion criteria for including studies in this paper were: (1) publication in the English language, (2) conducted in the USA, (3) a primary research paper evaluating any physical activity intervention, (4) publications in peer reviewed journals between January 1988 and April 2011, and (5) the target audience for intervention was >35% Hispanics (over 18 years). Exclusion criteria were articles in languages other than English and case studies. Studies were not required to be randomized controlled trials (RCTs) because this is a relatively new area of research, and due to the relatively small amount of studies targeting this specific population, all were included as a first step in understanding the existing evidence of interventions targeting physical activity in Latinos and Hispanics.

3.3. Data Extraction. Data from studies were extracted independently by two researchers using a standardized form developed by the authors (available on request). It was determined that the first author would be assigned to be the data extractor who completed the data extraction form, and the second author would be the data checker who confirmed that the data on the extraction form were correct. Any disagreements were examined and the agreed final data were recorded. Extracted data included lead author, publication year, age of participants, percentage of Hispanic participants, theoretical framework used to guide intervention design and implementation, design, primary and secondary outcomes, measures used to obtain collected data, description of intervention, intervention frequency and duration, and main findings. These variables are summarized in Table 1.

3.4. Data Analysis. No statistical analysis or meta-analysis was conducted. Thus, the existing analysis reported in the reviewed articles was extracted and reported in a systematic format. In accordance with reporting guidelines for systematic reviews, a PRISMA checklist was used for this paper.

4. Results

4.1. Included Studies. Over 700 articles were originally identified using the aforementioned search criteria. After duplicates were removed, 507 articles were screened independently by both authors. Of those, 54 full-text articles were assessed for eligibility, resulting in 20 interventions to be included in this paper. See flow diagram in Figure 1 for a summary of the systematic search. The included 20 interventions have been summarized in Table 1, giving a description of the target population, measures used, the intervention and design, and salient findings. The interventions have been arranged alphabetically by first author's last name.

4.2. Design and Sample. This paper was limited to interventions in which the population included greater than or equal to 35% Hispanic adults. Nine of the interventions included a 100% Hispanic population [3, 18, 27–33]; while the others ranged from 70–80% Hispanics ($n = 6$) [34–39] and 40–50% ($n = 4$) [28, 40–42]. The age of participants in the interventions ranged from 18 to 95 years, although 85% ($n = 17$) targeted middle-aged adults. Half of the interventions ($n = 10$) specifically targeted females [18, 28, 30, 32–35, 38, 39, 42], which may reflect the increased prevalence of obesity among Hispanic women [6]. In addition, several of the interventions recruited specific populations including low income ($n = 6$) [3, 18, 30, 32, 35, 43], sedentary ($n = 4$) [18, 28, 32, 40], obese ($n = 3$) [28, 32, 39], those with diabetes ($n = 3$) [3, 27, 29], and individuals at risk for cardiovascular disease ($n = 1$) [33].

Considering the design of the studies reported, 65% ($n = 13$) were randomized controlled trials [18, 25, 28, 30, 32–36, 39, 41, 44, 45], in which participants were randomly assigned to the intervention or control group. Two of the interventions were quasiexperimental [40, 42], which did not randomize the participants, yet still had a control or comparison group. A nonexperimental design was also used in four of the interventions [3, 31, 37, 38], in which control and/or comparison groups were not delineated. In addition, one of the interventions [29] used a qualitative nonexperimental design.

The number of participants within each intervention was extremely varied. To differentiate, interventions were categorized from very small to extra large sample sizes. Three of the interventions were very small (under 20 [3, 28, 40]), six were small (20–75) [27–29, 34, 36, 45], five were medium (75–150) [30, 32, 38, 41, 42], five were large (150–300) [18, 31, 35, 39, 40], and one intervention was considered to have a very large sample size with 869 participants [33].

4.3. Theoretical Framework. Theory was widely incorporated into the interventions, with 75% ($n = 15$) reporting the use of some theoretical framework. social cognitive theory ($n = 5$) [30, 32, 35, 39, 42] and the transtheoretical model ($n = 5$) [32–34, 37, 40] were used most frequently. Other mentioned theories included operant learning theory [18], grounded theory [29], social science [31], social-ecological model [3], self-management model [44], and reversal theory [41]. One intervention integrated the use of multiple theories, reporting the use of both social cognitive theory and the transtheoretical model [32]. Yet, 25% of the interventions ($n = 5$) did not mention using a theoretical framework to guide the intervention [27, 28, 36, 38, 45].

4.4. Intervention Approach. Community-based settings were the most abundant ($n = 14$), although clinical settings ($n = 2$) [25, 28], family and home-based ($n = 3$) [30, 34, 42], and faith-based settings ($n = 1$) [36] were also represented. Duration of the interventions ranged from one to three sessions ($n = 2$) [31, 33] to twelve months ($n = 2$) [35, 39]. The duration of 90% of the interventions lasted less than one year; 1.5 to 2 months ($n = 6$) [34, 36, 41, 42, 44, 45], three to four months ($n = 6$) [3, 25, 29, 30, 37, 38], six months ($n = 3$) [18, 32, 40], and 9 months ($n = 1$) [44]. Duration within sessions also varied with 20-30-minute phone calls [42] to 90-minute educational and group-led exercise sessions [18].

Table 1: Summary of Physical Activity Interventions in Hispanic Adults.

Study	Age/% of Hispanic participants	Theory	Design & sample	Measures	Intervention	Duration	Salient findings
Albright et al. [34]; Collins et al. [54]	18–66 years; 70% Mexican American/Latino women	Transtheoretical Model	Two-group-repeated measures RCT; $N = 72$	Knowledge; perceived barriers to exercise; self-efficacy for PA; social support for exercise; motivational readiness for PA; processes of change; decisional balance; 7-day PA recall; acculturation; BMI; CVD risk factors	Eight 1-hour weekly behavioral skill building sessions; focused on overcoming barriers, setting short-term goals, and developing a PA program; cultural tailored curriculum including ethnically matched health educators; home-based randomized trial began after the series of classes and included either mail support or ongoing PA counseling via telephone and mail (14 calls over 10 months)	8 weeks then 10 months	After preintervention 8-week preparatory course, there was a significant increase in knowledge, perceived social support, walking minutes per week, and total cognitive and behavioral processes ($P < .01$). After 10 months of a home-based intervention, women in the phone + mail counseling condition had a significantly greater increase in estimated total energy expenditure compared to women in the support condition ($P < .05$)
Avila & Hovell [45]	40–44 years	Not mentioned	Two-group-repeated measures RCT; $N = 44$	Attitudes; beliefs; knowledge of exercise; MVPA; BMI; BP; glucose; cholesterol; waist/hip circumference; 1-mile walk and estimated VO_2 max	Eight 1-hour sessions consisting of self-change behavioral modification; assistance from an assigned buddy (social support); stretching and walking component (led for 20 mins. of walking during each session) conducted by bicultural Spanish speaking physician	8 weeks	Statistically significant ($P < .05$) decrease compared to control group for BMI, waist-to-hip ratio, and cholesterol; significant increases ($P < .05$) for VO_2 max, exercise rate frequency, self-efficacy, fitness level, and knowledge
Bopp et al. [36]	Mean age = 42.5 years (SD = 12.1); 81.1% of Mexican descent	Not mentioned	Three-group RCT (2 intervention, 1 comparison); $N = 50$	Process evaluation outcomes; PA knowledge; height; weight; program barriers; activity awareness	Faithful Footsteps Program; Faith-based physical activity intervention; culturally and spiritually relevant educational materials and activities developed promoting the health benefits of PA; team-based walking contest to promote social support for PA; health "fiesta" provided hands-on educational opportunities for PA	8 week	66% of participants identified health reasons for participating in PA (compared to 36%); 47% accurately described PA recommendations (versus 16%)

Table 1: Continued.

Study	Age/% of Hispanic participants	Theory	Design & sample	Measures	Intervention	Duration	Salient findings
Castenada et al. [27]	Mean age = 66 years; all Hispanic, Caribbean descent (84–90%)	Not mentioned	Two-group-repeated measures RCT; over 55 years; type 2 diabetes; $N = 62$	Glycemic and metabolic control; BMI; WHR; % body fat; 7-day PA recall; muscle strength with 1RM	Structured 45 mins. exercise session 3 times/week; progressively increased intensity	16 weeks	Leisure and household physical activity levels significantly improved in intervention group $P < .001$); improved glycemic control, decreased diabetes medications
Castro et al. [44]	24–55 years; 45.3% Hispanic	Self-management model	Two-group-repeated measures RCT; $N = 53$	PA minutes per week; barriers, enjoyment; self-efficacy; social support	Walking program with one session per week; participants given written materials and health and weekly phone counseling sessions; focusing on informational control, education, social support, motivation, problem-solving, and improving self-efficacy	6 weeks	At 5-month followup, PA, barriers, enjoyment, and self-efficacy were not significant; increase in social support was significant ($P < .01$); both conditions increased walking minutes per week ($P < .001$)
Chen et al. [42]	23–54 years; 44.5% Hispanic women	Social cognitive theory	Two group by three repeated measures quasiexperimental design (randomized to comparison or treatment); $N = 128$	Self-reported walking; subsample-used accelerometers	Home-based behavioral intervention to promote walking; intervention group received six phone calls (20–30 mins.) with counseling versus educational phone calls intended to increase self-efficacy, assess barriers, problem solve to promote social support	8 weeks	Both conditions increased self-reported walking at the 2 months after test($P < .88$), with mean change of 86 and 81 mins./week for behavioral and educational group, respectively
Grass et al. [38]	18–55 years; 72% Hispanic women	Not mentioned	Nonexperimental-repeated measures design; $N = 130$	PA minutes per week; PA barriers	Participatory action research; four sessions over 3 months of "walking clubs"; family focused to influence social support; written materials in English and Spanish	3 months	No significance in PA; PA barriers significance ($P < .05$)

Table 1: Continued.

Study	Age/% of Hispanic participants	Theory	Design & sample	Measures	Intervention	Duration	Salient findings
Hayashi et al. [33]	40–64 years; 100% Hispanic Women	Transtheoretical model	RCT at 4 sites; lower income under or uninsured; at risk for CVD; $N = 869$	Stage of readiness questionnaire; cholesterol, BP, BMI, coronary heart disease risk; PA level/ intensity/barrier	Wisewoman; delivered by community health workers who were bilingual and bicultural; focused on health behavior counseling	3 lifestyle sessions (30–45 mins.)	Improvement in PA readiness for change in 68% of intervention group; achieving a high degree of improvement in PA was twice as likely; improvement in estimated 10-year CHD risk
Hovell et al. [18]	18–55 years; 100% Hispanic Women	Operant learning theory	Two-group-repeated measures RCT; low income; sedentary immigrants; $N = 151$	Physical activity; aerobic fitness VO_2 max; height; weight; BP; glucose; insulin; lipid measurements	Three 90-minute sessions per week of supervised aerobic dance in a community setting; 5 : 1 participant to staff ratio; bilingual Aerobic instructor; 30-mins. of exercise/diet education after each session including culturally appropriate materials; problem-solve barriers; assigned exercise buddy	6 months	More vigorous exercise and walking at posttest for intervention group ($P < .001$); meeting ACSM guidelines increased from 19.1% to 63.2% in intervention group compared to control group (13.6% to 16.7%); sig increase in VO_2 max ($P < .01$)
Ingram et al. [29]	33–95 years; 100% Hispanic	Grounded theory	Qualitative (focus groups); w/diabetes; $N = 20$	Focus group explored themes related to self-efficacy and social support (conducted in Spanish)	Animadora study; community-based intervention to promote walking; series of walking groups led by individuals who had demonstrated success and expressed desire to help others; met 3 times/week	12 weeks	Social support expressed as commitment and companionship; walkers demonstrated a high level of self-efficacy for walking; development of group identity/social cohesion was a motivator to walk
Keele-Smith [41]	18–59 years; staff and students at New Mexico University; 42% Hispanic	Reversal theory	Two-group-repeated measures RCT; $N = 149$	PA frequency and duration; weight, body fat; exercise motivation; social support	Participants given brochure highlighting general information about exercise; individualized-written exercise prescription developed based on baseline data; one-on-one weekly educational seminars 30–45 mins.; monitoring only group that received weekly phone calls	5 weeks	More participants in intervention group were meeting PA recommendations; no significant differences in weight, body fat; consistent exercisers had significantly higher motivation scores than did inconsistent exercisers

TABLE 1: Continued.

Study	Age/% of Hispanic participants	Theory	Design & sample	Measures	Intervention	Duration	Salient findings
Keller and Cantue [28]	45–70 years; 100% Hispanic women	Not Mentioned	Two-group-repeated measures RCT; women who were postmenopausal, obese, and sedentary; $N = 18$	bioelectric impedance and BMI; anthropometric measures; total serum cholesterol; PAR; PA log; community/friend/family assessment for exercise survey; acculturation scale	Camina por Salud; clinical feasibility study designed to evaluate the effects of two frequencies of walking (3 versus 5 days/week); 30 minutes at the pace of a 20-minute mile (3.2-MET intensity	36 weeks	Significiant differences in BMI reduction, ($P = .001$); No significiant difference in anthropometric and blood lipid results; No significiant relationship between the mins. walked/week and acculturation or neighborhood characteristics. For Group I, there was a strong correlation between mins. walked and social support scores ($r = .99$, $P = .04$)
Leeman-Castillo et al. [31]	31–50 years; 100% Hispanic	Social science theory	Nonexperimental two-group-repeated measures design; Spanish & English speaking recruited ≥21 years; $N = 299$	Self-report PA	LUCHAR; Community-based health kiosk program, English or Spanish; users receive personalized feedback from computerized role models that guide them in establishing goals; printout at the completion of the program includes personal program summary and referrals for local resources	1-session; 2-month followup for risk assessment	Significant increase in participants meeting PA recommendations in community setting (33% to 49%) and clinic setting (45% to 65%) at 2-month followup
Martyn-Nemeth et al. [3]	30–65 years; 100% Hispanic	Social ecological model	Nonexperimental one-group-repeated measures design; w/type 2 diabetes; low income; $N = 16$	Hemoglobin A1C, lipids, psychological well-being; BMI; daily exercise log	Community-based, culturally designed exercise program through dance (60 mins.) received weekly exercise appointment cards	12 weeks	80% of the reported becoming physically active at least 6 days per week or more; no significiant change in BMI; trend toward improved psychological well-being & diabetes measures
Mier et al. [37]	Mean age = 32.4 years; 93.8% Mexico country of origin	Transtheoretical model	Nonexperimental one-group-repeated measures design; $N = 16$	Physical walking level; depressive symptoms; stress; BMI	Spanish handbook (Let's Walk) developed to include information which was culturally appropriate used individualized problem-solving and self-management strategies; use of social support	12 weeks	Significant differences for walking MET ($P < .02$); level of depressive symptoms and stress were significantly reduced ($P < .05$)

TABLE 1: Continued.

Study	Age/% of Hispanic participants	Theory	Design & sample	Measures	Intervention	Duration	Salient findings
Olvera et al. [30]	28–48 years; 100% Hispanic mother-daughter pairs	Social cognitive theory	Two-arm experimental design; lower income mother/daughter pairs; $N = 46$ pairs	Acculturation scale; BMI; shuttle run test or rockport walk test; accelerometers; SPAN survey; nonexercise PA rating	Bounce; family-based program delivered in community and school settings; 3-week structured group aerobic, sport sessions, or free play recreational activities; 1-week behavioral counseling session	12 weeks	No significiant differences in mother's physical fitness or PA levels; no significiant differences in BMI; although daughters did exhibit significant changes in physical fitness and PA levels ($P < .05$)
Pekmezi et al. [32]	18–65; 100% Hispanic women	Transtheoretical model; social cognitive theory	Two-group-repeated measures RCT; low-income, acculturated, majority overweight/Obese; inactive; $N = 93$	Self-report PA, 7-day PA recall; height, weight; social support; environmental access scale; CES-D scale; stage of change	Seamos activas; emphasized behavioral strategies such as goal-setting, monitoring, problem-solving, barriers, increasing social support, and rewarding oneself for meeting PA goals; monthly educational materials mailed based on individual-level-tailored feedback	6 months	MVPA increased from 16.56 mins./week to 147.27 min.; significiant increase in cognitive and behavioral processes of change ($P < .01$)
Poston et al. [39]	Mean age = 39.2 years; 70% USA. born Hispanic women	Social cognitive theory	RCT prospective block design (preestablished social groups); overweight or obese; $N = 269$	7-day PAR; BMI; WHR; blood lipids; BP; social support; health locus of control	One session per week for 12 months focused on influence of education, use of social support networks, dealing with negative influences, and restructuring personal environment; instructors were bilingual; bilingual materials; participated in 30 mins. of walking during the weekly meeting and walking clubs set up during the week	12 months	Intervention participants were not more active than controls at 6 or 12 months; no significant changes in BMI, PA recommendations, and blood lipids; significantly fewer participants who met the activity goal in the treatment group compared to wait-list control group at baseline (22% versus 25%)

Table 1: Continued.

Study	Age/% of Hispanic participants	Theory	Design & sample	Measures	Intervention	Duration	Salient findings
Staten et al. [35]	Mean age = 57.2 years; 74% Hispanic women	Social cognitive theory	Three-group (interventions) randomized experimental design; uninsured over 50 years; $N = 217$	BMI; WHR; cholesterol; glucose; activity frequency questionnaire	One group received provider counseling (PC) (active control); 2nd group received health education classes and a monthly newsletter as well as PC (PC + HE); 3rd group received all of the above and social support provided by community health workers (PC + HE + CHW); CHW were bilingual Hispanic women; CHW led bimonthly walks and encouraged participants to find walking partners, build social support	12 months	All groups showed significant increase in MVPA with no significant differences between groups; BP decreased significiant among PC + HE + CHW ($P < .05$) and PC + HE; no significiant change in BMI
Yan et al. [40]	Mean age = 72.9 years; 50.5% Hispanic	Transtheoretical model	Quasiexperimental design (intervention and small wait-list comparison); over 50 years; sedentary; $N = 208$	Participation rates; physical performance	Active start: 1 hour per week in a group setting to set goals, identify barriers, and establish social support system; after week 4, participants met 3 times/week for 45 mins.; exercises were performed to culturally preferred music; given safe exercises at home handout	6 months	Significant improvements in fitness testing measures among intervention group, including Hispanics within this group ($P < .001$)

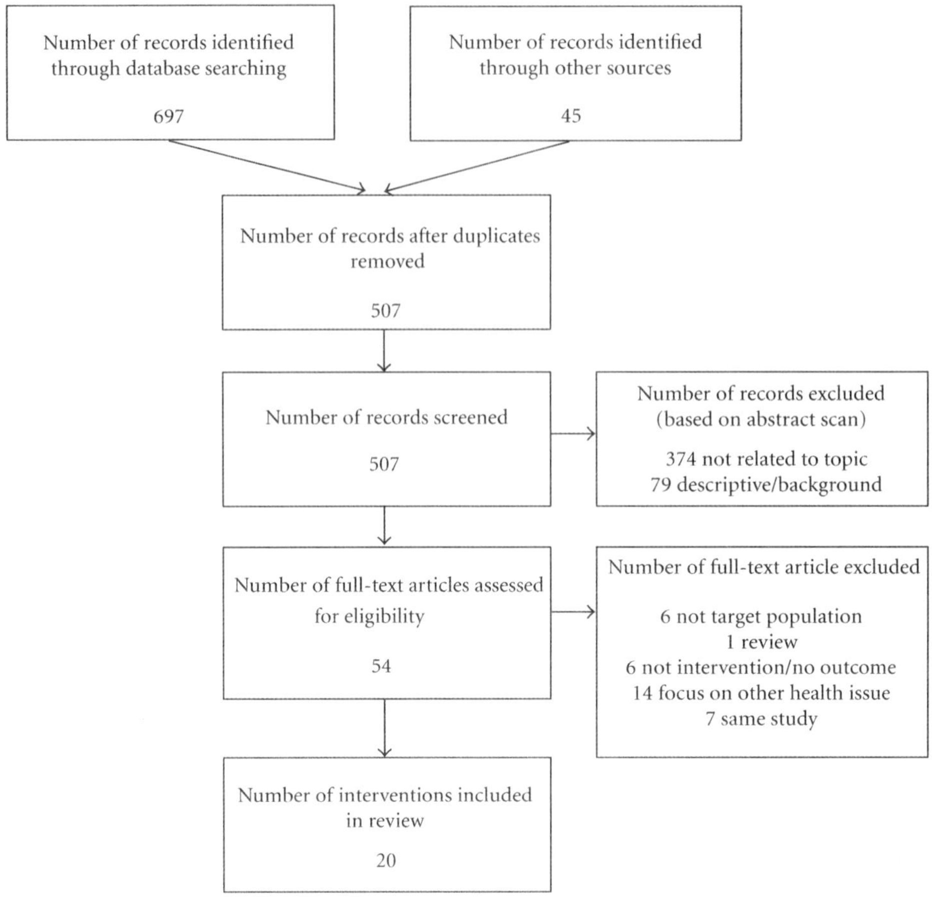

Figure 1: Summary of search results.

A variety of strategies were used within the design and implementation of each of the interventions. Increasing social support was a focal point in a 65% ($n = 13$) of the interventions [18, 29, 30, 32, 35–40, 42, 44, 45]. Building on this concept, 45% ($n = 9$) of the interventions used walking groups [28, 29, 35, 36, 38, 39, 42, 44, 45], 30% ($n = 6$) incorporated group aerobics/dance or structured activities [3, 18, 25, 27, 30, 40]. It was also important to use culturally appropriate activities and materials throughout the interventions, as reported in 45% ($n = 9$) of the interventions [3, 18, 33, 34, 36–40]. This included the use of bilingual instructors ($n = 6$) in 30% of the interventions [18, 33–35, 39, 45]. Self-management strategies including goal-setting and problem solving were used in 30% of the interventions ($n = 6$) [31, 32, 34, 37, 40, 45]. Behavioral counseling was also used as a behavior change strategy ($n = 4$) [30, 33–35], with 15% ($n = 3$) [34, 42, 44] of the interventions building in counseling via telephone. In addition, the use of personalized programs and individualized programs was incorporated into 15% ($n = 3$) [31, 32, 41] of the interventions.

4.5. Intervention Outcomes and Measures. For 90% of the interventions ($n = 18$), behavior change related to physical activity was measured, whether it was by self-report via logs or checklists ($n = 9$) [3, 31, 35, 37, 38, 41, 42, 44, 45], a 7-day recall ($n = 6$) [18, 25, 28, 32, 34, 39], or through the use of pedometers ($n = 1$) [3] or accelerometers ($n = 2$) [30, 42]. Body mass index (BMI) was measured in 55% ($n = 11$) of the interventions [3, 27, 28, 32–37, 39, 45], although it was not necessarily used as the primary outcome measure in each intervention. Other measures included clinical tests related to diabetes and/or cardiovascular disease ($n = 9$) [3, 18, 27, 28, 34, 35, 39, 43, 45], other anthropometric measures ($n = 6$) [27, 35, 39, 41, 44, 45], social support questionnaires ($n = 6$) [28, 32, 34, 39, 41, 44], measures of acculturation ($n = 2$) [28, 34], stage of change/motivation ($n = 4$) [33, 34, 41, 43], fitness testing ($n = 4$) [18, 27, 30, 45], physical activity attitudes/knowledge/awareness ($n = 4$) [34, 36, 44, 45], self-efficacy for physical activity ($n = 2$) [34, 44], and psychological well-being ($n = 2$) [3, 37].

It is important to recognize that 95% ($n = 19$) of the interventions reported success in some manner (i.e., change in physical activity, knowledge, fitness, etc.). Of those measuring physical activity as an outcome, 72% ($n = 13$) indicated an improvement.[3, 18, 25, 30–32, 34, 35, 37, 41, 42, 44, 45] Five interventions reported an increase in minutes walking and/or associated METS [18, 34, 37, 42, 44]. Three interventions reported an increase in individuals meeting recommended physical activity levels [3, 31, 41].

Two interventions indicated an increase in MVPA [32, 35] and one an increase in VPA [18].

As indicated earlier, there were other measures of success for the interventions. Four of the interventions reported an improvement in either physical activity knowledge or awareness [32, 34, 36, 45]. Social support reportedly increased in 83% ($n = 5$) of the interventions which measured it in some capacity [18, 28, 29, 34, 44]. Improved psychological well-being including decreased stress and depressive symptoms was reported in two of the interventions [3, 37]. Fitness assessments improved in three of the interventions [18, 40, 45]. Clinical measures related to diabetes and/or cardiovascular disease also reportedly improved in three of the interventions [25, 33, 35]. Self-efficacy for physical activity had significant improvements in two of the interventions [29, 45]. Finally, two of the interventions reported a significant decrease in BMI at followup [28, 45]. Yet, it is important to note that only 25% ($n = 5$) of the interventions conducted a follow-up measure; two at 2 months [31, 34], one at 6 months [36], and two at 12 months [18, 33]. Sustainability of behavior change related to physical activity outcomes was not indicated among these five interventions.

5. Discussion

The purpose of this systematic review was to summarize the existing evidence related to physical activity interventions with the goal of obesity prevention in Hispanic adults, published between January 1988 and April 2011, in order to determine the benefits and limitations of selected strategies. Based on a review of the resulting 20 interventions, it is evident there is a need for more interventions that specifically target high-risk ethnic populations, including Hispanics. This paper was limited to interventions in which the population included more than 35% Hispanic adults; however, almost half of the interventions were comprised of 100% Hispanic individuals, and 80% of the interventions included over 70% Hispanics among the target population. This was similar to results found in a review (of lifestyle behaviors) by Villarruel and colleagues in 2007 in which 82% of the adult interventions reported samples comprised of 75%–100% Hispanics [26]. There is a need for future interventions which specifically target the Hispanic population, as a homogenous makeup of participants increases the capability of addressing specific language and cultural needs of the population [36].

Half of the interventions targeted females specifically, which makes sense due to the increased prevalence of obesity among Hispanic women [6]. Furthermore, over 70% of Hispanic women report that they do not participate in leisure time physical activity [14], thereby increasing the risk for overweight and obesity. In addition, interventions recruited specific populations including low income [3, 18, 30, 32, 33, 35], sedentary [18, 40, 43], obese [28, 32, 39], those with diabetes [3, 27, 29], and individuals at risk for cardiovascular disease [33]. Targeting these subgroups is important considering physical activity that is an essential component of diabetic care, associated with a decline in cardiovascular disease risk [3], and directly linked to the prevalence of obesity [46]. In fact, based on their results, Castaneda and colleagues suggest that adopting a more physically active lifestyle has potential to reduce diabetes medication by patients and deserves further investigation [27]. Consequently, it is important to consider that these interventions were primarily designed for their target population, and thus results may not be generalizable to all subgroups of the Hispanic population.

Community-based interventions were the most prevalent, which makes sense when targeting the Hispanic population, as it has been reported that a sense of community and social support are extremely important within their culture [11]. Considerations in working with this population include finding innovative, community-based strategies to recruit and retain individuals [34]. Incorporating community collaboration into the interventions improved the reach of the program and showed community buy-in, which essentially built trust and rapport with the participants [31]. Olvera and colleagues structured their community-based intervention to take advantage of the already existing community resources [30]. Similarly, Leeman-Castillo and colleagues gave individuals referrals for local community resources to support their goal(s) and said the support of the community was integral to the success of such an approach [31]. Yan and colleagues also indicated the importance of community agencies in recruitment and implementation of such programs [40]. Using community centers, parks, playgrounds, grocery stores, and schools engaged the participant, and set the program up for sustainability, which tends to be difficult with many physical activity programs, particularly among Hispanic individuals [30]. Of the 14 interventions which were community-based, all achieved positive outcomes but one [39]. Specifically, 78.6% of the community-based interventions improved physical activity [3, 18, 31, 32, 34, 35, 37, 41, 42, 44, 45].

Due to the varying nature of the intervention setting, the duration of each intervention, the target population, the theoretical frameworks used, and the strategies used for each intervention were extremely different. Ingrained into 65% of the interventions was the idea of social support. Within the Hispanic population, social support is described as having a friend who is supportive [18], knowing people who exercise or seeing people exercise [19], or being involved in a group exercise activity [20]. Interventions which built on the assumption that social support has been identified as a strong motivator of physical activity [3, 11, 17] found success, as 60% resulted in an increase in physical activity levels.

Keller and Cantue encouraged a planned walking group among a group of women. They found the women became *comadres* and provided each other with encouragement and support [28]. Martyn-Nemeth and colleagues uncovered similar trends and found social support increased the likelihood of participation in physical activity; an unintended benefit was the friendships which were formed throughout the duration of the intervention [3]. Another intervention also promoted walking; using groups led by individuals who had already demonstrated success and expressed a desire to help others found success [29]. Building on the potential impact of social support, combined with the importance the Hispanic community places on family, one intervention took advantage of natural interactions occurring in Latino mother-daughter pairs [30]. This unique relationship would be beneficial to improve physical activity among Hispanic women. Participants reported improved social support from family and friends initially after the intervention. However, at followup, Castro and colleagues found this decreased significantly [44]. When the intervention ended, the lack of contact with the counselor and potential loss of interest from family and friends may relate to the decrease in social support. This must be considered when designing future interventions, that is, how can the sense of social support be maintained?

When targeting underserved groups, it is necessary to incorporate individually tailored programs and those which participants find fun and enjoyable, to increase likelihood of action. Keele-Smith found that participants in the group receiving individually tailored exercise prescription were more likely to be consistent exercisers [41]. Motives behind individual choices and behaviors are important to consider when designing program, and seem to improve and/or maintain compliance, particularly with this ethnic population. Utilizing dance was considered an enjoyable, safe, and low-cost method to promote physical activity among Hispanic participants [3]. It was also found that a culturally tailored aerobic dance program increased vigorous physical activity, walking, and fitness levels in overweight Hispanic participants [18].

Culturally appropriate messages were incorporated into 45% of the interventions, including the use of focus groups to assist in the design and implementation and the creation of culturally relevant materials. The goal of Hispanic-specific interventions includes specificity of cultural values and beliefs and addressing widespread barriers among this population [29]. Participants responded favorably when receiving the intervention in Spanish and appreciated information addressing culture-specific barriers to physical activity for Latinos [32].

Interventions which included staff from the same ethnic group of the population reportedly improved recruitment [47]. The reason being that participants may feel more comfortable when they perceive individuals involved are familiar with their culture, and a sense of trust is increased. Community health workers have also been considered an important element of community empowerment strategies to address health disparities [48]. In one intervention, culturally competent community health workers played a key role in minimizing dropout rates, through encouragement and follow-up phone calls [33]. Community health workers were also used as a mean to facilitate understanding of messages previously provided by counselors and/or through health education, and this combination was found to be successful in promoting behavior change [35]. Chen and colleagues reported difficulty in attaining this when working with a diverse ethnic makeup. They said the lack of heterogeneity between counselors and participants could have reduced the effectiveness of their intervention [42]. These strategies must be considered to make the most impact on physical activity behaviors of the Hispanic population.

Theory-based health behavior change programs are thought to be more effective compared to those that do not use theory [49]. Of the included interventions, 75% incorporated the use of theory, with social cognitive theory [30, 32, 35, 39, 42] and the transtheoretical model [32–34, 37, 40] used most frequently. Theory-based programs aid in the development of measurable program outcomes, help in the design of interventions, provide a framework for effective programming strategies, and increase the likelihood of successful replication [50] and should therefore be considered when designing future interventions.

Duration of the interventions ranged from one session to twelve months. For these interventions, duration was not necessarily correlated with more impactful results. However, as recommended by Prochaska and colleagues [51], for sustaining behavior change, interventions should be at least 6 months in duration. Six of the reviewed interventions met that criteria, thus relapse prevention and maintenance efforts must be considered [52]. However, of those six interventions, only one included followup measures at twelve months [18]. Thus, sustainability of behavior change cannot be indicated. Future studies should consider long-term follow-up and incorporate relapse prevention strategies.

With all of the different primary outcome measures, only limited comparisons can be made across studies; however, results of these 20 interventions were promising. Of the interventions, 72% reported an increase in physical activity levels at postmeasurement. For example, Hovell and colleagues reported more vigorous exercise and walking, and meeting ACSM guidelines increased from 19% to 63% among participants [18]. Another significant increase in physical activity level occurred in the 6-month intervention emphasizing behavioral strategies; moderate-to-vigorous physical activity increased from 16.5 minutes per week to 147.3 minutes/week [32]. Two interventions reported a reduction in BMI, although significant findings were only found in the study which was 9 months in duration [28]. Social support increased the likelihood of overall participation in two of the interventions [28, 29], again reinforcing the importance of social support in this population. Results also showed improved psychological well-being [3], as well as, improved physical activity knowledge and awareness [36]. These varying measures of success are promising and showcase the feasibility and potential for physical activity interventions among the Hispanic population.

5.1. Limitations. It is important to note the limitations of this paper. This is a narrative review and not a quantitative meta analysis. Hence, comment on aspects such as effect sizes for all studies, correlation coefficients, and other quantitative measures cannot be made. Although various subsets of questions exist within this literature, the paper purpose was framed in a manner that was not so prespecified, allowing for a more iterative method of review. Further, the interventions included were limited to those in the English language, published between January 1988 and April 2011 and the location of study must have been in the United States. This precluded interventions from other countries which may have also targeted Hispanic adults. The rationale behind this was that many of the environmental influences Hispanic adults deal with who live in the United States vary compared to those living in other countries.

5.2. Recommendations for Improving Interventions. The success of the summarized physical activity interventions among Hispanic adults is quite promising considering the implications this has for future obesity prevention and other chronic disease prevention efforts. Even though there were varying types of interventions, lessons can be learned from those which are found to be the most successful. When designing an intervention for any population, it is important to consider what strategies will be most effective in increasing the likelihood of participation. This is particularly important with a population which might be less likely to follow-through with such programs. Typically, participation rates decrease significantly with the Hispanic population [30]. This necessitates the importance of choosing activities that are appealing and fun, as well as, culturally relevant [18]. Walking programs can increase physical activity among socioeconomically disadvantaged groups; yet they are low-cost, culturally appropriate, and community based [37], all of which tie into those strategies found to be most effective in the Hispanic population.

Interventions among Hispanic populations should build on their sense of culture and incorporate means of social support to increase physical activity levels [29]. Sense of commitment, self-efficacy, and a strong sense of group identity and cohesion were all important factors in Hispanic adults participating in the physical activity interventions [29]. Building in educational opportunities as well as the ability for participants to enhance self-management skills resulted in participants being more likely to achieve positive benefits, particularly those related to an increase in physical activity levels.

Much of the improvement in the benefits achieved during the interventions tends to be lost in follow-up measures. As a result, there is a need to continue support once the intervention is complete; changes in community-wide policies may include supportive social norms and community-based resources [18]. With such a focus on individual-level variables as primary outcomes, these do not necessarily provide a full understanding of the potential for long-term community mobilization and change. Castro and colleagues recognize the complexity in changing physical activity behaviors, particularly in previously sedentary individuals. They acknowledge that future studies must consider environmental factors and other social and cognitive factors such as competing demands, stressful life events, role models, for physical activity, and normative and cultural beliefs about the importance of physical activity [44]. Evaluation of community level indicators is needed to demonstrate changes in community capacity, resource identification, and environmental change [53].

6. Conclusion

Considering the lack of physical activity among Hispanic American, and the associated barriers, the institute of medicine has expressed an urgent need to initiate interventions which influence obesity-related behaviors among diverse ethnic groups [24]. The lack of research in this area is of particular concern since the issue of lifestyle behaviors is likely to become a more prominent public health concern, as the Hispanic population continues to increase in the United States [26]. Greater attention needs to be given to the needs of such underserved populations [13].

Although it is critical to impart individual level behavior change, it is also crucial to address broader policy and environmental-level changes, as to impact individuals and communities. In fact, Healthy People 2020 recommends increasing legislative policies for the built environment that enhance access to and availability of physical activity opportunities [4]. Future interventions must attempt to combine such health promotion efforts to have a greater impact [25].

References

[1] Office of Minority Health and Health Disparities, U.S. Census Bureau facts for features: Hispanic heritage monthly, September-October, 2010.

[2] United States Census Bureau, Hispanic population of the United States, 2009, http://www.census.gov/population/www/socdemo/hispanic/hispanic_pop_presentation.html.

[3] P. A. Martyn-Nemeth, G. A. Vitale, and D. R. Cowger, "A culturally focused exercise program in hispanic adults with type 2 diabetes: a pilot study," *Diabetes Educator*, vol. 36, no. 2, pp. 258–267, 2010.

[4] United States Department of Health and Human Services, *Healthy People 2020*, United States Department of Health and Human Services, Washington, DC, USA, 2010.

[5] K. M. Flegal, M. D. Carroll, C. L. Ogden, and L. R. Curtin, "Prevalence and trends in obesity among US adults, 1999–2008," *Journal of the American Medical Association*, vol. 303, no. 3, pp. 235–241, 2010.

[6] Centers for Disease Control and Prevention, "Health disparities experienced by Hispanics—United States," *Morbidity and Mortality Weekly Report*, vol. 53, pp. 935–937, 2004.

[7] World Health Organization, *Obesity and Overweight*, WHO, Geneva, Switzerland, 2003.

[8] Centers for Disease Control and Prevention, *The Burden of Chronic Diseases and their Risk Factors: National and State Perspectives*, US Department of Health and Human Services & CDC, Atlanta, GA, USA, 2004.

[9] American Heart Association, Statistical fact sheet—risk factors: overweight and obesity, 2003, http://www.americanheart.org/.

[10] D. K. Pandey, D. R. Labarthe, D. C. Goff, W. Chan, and M. Z. Nichaman, "Community-wide coronary heart disease mortality in Mexican Americans equals or exceeds that in non-Hispanic whites: the Corpus Christi heart project," *American Journal of Medicine*, vol. 110, no. 2, pp. 81–87, 2001.

[11] N. Mier, A. A. Medina, and M. G. Ory, "Mexican Americans with type 2 diabetes: perspectives on definitions, motivators, and programs of physical activity," *Preventing Chronic Disease*, vol. 4, no. 2, p. A24, 2007.

[12] United States Department of Health and Human Services, *Physical Activity Guidelines for Americans, 2008*, USGP Office, Washington, DC, USA, 2008.

[13] C. J. Neighbors, D. X. Marquez, and B. H. Marcus, "Leisure-time physical activity disparities among Hispanic subgroups in the United States," *American Journal of Public Health*, vol. 98, no. 8, pp. 1460–1464, 2008.

[14] C. J. Crespo, E. Smit, O. Carter-Pokras, and R. Andersen, "Acculturation and leisure-time physical inactivity in Mexican American adults: results from NHANES III, 1988–1994," *American Journal of Public Health*, vol. 91, no. 8, pp. 1254–1257, 2001.

[15] T. Juarbe, X. P. Turok, and E. J. Pérez-Stable, "Perceived benefits and barriers to physical activity among older Latina women," *Western Journal of Nursing Research*, vol. 24, no. 8, pp. 868–886, 2002.

[16] I. A. López, C. A. Bryant, and R. J. McDermott, "Influences on physical activity participation among Latinas: an ecological perspective," *American Journal of Health Behavior*, vol. 32, no. 6, pp. 627–639, 2008.

[17] J. Wilbur, P. J. Chandler, B. Dancy, and H. Lee, "Correlates of physical activity in urban Midwestern Latinas," *American Journal of Preventive Medicine*, vol. 25, no. 3, pp. 69–76, 2003.

[18] M. F. Hovell, M. M. Mulvihill, M. J. Buono et al., "Culturally tailored aerobic exercise intervention for low-income Latinas," *American Journal of Health Promotion*, vol. 22, no. 3, pp. 155–163, 2008.

[19] M. P. Gallant, "The influence of social support on chronic illness self-management: a review and directions for research," *Health Education and Behavior*, vol. 30, no. 2, pp. 170–195, 2003.

[20] K. R. Evenson, O. L. Sarmiento, K. W. Tawney, M. L. Macon, and A. S. Ammerman, "Personal, social, and environmental correlates of physical activity in North Carolina Latina immigrants," *American Journal of Preventive Medicine*, vol. 25, supplement 1, pp. 77–85, 2003.

[21] A. Bandura, "Self-Efficacy," in *Encyclopedia of Human Behavior*, V. S. Ramachaudran, Ed., vol. 4, Academic Press, New York, NY, USA, 1994.

[22] A. A. Eyler, R. C. Brownson, S. J. Bacak, and R. A. Housemann, "The epidemiology of walking for physical activity in the United States," *Medicine and Science in Sports and Exercise*, vol. 35, no. 9, pp. 1529–1536, 2003.

[23] E. McAuley, G. J. Jerome, S. Elavsky, D. X. Marquez, and S. N. Ramsey, "Predicting long-term maintenance of physical activity in older adults," *Preventive Medicine*, vol. 37, no. 2, pp. 110–118, 2003.

[24] Institute of Medicine, *Progress in Preventing Childhood Obesity: How Do We Measure Up?* National Academies Press, Washington, DC, USA, 2006.

[25] M. Sharma, "Physical activity interventions in Hispanic American girls and women," *Obesity Reviews*, vol. 9, no. 6, pp. 560–571, 2008.

[26] A. M. Villarruel and D. Koniak-Griffin, "Lifestyle behavior interventions with Hispanic children and adults," *Annual Review of Nursing Research*, vol. 25, pp. 51–81, 2007.

[27] C. Castaneda, J. E. Layne, L. Munoz-Orians et al., "A randomized controlled trial of resistance exercise training to improve glycemic control in older adults with type 2 diabetes," *Diabetes Care*, vol. 25, no. 12, pp. 2335–2341, 2002.

[28] C. S. Keller and A. Cantue, "Camina por Salud: walking in Mexican-American women," *Applied Nursing Research*, vol. 21, no. 2, pp. 110–113, 2008.

[29] M. Ingram, M. Ruiz, M. T. Mayorga, and C. Rosales, "The Animadora Project: identifying factors related to the promotion of physical activity among Mexican Americans with diabetes," *American Journal of Health Promotion*, vol. 23, no. 6, pp. 396–402, 2009.

[30] N. Olvera, J. A. Bush, S. V. Sharma, B. B. Knox, R. L. Scherer, and N. F. Butte, "BOUNCE: a community-based mother-daughter healthy lifestyle intervention for low-income latino families," *Obesity*, vol. 18, supplement 1, pp. S102–S104, 2010.

[31] B. Leeman-Castillo, B. Beaty, S. Raghunath, J. Steiner, and S. Bull, "LUCHAR: using computer technology to battle heart disease among latinos," *American Journal of Public Health*, vol. 100, no. 2, pp. 272–275, 2010.

[32] D. W. Pekmezi, C. J. Neighbors, C. S. Lee et al., "A culturally adapted physical activity intervention for Latinas. A randomized controlled trial," *American Journal of Preventive Medicine*, vol. 37, no. 6, pp. 495–500, 2009.

[33] T. Hayashi, L.A. Chaput, D.A. Rocha, and M. Hernandez, "Lifestyle intervention, behavioral changes, and improvement in cardiovascular risk profiles in the California WISEWOMAN project," *Journal of Women's Health*, vol. 19, no. 6, pp. 1129–1138, 2010.

[34] C. L. Albright, L. Pruitt, C. Castro, A. Gonzalez, S. Woo, and A. C. King, "Modifying physical activity in a multiethnic sample of low-income women: one-year results from the IMPACT (Increasing Motivation for Physical ACTivity) project," *Annals of Behavioral Medicine*, vol. 30, no. 3, pp. 191–200, 2005.

[35] L. K. Staten, K. Y. Gregory-Mercado, J. Ranger-Moore et al., "Provider counseling, health education, and community health workers: the Arizona WISEWOMAN project," *Journal of Women's Health*, vol. 13, no. 5, pp. 547–556, 2004.

[36] M. Bopp, E. A. Fallon, and D. X. Marquez, "A faith-based physical activity intervention for Latinos: outcomes and lessons," *American Journal of Health Promotion*, vol. 25, no. 3, pp. 168–171, 2011.

[37] N. Mier, J. Tanguma, A. V. Millard, E. K. Villarreal, M. Alen, and M. G. Ory, "A pilot walking program for Mexican-American women living in colonias at the border," *American Journal of Health Promotion*, vol. 25, no. 3, pp. 172–175, 2011.

[38] K. Grass, P. Tello, and G. He, "Physical activity training for weight loss in Latinas: a controlled trial," *Journal of Health Education*, vol. 30, supplement 2, pp. S13–S17, 1999.

[39] W. S. C. Poston, C. K. Haddock, N. E. Olvera et al., "Evaluation of a culturally appropriate intervention to increase physical activity," *American Journal of Health Behavior*, vol. 25, no. 4, pp. 396–406, 2001.

[40] T. Yan, K. H. Wilber, R. Aguirre, and L. Trejo, "Do sedentary older adults benefit from community-based exercise? results from the active start program," *The Gerontologist*, vol. 49, no. 6, pp. 847–855, 2009.

[41] R. Keele-Smith, "Evaluation of individually tailored interventions on exercise adherence," *Western Journal of Nursing Research*, vol. 25, no. 6, pp. 623–640, 2003.

[42] A. H. Chen, J. F. Sallis, C. M. Castro et al., "A home-based behavioral intervention to promote walking in sedentary ethnic minority women: project WALK," *Women's Health*, vol. 4, no. 1, pp. 19–39, 1998.

[43] J. P. Elder, G. X. Ayala, and S. Harris, "Theories and intervention approaches to health-behavior change in primary care," *American Journal of Preventive Medicine*, vol. 17, no. 4, pp. 275–284, 1999.

[44] C. M. Castro, J. F. Sallis, S. A. Hickmann, R. E. Lee, and A. H. Chen, "A prospective study of psychosocial correlates of

physical activity for ethnic minority women," *Psychology and Health*, vol. 14, no. 2, pp. 277–293, 1999.

[45] P. Avila and M. F. Hovell, "Physical activity training for weight loss in Latinas: a controlled trial," *International Journal of Obesity*, vol. 18, no. 7, pp. 476–482, 1994.

[46] United States Department of Health and Human Services, *Overweight and Obesity*, United States Department of Health and Human Services, Washington, DC, USA, 2007.

[47] M. D. P. Rocha-Goldberg, L. Corsino, B. Batch et al., "Hypertension improvement project (HIP) Latino: results of a pilot study of lifestyle intervention for lowering blood pressure in Latino adults," *Ethnicity and Health*, vol. 15, no. 3, pp. 269–282, 2010.

[48] M. A. Farrell, T. Hayashi, R. K. Loo et al., "Clinic-based nutrition and lifestyle counseling for hispanic women delivered by community health workers: design of the california WISEWOMAN study," *Journal of Women's Health*, vol. 18, no. 5, pp. 733–739, 2009.

[49] J. E. Painter, C. P. C. Borba, M. Hynes, D. Mays, and K. Glanz, "The use of theory in health behavior research from 2000 to 2005: a systematic review," *Annals of Behavioral Medicine*, vol. 35, no. 3, pp. 358–362, 2008.

[50] K. Glanz, B. Rimer, and F. M. Lewis, *Health Behavior and Health Education: Theory, Research, and Practice*, Jossey-Bass, 3rd edition, 2002.

[51] J. O. Prochaska, C. Redding, and K. E. Evers, "The transtheoretical model and stages of change," in *Health Behavior and Health Education: Theory Research and Practice*, R. B. GlanzK and F. M. Lewis, Eds., Jossey Bass, San Francisco, Calif, USA, 3rd edition, 2002.

[52] M. Rose-Colley, J. M. Eddy, and E. D. Glover, "Relapse prevention: implications for health promotion professionals," *Health Values*, vol. 13, no. 5, pp. 8–13, 1989.

[53] A. Perez, J. Fleury, and C. Keller, "Review of intervention studies promoting physical activity in hispanic women," *Western Journal of Nursing Research*, vol. 32, no. 3, pp. 341–362, 2010.

[54] R. Collins, R. E. Lee, C. L. Albright, and A. C. King, "Ready to be physically active? The effects of a course preparing low-income multiethnic women to be more physically active," *Health Education and Behavior*, vol. 31, no. 1, pp. 47–64, 2004.

11

Contaminated Sites in Europe: Review of the Current Situation Based on Data Collected through a European Network

Panos Panagos, Marc Van Liedekerke, Yusuf Yigini, and Luca Montanarella

European Commission, Joint Research Centre, Institute for Environment and Sustainability, Via E. Fermi 2749, 21027 Ispra, Italy

Correspondence should be addressed to Panos Panagos; panos.panagos@jrc.ec.europa.eu

Academic Editor: Piedad Martin-Olmedo

Under the European Union (EU) Thematic Strategy for Soil Protection, the European Commission has identified soil contamination as a priority for the collection of policy-relevant soil data at European scale. In order to support EU soil management policies, soil-related indicators need to be developed which requires appropriate data collection and establishment of harmonized datasets for the EU Member States. In 2011-12, the European Soil Data Centre of the European Commission conducted a project to collect data on contaminated sites from national institutions in Europe using the European Environment Information and Observation Network for soil (EIONET-SOIL). This paper presents the results obtained from analysing the soil contaminated sites data submitted by participating countries. According to the received data, the number of estimated potential contaminated sites is more than 2.5 million and the identified contaminated sites around 342 thousand. Municipal and industrial wastes contribute most to soil contamination (38%), followed by the industrial/commercial sector (34%). Mineral oil and heavy metals are the main contaminants contributing around 60% to soil contamination. In terms of budget, the management of contaminated sites is estimated to cost around 6 billion Euros (€) annually.

1. Introduction

Soil contamination creates a significant risk to human health. For instance, heavy metals from industrial waste contaminate drinking water, soil, fodder, and food [1]. Also, the large volume of waste and the intense use of chemicals during past decades have resulted in numerous contaminated sites across Europe. Contaminated sites could pose significant environmental hazards for terrestrial and aquatic ecosystems as they are important sources of pollution which may result in ecotoxicological effects [2].

Emissions of hazardous substances from local sources could deteriorate soil and groundwater quality. Management of contaminated sites aims at assessing the adverse effects caused and taking measures to satisfy environmental standards according to current legal requirements. Additionally, the impact of soil contamination to health and more specifically the main epidemiological findings relevant to CS are briefly presented below.

The implication of soils to human health is direct such as ingestion, inhalation, skin contact, and dermal absorption. Some epidemiological examples include geohelminth infection and potentially harmful elements via soil ingestion, cancers caused by the inhalation of fibrous minerals, hookworm disease, and podoconiosis caused by skin contact with soils [3]. Elliott et al. (2001) [4] have found small excess risks of congenital anomalies and low and very low birth weights in populations living near landfill sites.

Soil contamination is mainly located close to waste landfills, industrial/commercial activities diffusing heavy metals, oil industry, military camps, and nuclear power plants. As European society has grown wealthier, it has created more and more rubbish. Each year in the EU, 3 billion tonnes of solid wastes are thrown away (some 90 million tonnes of them are hazardous). This amounts to about 6 tonnes of solid waste for every man, woman, and child (Eurostat, Environmental Data Centre on Waste [5]).

The main anthropogenic sources of heavy metals exist in various industrial point sources, for example, present and former mining activities, foundries, smelters, and diffuse sources such as piping, constituents of products, combustion of by products, and traffic related to industrial and human activities [6].

In the US, the army alone has estimated that over 1.2 million tons of soils have been contaminated with explosives, and the impact of explosives contamination in other countries in the world is of similar magnitude [7]. In recent years, growing concerns about the health and ecological threats posed by manmade chemicals have led to studies of the toxicology of explosives, which have identified toxic and mutagenic effects of the common military explosives and their transformation products [8]. Papp et al. (2002) [9] have studied the significant radioactive contamination of soil around a coal-fired thermal power plant.

Different contaminants have different effects on human health and the environment depending on their properties. The contaminant effect depends on its potential for dispersion, solubility in water or fat, bioavailability, carcinogenicity, and so forth. Chlorinated hydrocarbons (CHCs) are used mainly for the manufacturing of synthetic solvents and insecticides. They are environmental contaminants that bioaccumulate and hence are detected in human tissues. Epidemiological evidence suggests that the increased incidence of a variety of human cancers, such as lymphoma, leukemia, and liver and breast cancers, might be attributed to exposure to these agents [10].

Mineral oil large-scale use and various applications lead in many cases to environmental contamination [11]. Such contamination may be a consequence of petroleum transport, storage and refining, or accidents [12]. From a quantitative perspective, mineral oil is probably the largest contaminant in our body. That humans can tolerate this contaminant without health concerns has not been proven convincingly. The current Editorial of the European Journal of Lipid Science and Technology concludes that this proof either has to be provided or we have to take measures to reduce our exposure (from all sources, including cosmetics and pharmaceuticals) and the environmental contamination.

Polycyclic aromatic hydrocarbons (PAHs) are semi-volatile, chemically stable, and hydrophobic organic compounds which are ubiquitous in the environment and good markers of urban activities. PAHs are related with anthropogenic toxic element contamination [13].

Heavy metals have been used by humans for thousands of years. Although several adverse health effects of heavy metals have been known for a long time, exposure to heavy metals continues and is even increasing in some parts of the world, in particular in less developed countries, though emissions have declined in most developed countries over the last 100 years [14]. Any metal (or metalloid) species may be considered a "contaminant" if it occurs where it is unwanted, or in a form or concentration that causes a detrimental human or environmental effect. Metals/metalloids include lead (Pb), cadmium (Cd), mercury (Hg), arsenic (As), chromium (Cr), copper (Cu), selenium (Se), nickel (Ni), silver (Ag), and zinc (Zn). Other less common metallic contaminants include aluminium (Al), cesium (Cs), cobalt (Co), manganese (Mn), molybdenum (Mo), strontium (Sr), and uranium (U) [15].

According to WHO, priority should be given to the pollutants on the basis of toxicity, environmental persistence, mobility, and bioaccumulation [16]. Many of the heavy metals such as cadmium, arsenic, chromium, nickel, dioxins, and PAHs are considered to be carcinogenic, based on animal studies or studies of people exposed to high levels [17]. In addition to carcinogenicity, many of these substances can produce other toxic effects (depending on exposure level and duration) on the central nervous system, liver, kidneys, heart, lungs, skin, reproduction, and so forth.

The toxicity and fate of phenolic pollutants in the contaminated soils are associated with the oil-shale industry [18]. Phenol has been shown to cause liver and kidney damage, neurotoxic effects, and developmental toxicity in laboratory animals (Environment Agency, 2009).

The most common source of cyanide contamination is former gas work sites. However, cyanide contamination is also associated with electroplating factories, road salt storage facilities, and gold mining tailings [19]. Cyanide toxicity results from inhibition of cytochrome oxidase thereby limiting the absorption of oxygen at the cellular level. The central nervous system is a major target of acute cyanide toxicity, with a short period of stimulation evidenced by rapid breathing, followed by depression, convulsions, paralysis, and possibly death [20].

Benzene, toluene, ethylbenzene, and xylene (BTEX) are classified as hazardous air pollutants (HAPs) [21]. Exposure to HAPs can cause a variety of health problems such as cancerous illnesses, respiratory irritation, and central nervous system damage [22].

The objective of relevant EU policies is to achieve a quality of the environment where the levels of manmade contaminants on sites do not give rise to significant impacts or risks to human health and ecosystems. The most recent developments in soil policy at European level are the introduction of the thematic strategy for the protection of soils [23] and the proposed soil framework directive [24]. Soil contamination is recognised as one of the eight soil threats expressed in the thematic strategy and the proposed directive. As there was not a consensus for the establishment of the soil framework directive, legal requirements for the general protection of soil have not been agreed at EU level and only exist individually in most Member States. However, the integrated pollution and prevention control directive [25] requires that operations falling under its scope do not create new soil contamination. Other EU directives such as the water framework directive [26] and the waste directive [27], not aimed directly at soil protection, provide indirect controls on soil contamination [28]. Notwithstanding these controls, some significant new site contamination still occurs as a result of accidents [29] and illegal actions. While the creation of new contaminated sites is constrained by regulation, a very large number of sites exist with historical contamination that may present unacceptable risks and these sites require management. One example is the environmental disaster following flooding by red sludge in the Ajka region in Hungary [30]. However, the research and political arena regarding land contamination no longer consider only a few incidents that lead to severe soil contamination, but rather look at it as a wide spread environmental problem.

In 2001, the European Environment Agency (EEA) in cooperation with EEA affiliated countries started to develop a core set of policy relevant indicators, among which the indicator "Progress in the Management of Contaminated Sites" (CSI015) was the only one related to soil. Since then, data collections in relation to this indicator were launched four times by EEA [31], the last one in 2006, with contribution from member countries of the European Environment Information and Observation Network (EIONET) [32]. In the period 2011-2012, the European Soil Data Centre (ESDAC) [33] organized a similar campaign in order to update the CSI015. This indicator quantifies the progress in the management of local contamination, identifies sectors with major contribution to soil contamination, classifies the major contaminants, and finally addresses issues of budgets spent for remediation. The indicator is very important for policy makers as it tracks progress in the management of contaminated sites and the provision of public and private money for remediation. With this indicator, a number of activities causing soil pollution can be clearly identified across Europe. The indicator also supports the implementation of existing legislative and regulatory frameworks (integrated pollution prevention and control directive, landfill directive, water framework directive) as they should result in less new contamination of soil.

The present study presents an overall picture in Europe concerning contaminated sites and does not focus on individual countries. Instead, there are many other studies, such as the one of Ferguson (1999) [34], that present the inventories of contaminated sites for individual countries. The overall objective of this paper is to make an overview of the current situation of contaminated sites in Europe. Specifically, the study intends to

(i) focus on contaminated sites caused by industrial activities;

(ii) review the type of sources;

(iii) respond to the main policy questions addressed in the indicator CSI015.

2. Materials and Methods

The study makes an assessment of the data collected through EIONET and then focuses on the data related to contamination as a consequence of industrial activities.

2.1. EIONET-CSI Data. The contaminated sites data (denoted as EIONET-CSI from now on) were collected and managed by the European Soil Data Centre (ESDAC). The data were collected in 2011-2012 through the EIONET network which consists of representative organizations from 38 European countries for a number of environmental themes [35]. The appointed organisations for the theme "soil" are lead institutions in the soil domain at national level, and they provide official country data on specific requests related to soil by ESDAC.

The geographical coverage of EIONET includes 27 Member States of the European Union together with Iceland, Liechtenstein, Norway, Switzerland, Turkey, and the West Balkan cooperating countries: Albania, Bosnia, Herzegovina, Croatia, the former Yugoslav Republic of Macedonia, Montenegro, and Serbia as well as Kosovo under the UN Security Council Resolution 1244/99. Similar data on contaminated sites have been collected in 2001, 2002, 2003, and 2006. The data were collected through a standard questionnaire and then compiled in a centralized database. The questionnaire was designed such that received data could feed the compilation of the indicator, the CSI015 indicator. There is no legal obligation for the EIONET member countries to submit data, and their contribution is on a voluntary basis.

2.2. Terms and Definitions. In order to minimize the differences in interpretation by individual countries of certain terms used in the questionnaire, ESDAC provided the following definitions according to EEA [31].

(i) "Contaminated site" (CS) refers to a well-defined area where the presence of soil contamination has been confirmed and this presents a potential risk to humans, water, ecosystems, or other receptors. Risk management measures (e.g., remediation) may be needed depending on the severity of the risk of adverse impacts to receptors under the current or planned use of the site.

(ii) "Potentially contaminated site" (PCS) refers to sites where unacceptable soil contamination is suspected but not verified, and detailed investigations need to be carried out to verify whether there is unacceptable risk of adverse impacts on receptors.

(iii) "Management of contaminated sites" aims to access and, where necessary, reduce to an acceptable level the risk of adverse impacts on receptors (remediate). The progress in management of CS is traced in 4 management steps starting with preliminary study, continuing with preliminary investigation, followed by site investigation, and concluding with implementation of site remediation (reduction of risk).

There is an important definition in terminology which allows the readers of the article to distinguish between "estimated" and "identified" sites. The questionnaire asked the countries to provide estimations on how many CSs and PCSs may be situated in their territory. Data on estimated CS and PCS is based on studies or expert judgment. The questionnaire also asked for identified number of CS and PCS. In this case, the countries report data for which they actually posses available information about local soil properties and hydrology.

2.3. Other Datasets. For a more comprehensive assessment, a number of auxiliary official Eurostat datasets [35] were used such as the countries' populations, the surface area, the gross domestic product (GDP), and the number of enterprises in the industrial/services sectors. Those datasets are used for developing statistics with parameters that include the surveyed population, the surveyed area, the density of CS and

PCS, the contribution (%) of various industrial sectors to contamination, and the proportion of budget spent for management of CS.

2.4. Methodology. The study is based on the received data from the countries that participated in the survey, replying to the questionnaire available in the European Soil Portal [36]. The questionnaire has a user-friendly format as a Microsoft Excel file and contains 5 main sections: "management of contaminated sites," "contribution of polluting activities to local soil contamination," "environmental impacts," "expenditures," "remediation targets and technologies." Each section includes between 1 and 5 questions requesting the "user" to submit the data for each of the available options. The questionnaire was requesting numerical values (not classes or vague responses) which allowed making aggregations depending on the policy question that was to be addressed. Two example questions are the following: percentage (%) of sites, where risk reduction measures are completed; expenditures in million euro per capita per year. As a support, a guidelines document was available with detailed explanation for each of the questions and the possible options plus example responses based on previous data collection exercises.

Each country represented by its designated EIONET National Reference Centre for soil provided its best assessment based on available data. The data collection campaign was launched in October 2011 and ended in February 2012.

3. Results

Even if the questionnaire included other data and information, this paper mainly focuses on the local contamination analysis, the type of contamination (which sectors are contributing the most), the distribution of the main contaminants, and the budget spent for remediation. The management of CS will not be analysed in detail as each country follows a different approach concerning the management steps. The analysis is performed in the study area as a whole and not at country level. It should be noted that quite different interpretations of the abovementioned definitions have been applied by individual countries.

3.1. Extent of Local Contamination in Europe. Data on soil contamination per country is a necessary input in order to estimate the scale of soil contamination in Europe. The majority of the addressed countries (33 out of 38 countries), corresponding to 80% of the total population, have responded with data on the identified number of PCS and CS (Figure 1(a)). The missing five countries were Bosnia, Herzegovina, Poland, Portugal, Slovenia, and Turkey. According to Figure 1(a), around 1,170,000 PCSs have been identified in Europe till 2011. More than 10% of them or around 127,000 have been identified or confirmed as CSs. The ratio of remediated sites (RSs) to CSs is around 45% as more than 58,000 CSs have already been remediated (Figure 1(a)). The data gap for the 5 missing countries can be covered by employing the density of PCS (2.4 PCS/1,000 capita) and CS (2.62 CS/10,000 capita) (Table 1). Applying the average of 2.4 identified PCS per 1,000 capita for the 5 missing countries, the identified PCS for the whole Europe (38 countries) is estimated to be around 1,470,000. Applying the average of 2.62 identified CS per 10,000 capita (Table 1, column (a)) for the missing 5 countries, the identified CS can be raised to 160,000.

Apart from the identified PCS and CS, countries have been asked to provide their estimations for those 2 figures. A subset of 12 countries out of the 33 participating ones has provided estimations about the PCS (Table 1, column (b)). As a rule of thumb, the estimations are greater than the identified ones. According to their estimations, 740,000 PCSs may exist in their territory with a density of 4.2 PCS/1,000 capita. Those 12 countries have reported 520,000 PCSs which result that the ratio "*identification to estimation*" for PCS is around 70%. Two types of extrapolations can be performed in order to estimate the total number of PCS. In the first one, the average value of 4.2 PCS/1,000 capita is applied to the total population of the 38 countries, and the total number of estimated PCS is then around 2,553,000 (Figure 1(b)). In the second extrapolation method, the ratio "*identification to estimation*" for PCS (70%) is applied to the countries which were unable to provide estimations; then the approximate number of PCS can be estimated to be 2,087,000.

Another subset of 11 countries (not a sub group of the previous 12) covering 10% of total population has provided estimations about CS. They estimated more than 32,000 CSs with a density of 5.7 CS/10,000 capita (Table 1, column (c)). Those 11 countries have reported 10,036 identified CSs which result that the ratio "*identification to estimation*" for CS is 30.7%. The first method of extrapolation is to apply the average density to the rest of the population (90%), where data does not exist. According to this estimation, the number of CS in Europe is estimated to be around 342,000 which accounts for 14% of the total estimated PCS (Figure 1(b)). In the second extrapolation method, the ratio "*identification to estimation*" for CS (30.7%) is applied to the whole population, and the estimated number of CS becomes more than 516,000. When comparing to the last survey of 2006, the estimated number of PCS was around 3 million, and the estimated number of CS was around 250,000.

The high variability of the data reported can be seen in Figure 2. The huge differences in the density rates represent the situation of PCS per country and how countries interpret the term of "potential contamination." Interpreting the metadata that come with the received data, PCSs are understood in a different way. For instance, Luxemburg, Belgium, Netherlands, and France include potentially polluting activities in their PCS figures, and this is the reason for high density of PCS in those countries (Figure 2). Other countries such as Austria, Hungary, and Norway include in their PCS figures only the sites where there is an evidence of potential contamination. Another factor contributing to this high variability is the granularity of a site. Some countries report sites which are important at national level, while others include also small sites such as storage tanks.

3.2. Sectors Contributing Most to Soil Contamination. Soil contamination is the result of various sectors and activities. The countries were asked to allocate a percentage of contribution of each sector to local soil contamination based on

Table 1: Estimated and identified PCS and CS.

	Identified PCS and CS (a)	Estimated PCS (b)	Estimated CS (c)	Total (d)
Countries	33	12	11	38
Surveyed population	487,152,449	177,412,672	57,568,148	612,117,243
Surveyed surface area (km^2)	4,460,305	1,552,984	833,188	5,772,075
Surveyed of total population	79.6%	29.0%	9.4%	
Surveyed of total area	77.3%	26.9%	14.4%	
PCS	1,169,649	739,968		2,553,000*
PCS/1000 capita	2.4	4.2		
CS	127,475		32,601	342,000*
CS/10,000 capita	2.62		5.7	
Remediated sites (RSs)	58,336			
RS/10,000 capita	1.20			

*Based on extrapolated data.

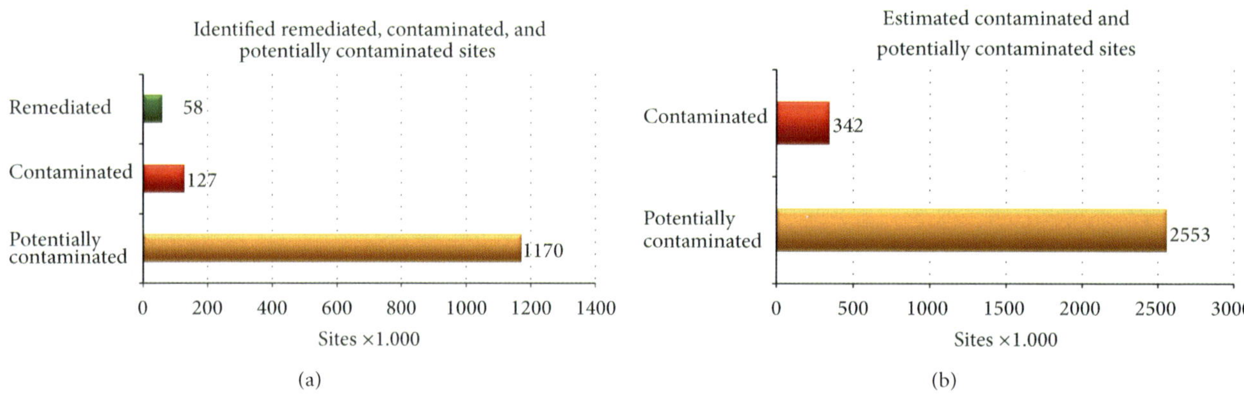

Figure 1: (a) Number of identified remediated (RS), potentially (PCS), and contaminated Sites (CS) reported by 33 countries. (b) Number of estimated potentially (PCS) and contaminated sites (CS) extrapolated to 38 countries.

the occurrence of incidents. The following seven categories of activities were proposed:

(i) waste disposal (municipal waste disposal and industrial waste disposal).

(ii) industrial and commercial activities (mining, oil extraction and production, and power plants).

(iii) military (military sites and war affected zones).

(iv) storages (oil storage, obsolete chemicals storage, and other storages).

(v) transport spills on land (oil spill sites and other hazardous substance spills sites).

(vi) nuclear.

(vii) other sources.

Responses related to contributing sectors were received from 22 countries which correspond to circa 53% of the total study population. Waste disposal and treatment contribute to more than 37% of soil contamination. Inside this category, municipal waste and industrial waste contribute to similar shares. The industrial and commercial activities contribute to 33.3% share, followed by storage (10.5%), while of the rest have a contribution of 19.1%. Nuclear operations contribute only 0.1%, but contamination from major nuclear players (e.g., scores from nuclear power stations) was not taken into account by some countries. The data cannot be compared to 2006 survey as the sample of countries that responded is dissimilar.

A special focus is given to the industrial and commercial sectors causing soil contamination. The countries were asked to assign percentages in each specific industrial sector which contributes to soil contamination. The responses of 17 countries covering 44% of the total study population suggested that the production sector contributes to around 60% of soil contamination, while the service sector has a share of 33% and the mining sector contributes to around 7% (Figure 3).

A closer look at the production sector reveals that the textiles, leather, wood, and paper industries are of minor importance for local soil contamination (circa 5%), while metal industries are most frequently reported to be important sources of contamination (13%) followed by chemical industry (8%), oil industry (7%), and energy production (7%) that sum up the 35% of the production sector, while all of the rest

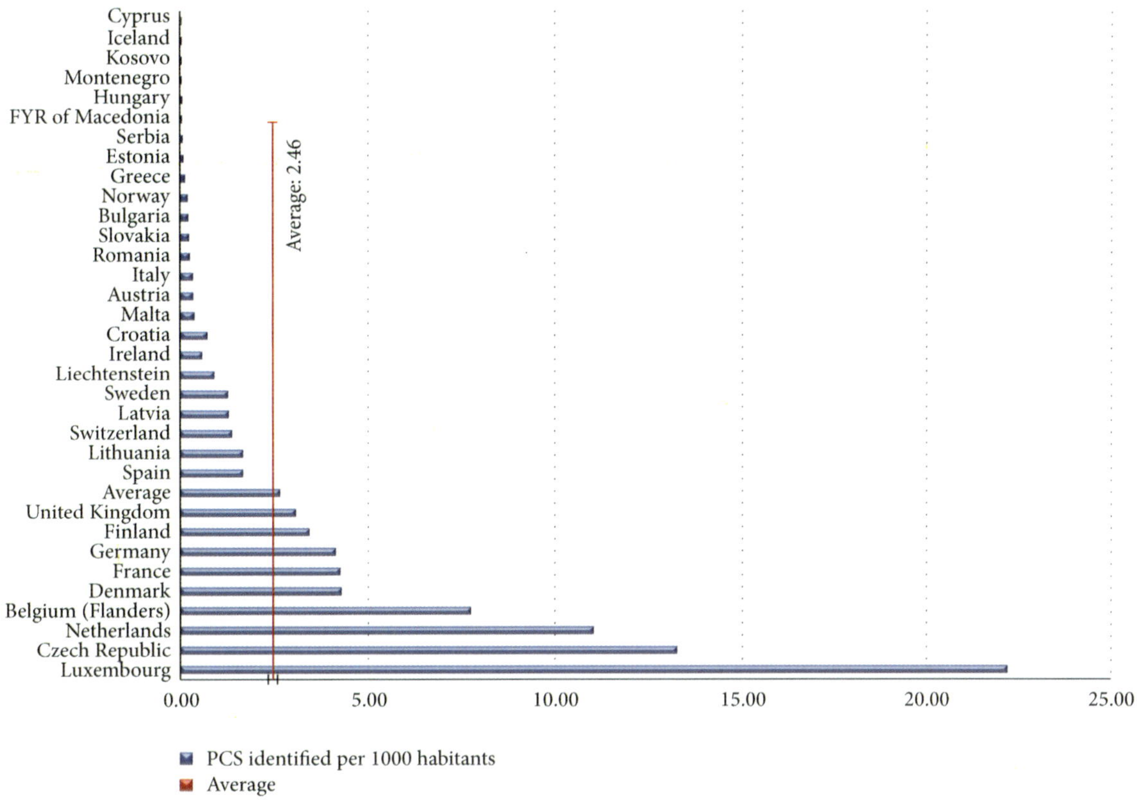

FIGURE 2: Density (identified PCS/1,000 capita) in 33 countries.

(25%) are distributed in 6 categories. For the service sector, gasoline stations are the most frequently reported sources of contamination (15%) followed by the car service stations (around 6%).

The Eurostat data on sectoral breakdown of manufacturing (NACE [37]) sums up the total number of enterprises in the EU to 2.041 million. The Eurostat industrial sectors do not correspond one-to-one with the industrial production sectors considered in the EIONET-CSI questionnaire (Table 2, column (a)). Some grouping of the Eurostat sectors (plus sign in column (c)) has taken place to make the correspondence. Note that the Eurostat data for the mining sector was embedded in the Eurostat category "other manufacturing." From the values in columns d and b, a new value (column (e)) is computed that expresses how many enterprises of an industrial sector contribute to 1 percent of the local contamination coming from that sector. The smaller the number, the more one site contributes to industrial contamination. The resulting figures show for instance that mining sites are individually heavier polluters compared to other sectors. Instead, the electronic industry enterprises pollute less compared to the shown sectors (Table 2).

3.3. Main Contaminants. The countries were asked to allocate a percentage for the proposed contaminant categories based on the occurrence of soil contamination. Distinctions were made between contaminants affecting the solid matrix (soil, sludge, and sediments) and the liquid matrix (groundwater, surface waters, and leachate). The following eight categories of contaminants were proposed both for solid and liquid matrices:

(i) chlorinated hydrocarbons (CHCs).

(ii) mineral oil.

(iii) polycyclic aromatic hydrocarbons (PAHs).

(iv) heavy metals.

(v) phenols.

(vi) cyanides.

(vii) aromatic hydrocarbons (BTEX: benzene, toluene, ethyl benzene, and xylene).

(viii) others.

The responses were received from 16 countries which correspond to about 40% of the total study population. The analysis based on these responses is of key importance for research and development, the remediation market, and related industries. For instance, if a specific compound is known to be a major soil contaminant, it may be worthwhile to develop new detection methods (i.e., in situ detection) and more efficient remediation techniques.

The distribution of the contaminants affecting soil is similar to the one of groundwater. The main contaminant categories are heavy metals and mineral oil contributing jointly to around 60% in soil contamination and 53% of the groundwater contamination (Figure 4). On the contrary, the phenols

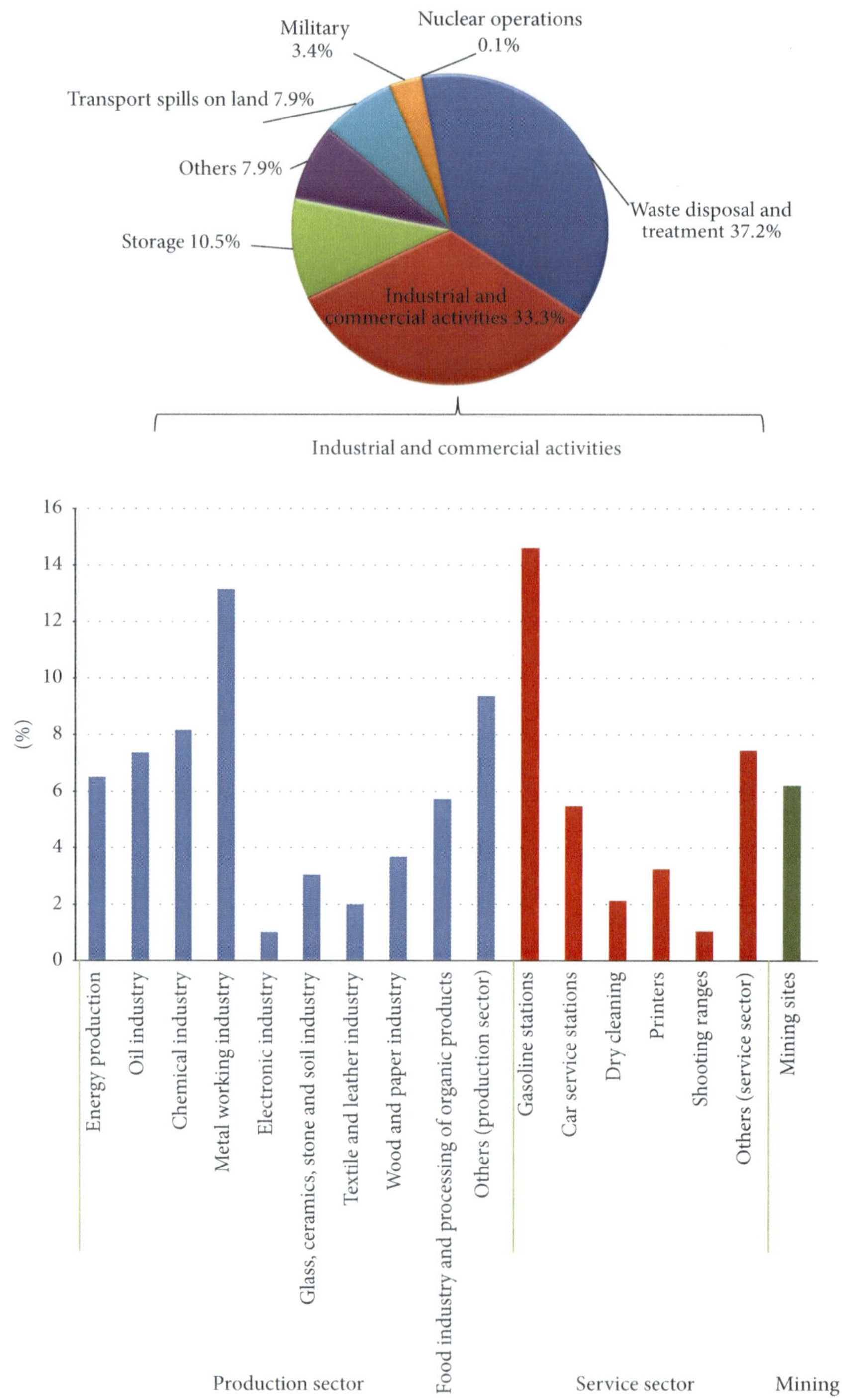

FIGURE 3: Distribution of sectors contributing to soil contamination in Europe with special focus to industrial/commercial activities.

and cyanides have an insignificant contribution to total contamination. The remaining four categories (BTEX, CHC, PAH, and others) have similar contributions to soil contamination varying between 8 and 11% and summing up to 40%. In the groundwater contamination, their contribution is around 45% ranging from 6% for PAH to 15% for BTEX. The current distribution is similar to the one proposed after the analysis of the 2006 surveyed results.

3.4. Budget Allocated. The cost of managing the CS is an important element taken into account by policy makers. The questionnaire included parts to investigate annual estimation of expenditures, share of private/public money, and share of total expenditure. This is a very important aspect as one of the most criticised issues in the proposed European soil framework directive [24] was the required estimate of annual cost for management of CS. According to the impact

TABLE 2: Comparison of sectoral contribution to industrial contamination against the total number of enterprises.

Industrial/service sector	Sector contribution to industrial contamination (production)	Manufacturing sector	Number of enterprises (1,000)	Number of enterprises (1,000) contributing to 1% of industrial contamination
(a)	(b)	(c)	(d)	(e)
Chemical industry	8.2%	Chemicals plus rubber and plastic products	97.2	11.9
Metal working industry	13.1%	Basic metals plus fabricated metal products	381.2	29.1
Textile and leather industry	2.0%	Textiles plus wearing apparel plus leather	225.4	112.7
Wood and paper industry	3.7%	Wood and paper	191.8	51.8
Food industry and processing of organic products	5.7%	Food products plus beverages	273.8	48.0
Electronic industry	1.0%	Computer, electronic, plus electrical equip.	94.1	94.1
Mining sites	6.2%	Mining	18.2	2.9
Total	39.9%	Total	1281.7	

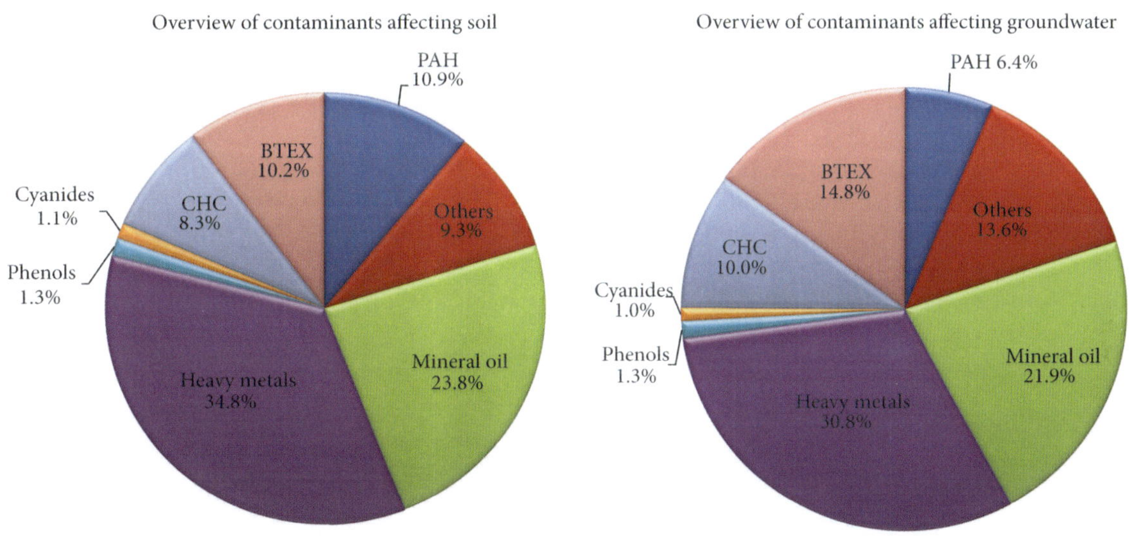

FIGURE 4: Distribution of contaminants affecting soil and groundwater in Europe.

assessment of the proposed directive, there was a wide-ranging estimate from 2.4 to 17.3 billion Euros.

According to the responses of 11 countries covering 23% of the total population (139 million out of the 612 million inhabitants for the total area), 1,483.2 million euros (€) were spent annually for the management of CS in these countries. In absolute terms, this is around 10.7€ per capita or 0.041% of the gross domestic product (GDP) for the 11 countries. The reported data show a small decrease in expenditure for management of CS compared to 2006 (12€ per capita).

If this sample of 11 countries is considered representative for the whole Europe, then the management of contaminated sites can be estimated to be 6,526 million euros (€) per year. Compared to the impact assessment of the proposed soil framework directive, this amount of money is probably a more precise estimate of the cost of the management of all identified CSs (including remediation).

Regarding the share of private/public money, 42% of the total expenditure comes from public budgets while the 58% from private investments. Another interesting aspect of the study is the share in the total expenditures for the management of CS for the different management steps. The vast majority (80.6%) is spent for the remediation measures while 15.1% is spent in site investigation and only 4.3% in after care measures and redevelopment of the sites. When considering the budget spent on remediation and the number or remediated sites (RSs) in the 11 reported countries, it is calculated that the average amount spent per RS annually is around 37.1 thousand euros (€) in a range varying from 7.5 thousand € to 232 thousand € annually. As the remediation of sites has a duration of more than 1 year, the majority (40%) of the reported remediation projects fall in the range 50,000 to 500,000€, while a considerable 26.5% of the reported cases fall in the range between 5,000 and 50,000€.

4. Discussion and Conclusions

In terms of estimations, around 1,170,000 PCSs have been identified which are circa 45% of the total estimated PCSs. Also, around 127,000 CSs have been already identified which are circa 27% of the total estimated 342,000 CSs. Moreover, around 46% of the total identified CSs have been remediated (58,300 RSs). The identified figures for CS, PCSs and RS are based on reported data from 33 countries, while the estimated CSs and PCSs have been extrapolated based on data from a limited sample (11 or 12 countries).

Notwithstanding the positive outcomes of the EIONET-CSI data collection, it could be noted that the data submitted were not homogeneous since there are differences in the way that countries interpret the terms of contaminated sites. As shown in Figure 2, there is a high variability between the data submitted by countries. This variability is explained by the large uncertainty both in terms of methodology and data. Some countries run their own CS management system which may not fit perfectly to the definition of the CSI015 indicator, and this contributes to methodology uncertainty. Moreover, the reported data are usually based on expert judgement which includes a high degree of uncertainly. The countries may interpret the data specifications in different ways, and this increases the heterogeneity in the data reported. The reported data on CSI015 indicator are based on the exceed of limits in concentrations of hazardous chemicals. However, common limits are unlikely to be established at the European level since they may be strongly influenced by local soil and geological properties.

An adequate response to the high data variability could be to make a pan-European training event with the participation of competent national EIONET authorities, with the objective to apply the same terminology in all countries in subsequent data collections. The heterogeneity of responses can also be decreased if the provided documentation is taken into account.

In general, there are difficulties in getting the data on soil contamination, but improvement in data availability and data quality over the years can be observed. At this moment, the resulting dataset is the best "picture" that can be achieved based on national data. The EIONET-CSI data collection has taken place 5 years after the previous one of 2006. This 5-year period between data collections seems to be more appropriate than the 2-year period applied in the past, since the data on CS are not changing considerably in such a relative short time.

The direct and indirect costs to a country for dealing with the problem of CS depend on the amount and characteristics of CS in its territory. Generally, the presence of CS can affect company profits, business confidence, and attractiveness to investors. It may also affect aspects of public health and ecosystem protection. The remediation cost of CS, even if only a very little percentage of GDP, seems to be a major issue, and investments to improve the land quality through remediation are not readily made. Countries should weigh the costs of dealing with local land contamination against benefits to public health, improvement of the environment (e.g., water quality), land regeneration, and sustainable use of soil.

Restrictions set by privacy law in Europe are a major obstacle to identification and management of land contamination. Status and data on private land are not easily accessible to public authorities as this may have some implications for the land owner. However, the situation of his land is affecting public health, water quality, and ecosystem services. In cases of proven soil contamination, public authorities could be allowed for intervention or even raise public awareness. The conflicts between public interest and privacy regarding land and in general environmental problems should be resolved at a legal basis.

The EIONET-CSI dataset will be supplemented with heavy metals data at European level. In 2009, 22,000 soil samples were taken in European Union countries during a soil survey named LUCAS [38]. Those soil samples have been analysed for some of the most important soil attributes such as soil organic carbon, and the results assist to estimate better the overall situation in Europe [39]. Currently, these soil samples are analysed for heavy metals, and the expected output results will facilitate better assessment of soil contamination in European Union. The LUCAS heavy metals dataset will face the issue of privacy which can overcome with the application of digital soil mapping for the development of interpolated maps. The combination of LUCAS heavy metals with EIONET-CSI will be an important step in assessing soil contamination in Europe.

The proposed datasets and the current study can be considered by public health professionals for epidemiological assessments. The study of human exposure pathways is a key issue on contaminated sites, and certainly the integration of EIONET-CSI datasets with epidemiological data would be a very important step forward in this direction. Moreover, as the majority of food is growing in soil, biomonitoring and other research should investigate the pathways and routes from producers to consumers.

Conflict of Interests

The authors confirm and sign that there is no conflict of interests with networks, organisations, and data centres referred in the paper. In specific, ESDAC is the European Soil Data Centre and is an integral part of the Joint Research Centre of the European Commission, to which the authors are affiliated. Moreover, the ESDAC is operated by the authors themselves, so there cannot be any conflict of interests whatsoever. Also, the authors have published the paper relevant to ESDAC [33]. European Environment Information and Observation Network for soil (EIONET-SOIL) is the network of soil organizations officially designated by the European countries that deliver, on request by ESDAC and on a voluntary basis, data on soil related topics, in this case, contaminated sites. Therefore, there cannot be any conflict of interests. Note that the contributing organizations of the EIONET-SOIL are explicitly acknowledged in the paper. Also, the authors have published a paper relevant to another data collection (soil organic carbon) in the past [32].

Acknowledgments

The authors would like to acknowledge the countries (persons and organizations) that contributed to data in the EIONET study: Albania (Loreta Sulovari of the Agency of Environment and Forestry; Erinda Misho of AEF); Austria (Stefan Weihs, Dietmar Mueller, and Sabine Rabl-Berger of the Umweltbundesamt GmbH Environment Agency Austria; Franz Buchebnerof the Bundesministerium für Land-und Forstwirtschaft, Umwelt und Wasserwirtschaft; Sebastian Holub of the Kommunalkredit Public Consulting GmbH); Belgium (Flanders) (Marijke Cardon and Els Gommeren of OVAM); Bosnia and Herzegovina (Hamid Custovic of the University of Sarajevo, Faculty of Agriculture and Food Sciences); Croatia (Andreja Steinberger and Željko Crnojević of the Croatian Environment Agency (CEA)); Cyprus (Chrystalla Stylianou and Neoclis Antoniou of the Department of Environment; Andreas Zissimos of the Geological Survey Department); Estonia (Peep Siim of the Ministry of Environment Water Department Project Bureau); Finland (Teija Haavisto of the Finnish Environment Institute); France (Véronique Antoni, Delphine Maurice, Farid Bouagal, Philippe Bodenez, and Claudine CHOQUET of the French Ministry in charge of ecology; Jean-François Brunet of BRGM; Antonio Bispo of ADEME); Germany (Joerg Frauenstein of the Umweltbundesamt); Hungary (Gabor Hasznos of the Ministry for Rural Development); Ireland (David Smith of the Environmental Protection Agency); Italy (Laura D'Aprile of ISPRA); Kosovo (Republic of Kosova) (Gani Berisha of the Ministry of Environment and Spatial Planning, Soil Protection Sector; Shkumbin Shala of the Hydrometeorological Institute, Kosova's Environmental Protection Agency); Lithuania (Virgilija Gregorauskiene of the Lithuanian Geological Survey); Former Yugoslav Republic of Macedonia (Margareta Cvetkovska of the Macedonian Environmental Information Center, Ministry of Environment and Physical Planning); Malta (Christina Mallia of the Environmental Permitting and Industry Unit of the Malta Environment and Planning Authority); Montenegro (Vesna Novakovic of the Environmental Protection Agency of Montenegro); Netherlands (Versluijs C. W. and Bogte J. J. of the RIVM); Norway (Per Erik Johansen of the Klima- og forurensningsdirektoratet); Poland (Joanna Czajka of the Chief Inspectorate for Environmental Protection); Slovakia (Katarina Paluchová of the Slovak Environmental Agency; Vlasta Jánová of the Ministry of the Environment of the Slovak Republic); Serbia (Dragana Vidojevic of the Ministry of Environment, Mining, and Spatial Planning, Environmental Protection Agency); Spain (Begoña Fabrellas of the Ministerio de Agricultura, Alimentación y Medio Ambiente); Switzerland (Christoph Reusser of the Federal Office for the Environment (FOEN)); United Kingdom (Mark Kibblewhite and Caroline Keay of Cranfield University). Special thanks should be expressed to Gondula Prokop (Environment Agency Austria) who conducted the operation of data collection and analysis on behalf of ESDAC.

References

[1] V. Rajaganapathy, F. Xavier, D. Sreekumar, and P. K. Mandal, "Heavy metal contamination in soil, water and fodder and their presence in livestock and products: a review," *Journal of Environmental Science and Technology*, vol. 4, no. 3, pp. 234–249, 2011.

[2] K. Fent, "Ecotoxicological effects at contaminated sites," *Toxicology*, vol. 205, no. 3, pp. 223–240, 2004.

[3] P. W. Abrahams, "Soils: their implications to human health," *Science of the Total Environment*, vol. 291, no. 1–3, pp. 1–32, 2002.

[4] P. Elliott, D. Briggs, S. Morris et al., "Risk of adverse birth outcomes in populations living near landfill sites," *British Medical Journal*, vol. 323, no. 7309, pp. 363–368, 2001.

[5] Eurostat, "Environmental Data Centre on waste," http://epp.eurostat.ec.europa.eu/portal/page/portal/waste/introduction.

[6] N. Guvenç, O. Alagha, and G. Tuncel, "Investigation of soil multi-element composition in Antalya, Turkey," *Environment International*, vol. 29, no. 5, pp. 631–640, 2003.

[7] T. A. Lewis, D. A. Newcombe, and R. L. Crawford, "Bioremediation of soils contaminated with explosives," *Journal of Environmental Management*, vol. 70, no. 4, pp. 291–307, 2004.

[8] J. S. Fuchs, M. L. Oneto, N. B. Casabé et al., "Ecotoxicological characterization of a disposal lagoon from a munition plant," *Bulletin of Environmental Contamination and Toxicology*, vol. 67, no. 5, pp. 696–703, 2001.

[9] Z. Papp, Z. Dezso, and S. Daróczy, "Significant radioactive contamination of soil around a coal-fired thermal power plant," *Journal of Environmental Radioactivity*, vol. 59, no. 2, pp. 191–205, 2002.

[10] A. F. Badawi, E. L. Cavalieri, and E. G. Rogan, "Effect of chlorinated hydrocarbons on expression of cytochrome P450 1A1, 1A2 and 1B1 and 2- and 4-hydroxylation of 17β-estradiol in female Sprague-Dawley rats," *Carcinogenesis*, vol. 21, no. 8, pp. 1593–1599, 2000.

[11] J. L. R. Gallego, J. Loredo, J. F. Llamas, F. Vázquez, and J. Sánchez, "Bioremediation of diesel-contaminated soils: evaluation of potential in situ techniques by study of bacterial degradation," *Biodegradation*, vol. 12, no. 5, pp. 325–335, 2001.

[12] P. Juteau, J.-G. Bisaillon, F. Lépine, V. Ratheau, R. Beaudet, and R. Villemur, "Improving the biotreatment of hydrocarbons-contaminated soils by addition of activated sludge taken from the wastewater treatment facilities of an oil refinery," *Biodegradation*, vol. 14, no. 1, pp. 31–40, 2003.

[13] X. L. Zhang, S. Tao, W. X. Liu, Y. Yang, Q. Zuo, and S. Z. Liu, "Source diagnostics of polycyclic aromatic hydrocarbons based on species ratios: a multimedia approach," *Environmental Science and Technology*, vol. 39, no. 23, pp. 9109–9114, 2005.

[14] L. Järup, "Hazards of heavy metal contamination," *British Medical Bulletin*, vol. 68, pp. 167–182, 2003.

[15] T. McIntyre, "Phytoremediation of heavy metals from soils," *Advances in Biochemical Engineering/Biotechnology*, vol. 78, pp. 97–123, 2003.

[16] WHO European Centre for Environment and Health, *Methods of Assessing Risk to Health from Exposure to Hazards Released from Waste Landfills*, WHO Regional Office for Europe, Lodz, Poland, 2000.

[17] B. L. Johnson, "Hazardous waste: human health effects," *Toxicology and Industrial Health*, vol. 13, no. 2-3, pp. 121–143, 1997.

[18] A. Kahru, A. Maloverjan, H. Sillak, and L. Põllumaa, "The toxicity and fate of phenolic pollutants in the contaminated soils associated with the oil-shale industry," *Environmental science and pollution research international*, vol. 1, pp. 27–33, 2002.

[19] P. Kjeldsen, "Behaviour of cyanides in soil and groundwater: a review," *Water, Air, and Soil Pollution*, vol. 115, no. 1–4, pp. 279–307, 1999.

[20] T. A. Gossel, *Principles of Clinical Toxicology*, Raven Press , New York, Ny, USA, 1984.

[21] US EPA, "National emissions standards for hazardous air pollutants: municipal solid waste landfills," Tech. Rep. 68/FR/2227, U.S. Environmental Protection Agency (US EPA), Office of Air Quality Planning and Standards, Washington, DC, USA, 2003.

[22] E. Durmusoglu, F. Taspinar, and A. Karademir, "Health risk assessment of BTEX emissions in the landfill environment," *Journal of Hazardous Materials*, vol. 176, no. 1–3, pp. 870–877, 2010.

[23] EC, "Communication from the Commission to the Council, the European Parliament, the European Economic and Social Committee of the Regions, Thematic Strategy for Soil Protection," COM(2006) 231 final, 2006.

[24] EC, "Proposal for a Directive of the European Parliament and of the Council establishing a framework for the protection of soil and amending Directive 2004/35/EC," Brussels, COM (2006) 232 final, 2006.

[25] IPPC, "Directive 2008/1/EC of the European Parliament and of the Council of 15 January 2008 concerning integrated pollution prevention and control," http://europa.eu/legislation_summaries/environment/waste_management/l28045_en.htm, 2008.

[26] WFD, *Directive 2000/60/EC of the European Parliament and of the Council Establishing a framework for the Community Action in the Field of Water Policy*, 2000.

[27] Waste, "Waste Framework Directive, or Directive 2008/98/EC of the European Parliament and of the Council of 19 November 2008 on waste," http://eur-lex.europa.eu/LexUriServ/LexUriServ.do?uri=CELEX:32008L0098:EN:NOT, 2008.

[28] K. Hinsby, M. T. Condesso de Melo, and M. Dahl, "European case studies supporting the derivation of natural background levels and groundwater threshold values for the protection of dependent ecosystems and human health," *Science of the Total Environment*, vol. 401, no. 1–3, pp. 1–20, 2008.

[29] J. Koarashi, M. Atarashi-Andoh, T. Matsunaga, T. Sato, S. Nagao, and H. Nagai, "Factors affecting vertical distribution of Fukushima accident-derived radiocesium in soil under different land-use conditions," *Science of the Total Environment*, vol. 431, pp. 392–401, 2012.

[30] D. Czövek, Z. Novák, C. Somlai et al., "Respiratory consequences of red sludge dust inhalation in rats," *Toxicology Letters*, vol. 209, no. 2, pp. 113–120, 2012.

[31] European Environment Agency (EEA), http://www.eea.europa.eu/data-and-maps/indicators/progress-in-management-of-contaminated-sites/progress-in-management-of-contaminated, 2011.

[32] P. Panagos, R. Hiederer, M. Van Liedekerke, and F. Bampa, "Estimating soil organic carbon in Europe based on data collected through an European network," *Ecological Indicators*, vol. 24, pp. 439–450, 2013.

[33] P. Panagos, M. Van Liedekerke, A. Jones, and L. Montanarella, "European Soil Data Centre: response to European policy support and public data requirements," *Land Use Policy*, vol. 29, no. 2, pp. 329–338, 2012.

[34] C. C. Ferguson, "Assessing risks from contaminated sites: policy and practice in 16 European Countries," *Land Contamination and Reclamation*, vol. 7, no. 2, pp. 87–108, 1999.

[35] Eurostat, "Directorate-General of the European Commission," http://epp.eurostat.ec.europa.eu/portal/page/portal/eurostat/home, 2013.

[36] Eusoils, "Data Collection on Contaminated Sites 2011," http://eusoils.jrc.ec.europa.eu/library/data/eionet/2011_Contaminated_Sites.htm, 2012.

[37] NACE Section, "Manufacturing statistics—NACE ver.2," http://epp.eurostat.ec.europa.eu/statistics_explained/index.php/Manufacturing_statistics_-_NACE_Rev._2, 2012.

[38] G. Toth, A. Jones, and L. Montanarella, "The LUCAS topsoil database and derived information on the regional variability of cropland topsoil properties in the European Union," *Environmental Monitoring and Assessment*, 2013.

[39] P. Panagos, C. Ballabio, Y. Yigini, and M. B. Dunbar, "Estimating the soil organic carbon content for European NUTS2 regions based on LUCAS data collection," *Science of the Total Environment*, vol. 442, pp. 235–246, 2013.

12

Active Commuting among K-12 Educators: A Study Examining Walking and Biking to Work

Melissa Bopp,[1] Tanis J. Hastmann,[2] and Alyssa N. Norton[1]

[1] *Department of Kinesiology, The Pennsylvania State University, University Park, PA 16802, USA*
[2] *Department of Physical Education, Exercise Science and Wellness, the University of North Dakota, Grand Forks, ND 58202, USA*

Correspondence should be addressed to Melissa Bopp; mjb73@psu.edu

Academic Editor: Ike S. Okosun

Background. Walking and biking to work, active commuting (AC) is associated with many health benefits, though rates of AC remain low in the US. K-12 educators represent a significant portion of the workforce, and employee health and associated costs may have significant economic impact. Therefore, the purpose of this study was to examine the current rates of AC and factors associated with AC among K-12 educators. *Methods.* A volunteer sample of K-12 educators ($n = 437$) was recruited to participate in an online survey. Participants responded about AC patterns and social ecological influences on AC (individual, interpersonal, institutional, community, and environmental factors). t-tests and ANOVAs examined trends in AC, and Pearson correlations examined the relationship between AC and dependent variables. Multiple regression analysis determined the relative influence of individual, interpersonal, institutional, community, and environmental levels on AC. *Results.* Participants actively commuted 0.51 ± 1.93 times/week. There were several individual, interpersonal, institutional, community, and environmental factors significantly related to AC. The full model explained 60.8% of the variance in AC behavior. *Conclusions.* This study provides insight on the factors that determine K-12 educators mode of commute and provide some insight for employee wellness among this population.

1. Background

Regular physical activity can improve the health and overall well-being of Americans of all ages [1]. However, current estimates indicate that the majority of adults aged 18–64 do not meet the recommended physical activity requirements of 150 minutes each week [2]. Physical activity provides numerous health benefits and reduces the risk for chronic disease morbidity and mortality. Additionally, there are a number of noted economic implications for low rates of physical inactivity [1, 3–6].

The benefits of overall physical activity are well documented. In addition to the obvious health benefits, engaging in physical activity is associated with less employee turnover [7], happier employees [8], reduced absenteeism [9], and reduced job stress [10]. Most importantly, physical activity is associated with reduced illness-related absenteeism [11]. Similarly, active transportation to and from school or a workplace, known as active commuting (AC), also provides numerous health benefits [12], including a reduced risk of obesity [13], cardiovascular disease [14], and all-cause mortality [15]. Despite these well-documented benefits, rates of AC remain low in the United States. Data from the National Health Interview Survey have shown that only 28% of individuals report walking anywhere as a mode of transportation [16], while Hu and Reuscher [17] have found that only 2.8% of individuals report walking to work. These rates remain quite low compared with Europe and Australia [18]. Comprehensively understanding the factors that influence AC will allow for targeting and tailored interventions to increase participation in this behavior.

Social ecological frameworks [19, 20] offer a comprehensive approach to understanding and changing physical activity behavior. Several studies have highlighted individual level influences on AC, including beliefs and attitudes [21–23], habit strength [24], and demographics [25]. Other research has examined social support [26] or the social environment [23] as possible influences on AC. Kaczynski and colleagues

[26] noted that the presence of physical support, measured by the availability of bike parking, storage policies, showers, or lockers at the workplace was associated with a threefold increase in actively commuting to work. Similar to other studies examining how the built and natural environment can influence physical activity participation [19, 27–29], environmental influences on walking and biking to work are also well documented [22, 23, 25, 30, 31].

Across the United States, there are more than 130,000 K-12 schools, serving more than 55 million children [32]. To serve these children, there are more than 3.2 million teachers in the US, with many hundreds of thousands of more support staff and administrators. In 2007-2008, it was estimated that of the $506.8 billion spent in public schools in the US, $303.2 billion were related to instruction and personnel, making employees a valuable resource in schools across the country. State and local governments shoulder the bulk of the financial burden with public education [32], and current economic conditions have resulted in some significant challenges in meeting the needs of the community with declining resources. One way to potentially reduce the enormous costs associated with educators and personnel would be to improve their health. As previously discussed, employees who are active have greater physical and mental health and less illness-related absenteeism compared to their lesser active counterparts [9, 11]. This information is corroborated by van Amelsvoort and colleagues, who showed that workers who engaged in leisure time physical activity twice or more per week reported significantly less sick absence compared to inactive workers [33]. One way to reduce illness-related absenteeism may be to increase employee active commuting. Therein the health and well-being of educators present some significant community level concern.

Although there has been evidence that AC has positive health effects on adults, there has not been much research on K-12 educators actively commuting to their workplace. Therefore, the purpose of this study was twofold: first, to analyze the patterns of AC and factors associated with teachers' AC and second, to extrapolate how these factors could improve the likelihood of teachers walking or riding their bike to work.

2. Methods

This cross-sectional survey was delivered online using the Qualtrics software program (Provo, UT, USA) from June–December 2011. This study was approved by the Institutional Review Board at Pennsylvania State University.

2.1. Participants. Individuals over the age of 18 years, employed full- or part-time outside of the home and physically able to walk or bike were eligible to take part in the survey. Recruitment took place primarily in the mid-Atlantic region of the US (PA, OH, WV, MD, NJ, and DE). Further details of the survey and non-K-12 educators are available elsewhere [34]. Websites of K-12 school districts in medium-large cities were examined for employee email addresses, and individuals were contacted directly via email. The email invitation description invited people to take part in a "commuting survey" in order to limit a volunteer bias of people who may have been more interested in active commuting methods. Survey invitations were emailed to $n =$ 2416 K-12 school district employees. Among the invitees, $n =$ 437 completed the survey, for a response rate of 18.1%.

2.2. Instruments

2.2.1. Individual Level

Commuting Patterns. Participants reported the number of times per week that they walked, biked, drove, and took public transportation to and from work. The number of individual trips via walking and biking was summed for number of active commuting trips/week.

Demographics and Medical. Participants reported their age, race/ethnic group (dichotomized as non-Hispanic White/other), marital status (dichotomized as married, partnered/not married, or partnered), number of children, sex, and number of cars in the household. Participants indicated from a list how many chronic diseases they had and reported their height and weight for body mass index (BMI) calculations. Respondents were asked to rate their current health status with a 5-point Likert scale from 1 (poor) to 5 (excellent).

Self-Efficacy. Participant's confidence with their cycling skills in urban areas was assessed with a single item using a 4-point Likert scale (1 = not at all confident to 4 = very confident).

AC Behavioral Beliefs. Respondents indicated their agreement using a 7-point Likert scale (1 = completely disagree to 7 = completely agree) with 13 statements about AC. Eight were related to AC and their physical or mental health (e.g., AC helps me control my weight can help me to relieve stress), and five were related to other AC benefits (e.g., AC is good for the environment helps me to save money). A total score was computed for all 13 items. This measure was based on a previously tested scale [35] and demonstrated excellent reliability in the present study ($\alpha = 0.91$).

Perceived Behavioral Control for AC. Participants indicated their agreement using a 7-point Likert scale (1 = completely disagree to 7 = completely agree) with six statements about why AC is difficult (e.g., AC is difficult because I am not committed to it because I am too tired) [36]. A total score was computed for the six items, and the scale showed good reliability ($\alpha = 0.84$).

2.2.2. Interpersonal

Coworker and Spouse AC Participation and Normative Beliefs. Participants responded with a Likert scale (1 = strongly disagree to 5 = strongly agree) to a question about their coworkers' AC behavior: "Most of my coworkers walk or bike to/from work." Respondents also reported the number of times/week their spouse walked or biked to/from work.

Coworker and spouse normative beliefs were assessed separately using a 5-point Likert scale to measure an individuals' level of agreement with four statements about their spouse/coworkers influence on their mode of travel to work. Items asked separately for spouse and coworkers but were worded identically. Items included "My spouse and I discuss issues related to walking and biking to work," "I value what my spouse thinks about the way I travel to/from work," "I have an opinion on the way my spouse travels to/from work," and "My spouse influences my choice on how I travel to/from work." Items were summed separately for spouse and coworkers and had good reliability (coworkers $\alpha = 0.76$, spouse $\alpha = 0.83$).

2.2.3. Institutional

Worksite Related. Participants were asked to report their employer's size and number of employer supports for AC (yes/no) from a list of seven items (incentives for AC, events related to AC, and flexible work hours, bike storage policies, bicycle parking, locker rooms, flexible dress code), which were summed. Participants indicated how much they perceived their employer supported AC using a 5-point Likert scale (1 = strongly disagree to 5 = strongly agree). Perceived problems for parking at work were assessed with three items about a lack of availability, high cost, and difficulty of parking. Parking items were summed with a greater score indicating more problems associated with parking.

2.2.4. Community

Community Factors. Participants reported (yes/no) on the availability of three supports for bicyclists in their community (e.g., bike racks on buses, covered bike parking, "share the road" signs), which were summed. Participants to indicate their agreement with five statements about perceived support for walking and biking using a 5-point Likert scale (1 = strongly disagree to 5 = strongly agree). Items were summed to create a perceived environmental supports score and included: town/city support for pedestrian or bicyclists issues, seeing others in their community walking/biking, and maintenance of sidewalks or bike lanes. Individuals were asked to rate their community's perceived pedestrian and bike friendliness from 1 (not pedestrian/bicycle friendly at all) to 5 (very pedestrian/bicycle friendly). Lastly, participants also indicated how long it would take them to walk or bike to work, dichotomized as ≤20 minutes and greater than 20 minutes.

2.2.5. Environmental

Barriers. Perceived environmental barriers were examined, with respondents rating the extent to which seven environmental features kept them from walking or biking to work (1 = strongly disagree to 5 = strongly agree). The items included a lack of on-street bike lanes, lack of off-street walking/biking paths, lack of sidewalks, speed/volume of traffic along route, perceived crime along route, difficult terrain, and bad weather.

2.3. Data Analysis. Basic descriptive statistics and frequencies were used to describe the sample. t-tests compared differences between older and younger participants. For categorical correlates of AC (e.g., gender), t-tests and analyses of variances (ANOVAs) were used to examine differences in rates of AC. For continuous variables (e.g., age, BMI, and perceived behavioral control), Pearson correlations were used to examine associations with AC. The variables with significant associations were included in a forced block entry multiple regression analysis to determine the relative influence of social ecological factors for AC. Specifically, five blocks of independent variables were forced into the model: individual, interpersonal, institutional, community, and environmental-level variables. All analyses were performed using IBM SPSS 20.0 (Armonk, NY, USA), and significance levels were set at $P < 0.05$.

3. Results

The characteristics of the sample are found in Table 1. Respondents were primarily middle aged (mean age 44.70 ± 11.11 years), female (79.9%), non-Hispanic White (93.4%), and overweight (BMI 26.40 ± 5.9 kg/m^2). On average participants actively commuted 0.51 ± 1.93 times/week, drove 8.77 ± 3.19 times/week, and took public transit 0.04 ± 0.68 times/week. Only 8.7% of participants reported actively commuting one or more times/week. Pearson correlations for AC are shown in Table 2.

3.1. Influences on Active Commuting. At the individual level, there were no differences for AC rates by sex, marital status, or race. BMI ($r = -0.11, P = 0.04$), number of cars in the household ($r = -0.18, P < 0.001$), and perceived behavioral control ($r = -0.44, P < 0.001$) were negatively related to AC, while self-efficacy for biking skills ($r = 0.14, P = 0.02$) and AC beliefs ($r = 0.13, P = 0.02$) was positively related to AC. At the interpersonal level, spouse AC ($r = 0.29, P < 0.001$), spouse normative beliefs ($r = 0.26, P < 0.001$), and coworker normative beliefs ($r = 0.24, P < 0.001$) were positively related to AC. Amount of employer support ($r = 0.14, P < 0.001$) and perceived ($r = 0.15, P < 0.001$) employer support was positively related to AC at the institutional level. At the community level those reporting less than a 20-minute walk ($t = 8.07, P < 0.001$) or bike ($t = 7.17, P < 0.001$) time to work were more likely to AC than those reporting a longer travel time. A lack of on-street bike lanes ($r = -0.15, P = 0.01$), lack of off-street walking/biking paths ($r = -0.20, P < 0.001$), lack of sidewalks ($r = -0.22, P < 0.001$), speed and volume of traffic along route ($r = -0.14, P = 0.01$), difficult terrain ($r = -0.18, P < 0.001$), and bad weather ($r = 0.13, P = 0.03$) were all negative environmental factors associated with AC. Since perceived walk time and bike time were highly related, only walk time was used in the full model.

The full model explained 60.8% of the variance in AC behavior (refer to Table 3). The individual block explained 42.0% of the variance ($F(6, 98) = 11.80, P < 0.001$) with perceived behavioral control ($\beta = -0.48, P < 0.001$) as a negative predictor. The interpersonal level block (2nd block)

TABLE 1: Characteristics of the sample of K-12 educators (n = 437).

Variable	n (%)	Mean (SD)
Individual level		
Age		44.7 (11.1)
Sex		
Male	77 (20.1)	
Female	283 (79.9)	
Marital status (% married/partnered)		
Married/partnered	297 (79.8)	
Single, divorced, widowed	75 (20.2)	
Race/ethnicity		
Non-Hispanic White	327 (93.4)	
All other racial/ethnic groups	23 (6.7)	
Number of children		0.63 (0.96)
Body mass index (kg/m^2)		26.4 (5.9)
Number of reported chronic diseases		0.62 (1.01)
Perceived health status (range: 1–5)		3.69 (0.80)
Number of cars in the household		3.26 (0.87)
Self-efficacy for bicycling skills (range: 1–4)		2.98 (1.53)
AC behavioral beliefs score (range: 13–91)		68.7 (13.66)
Perceived behavioral control for AC (range: 7–42)		29.06 (7.4)
Interpersonal level		
Spouse AC (times/week)		0.23 (1.4)
Spouse normative beliefs for AC (range: 4–20)		10.04 (4.07)
Perceived coworker AC (range: 1–5)		1.31 (0.61)
Coworker normative beliefs for AC (range: 4–20)		7.64 (3)
Institutional level		
Number of employer supports for AC (range: 0–7)		1.43 (1.42)
Perceived employer support for AC (range: 1–5)		2.03 (1.17)
Community level		
Perceived community support for AC (range: 5–25)		16.16 (4.82)
Perceived pedestrian friendliness for AC (range: 1–5)		3.27 (1.27)
Perceive bicycle friendliness for AC (range: 1–5)		3.07 (1.29)
Environment level (range 1–5)		
Lack of on-street bike lanes		3.15 (1.63)
Lack of off-street walking/biking paths		3.16 (1.62)
Lack of sidewalks		3.1 (1.64)
Speed and volume of traffic along route		3.36 (1.6)
Perceived crime along route		2.11 (1.43)
Difficult terrain		3.05 (1.54)
Bad weather		3.54 (1.45)

Note. AC: active commuting.

explained an additional 11.2% of the variance ($F(9, 95) = 11.99, P < 0.001$), with spouse AC ($\beta = 0.10, P = 0.001$) as a positive predictor. The third block (institutional level) explained an additional 0.1% of the variance in AC ($F(11, 93) = 9.65, P < 0.001$) with no significant predictors. The fourth block (community level) explained an additional 2.9% of the AC variance ($F(12, 92) = 9.83, P < 0.001$) with walk time as a negative predictor ($\beta = -0.18, P = 0.01$). The final block (environmental level) contributed another 4.6% ($F(18, 86) = 7.41, P < 0.001$), with lack of sidewalks ($\beta = -0.37, P = 0.03$) and speed and volume of traffic along route ($\beta = -0.30, P = 0.02$) as negative predictors.

4. Discussion

This study provides insight on the factors that determine whether K-12 educators choose to actively commute to work. The overall results of this study are important findings for the general health and well-being of educators and the individuals (i.e., students and staff) they influence. Few studies have

TABLE 2: Pearson correlations for active commuting and social ecological model variables.

Variable	r	P
Individual level		
Age	0.01	0.99
Body mass index (kg/m^2)	−0.109	**0.04**
Number of reported chronic diseases	−0.017	0.72
Perceived health status (range 1–5)	0.14	**0.008**
Number of cars in the household	−0.183	**<0.001**
Number of children	−0.07	0.21
Self-efficacy for bicycling skills (range: 1–4)	0.14	**0.02**
AC behavioral beliefs score (range: 13–91)	0.13	**0.02**
Perceived behavioral control for AC (range: 7–42)	−0.441	**<0.001**
Interpersonal level		
Spouse AC (times/week)	0.29	**<0.001**
Spouse normative beliefs for AC (range: 4–20)	0.26	**<0.001**
Perceived coworker AC (range: 1–5)	0.07	0.13
Coworker normative beliefs for AC (range: 4–20)	0.23	**<0.001**
Institutional level		
Number of employer supports for AC (range: 0–7)	0.14	**<0.001**
Perceived employer support for AC (range: 1–5)	0.15	**<0.001**
Community level		
Perceived community support for AC (range: 5–25)	0.06	0.27
Perceived pedestrian friendliness for AC (range: 1–5)	0.1	**0.06**
Perceive bicycle friendliness for AC (range: 1–5)	0.06	0.22
Environment level (range 1–5)		
Lack of on-street bike lanes	−0.15	**0.01**
Lack of off-street walking/biking paths	−0.2	**<0.001**
Lack of sidewalks	−0.22	**<0.001**
Speed and volume of traffic along route	−0.14	**0.01**
Perceived crime along route	−0.05	0.37
Difficult terrain	−0.18	**<0.001**
Bad weather	−0.13	**0.03**

Note. AC: active commuting; bold face indicates significance.

examined AC rates among this occupational class, yet there are significant health and economic outcomes associated with these findings. These results provide a number of possible implications for school health and employee health in school districts.

Public school districts providing health insurance are often saddled with the costs of rising healthcare expenditure, frequently accounting for a significant portion of the district's budget. For example, the State of New York reports that in 2007-2008 8.5% of an average school districts' expenditures were associated with health insurance [37]. Garrett and colleagues [6] have examined the direct costs to a health plan associated with physical inactivity. The findings suggested that 12% of mental health costs and 31% of chronic disease costs (colon cancer, cardiovascular disease, and osteoporosis) were attributable to a lack of physical activity participation. Actively commuting to work can increase the likelihood of individuals meeting current recommendations for physical activity [12, 27] which are associated with a decreased risk of chronic disease morbidity and mortality [1]. Olabarria and colleagues [38] showed significant positive health and economic outcomes when motorized trips were replaced by walking. Several reviews [39–41] have noted the cost-effectiveness of investments in worksite physical activity interventions, and school districts concerned with rising healthcare costs may consider interventions targeting AC as a method of improving health outcomes.

In addition to the potential health benefits garnered from regular physical activity, teachers who actively commute to school could potentially influence their students to live an active and healthy lifestyle. Few studies have examined teachers influence on their student's physical activity behaviors, however based on Social Cognitive Theory, this link between teachers AC and student physical activity would be well supported. Specifically, teachers serve as a role model to student's and have the potential to increase their self-efficacy for physical activity [42]. Providing vicarious experiences, such as AC modeling, to increase motivation is a strategy

Table 3: Hierarchical regression explaining variance in active commuting (AC).

Variable	B	SEB	β	R^2	ΔR^2
Step1: Individual influences				0.42	
Perceived health status	−0.05	0.26	−0.17		
Body mass index	0.03	0.04	0.05		
Perceived behavioral control for AC	−0.17	0.03	-0.48^{***}		
Self-efficacy for skills	−0.07	0.2	−0.03		
Number of cars in the household	−0.3	0.27	−0.09		
Step2: Interpersonal influences				0.53	0.11
Coworker normative beliefs for AC	0.07	0.07	0.08		
Spouse AC	0.4	0.11	0.27^{**}		
Spouse normative beliefs for AC	0.06	0.06	0.1		
Step3: Institutional influences				0.53	0.001
Perceived employer support for AC	−0.03	0.19	−0.01		
Number of employer supports for AC	0.04	0.16	0.02		
Step4: Community influences				0.56	0.03
Perceived walk time to work	−1.3	0.52	-0.1^{*}		
Step5: Environmental influences				0.61	0.05
Lack of on-street bike lanes	0.15	0.29	0.09		
Lack of off-street walking/biking paths	0.04	0.35	0.03		
Lack of sidewalks	−0.59	0.27	-0.37^{*}		
Speed and volume of traffic along route	0.5	0.2	0.3^{*}		
Difficult terrain	0.15	0.2	0.08		
Bad weather	−0.23	0.19	−0.12		

Note. $^{*}P < 0.05$, $^{**}P < 0.01$, and $^{***}P < 0.001$.

teachers could use to promote PA among children, which is a growing health concern with high rates of childhood obesity and sedentary behavior [43].

These findings in the present study indicated that the most influential factors for AC were individual level factors. Perceived behavioral control, AC beliefs, and self-efficacy for AC were significant predictors. It was apparent that the more barriers an individual endures, including lack of knowledge or skills or attitudes toward AC, the less likely they will actively commute. To address this barrier, there should be a focus on the individual level with theoretically based behavior-change strategies. Approaches could include goal setting, monitoring behavior, improving knowledge, and skills through educational approaches (e.g., instructional on health and financial reasons to bike to work, route selection, dealing with cargo and clothing, lighting, and traffic issues), all of which target self-efficacy and perceived behavioral control. Other individualized approaches could include teacher-tailored websites that offer encouragement, advice, and behavioral cues reminding teachers of the importance of their role modeling behavior.

On an interpersonal level, there was a positive correlation between the number of times a week a teacher actively commutes to work and the number of times their spouse actively commutes. These results corroborated with a review by Panter and Jones [23] that examined associations between social support from family and friends and active travel which demonstrated that social support was positively associated with active travel and biking to work. Although not found in the current study, other studies have found an association between an individual's AC participation and their coworkers' AC [26]. This suggests that it is essential to address social support and social norms when targeting AC participation. This could include the involvement of family in education and skill building strategies or building social support within the worksite for AC behavior.

Sallis and colleagues [27] have emphasized that changing built environments and developing pedestrian- and bicyclist-friendly policies can have a long-term impact on the people in those places and are related to rates of chronic disease, hypertension, and obesity. They also reveal that physical activity levels are driven by different built environment features and policies, which was evidence in the current study, with distance, infrastructure, and safety as significant concerns related to AC. This reinforces the approach of targeting the environment to be more pedestrian and bike friendly to have an impact on the amount of daily physical activity levels people in the community would obtain.

Although there were significant findings related to teachers active commuting to work through this study, there were some limitations within the process. First of all, the surveys were conducted through self-report and subjective measures. Self-report questionnaires are not always accurate, whereas some individuals may not report truthful or precise answers. Secondly, the sampling strategy of the study was not random. Additionally, the individuals who volunteered to participate may have had a bias towards the institution or the topic of the study. There was also not a strong response rate; though due to the use of electronic email as our recruitment method, we were not able to ascertain if individuals received the invitation to participate in their "inbox" compared with their "junk mail" box. However, the study still provides insight on teachers actively commuting to work and provides a baseline for future studies.

AC to work is an important source of daily physical activity; however, only a small percentage of teachers in our sample walk or rode their bike to work each day. Active commuting can improve the overall health and well-being of teachers, in addition to significant economic outcomes for school districts, making it an important public health and community issue. Furthermore, the physical activity behaviors of teachers can influence the behaviors of their students and increase the amount of students active commuting to school targeting childhood inactivity and obesity issues.

References

[1] Physical Activity Guidelines Advisory Committee, *Physical Activity Guidelines Advisory Committee Report, 2008*, US Department of Health and Human Services, Washington, DC, USA, 2008.

[2] Centers for Disease Control Prevention, "U.S. physical activity statistics: 2007 state demographic data comparison," 2012, http://www.cdc.gov/nccdphp/dnpa/physical/stats/index.htm.

[3] M. Pratt, C. A. Macera, and G. Wang, "Higher direct medical costs associated with physical inactivity," *The Physician and Sportsmedicine*, vol. 28, no. 10, pp. 63–70, 2000.

[4] G. A. Colditz, "Economic costs of obesity and inactivity," *Medicine and Science in Sports and Exercise*, vol. 31, supplement 11, pp. S663–S667, 1999.

[5] D. Chenoweth and J. Leutzinger, "The economic cost of physical inactivity and excess weight in American adults," *Journal of Physical Activity and Health*, vol. 3, no. 2, pp. 148–163, 2006.

[6] N. A. Garrett, M. Brasure, K. H. Schmitz, M. M. Schultz, and M. R. Huber, "Physical inactivity: direct cost to a health plan," *American Journal of Preventive Medicine*, vol. 27, no. 4, pp. 304–309, 2004.

[7] M. Cox, J. Shephard, and P. Corey, "Influence of an employee fitness programme upon fitness, productivity and absenteeism," *Ergonomics*, vol. 24, no. 10, pp. 795–806, 1981.

[8] O. Rosenfeld, G. Tenenbaum, H. Ruskin, and S.-T. Halfon, "Behavioural modifications following a physical activity programme in the Israeli pharmaceutical industry," *Australian Journal of Science and Medicine in Sport*, vol. 22, pp. 93–96, 1990.

[9] M. Odeen, L. H. Magnussen, S. Maeland, L. Larun, H. R. Eriksen, and T. H. Tveito, "Systematic review of active workplace interventions to reduce sickness absence," *Occupational Medicine*, vol. 63, no. 1, pp. 7–16, 2013.

[10] R. Norris, D. Carroll, and R. Cochrane, "The effects of aerobic and anaerobic training on fitness, blood pressure, and psychological stress and well-being," *Journal of Psychosomatic Research*, vol. 34, no. 4, pp. 367–375, 1990.

[11] B. H. Jacobson and S. G. Aldana, "Relationship between frequency of aerobic activity and illness-related absenteeism in a large employee sample," *Journal of Occupational and Environmental Medicine*, vol. 43, no. 12, pp. 1019–1025, 2001.

[12] R. J. Shephard, "Is active commuting the answer to population health?" *Sports Medicine*, vol. 38, no. 9, pp. 751–758, 2008.

[13] M. Lindström, "Means of transportation to work and overweight and obesity: a population-based study in southern Sweden," *Preventive Medicine*, vol. 46, no. 1, pp. 22–28, 2008.

[14] M. Hamer and Y. Chida, "Active commuting and cardiovascular risk: a meta-analytic review," *Preventive Medicine*, vol. 46, no. 1, pp. 9–13, 2008.

[15] L. B. Andersen, P. Schnohr, M. Schroll, and H. O. Hein, "All-cause mortality associated with physical activity during leisure time, work, sports, and cycling to work," *Archives of Internal Medicine*, vol. 160, no. 11, pp. 1621–1628, 2000.

[16] J. Kruger, S. A. Ham, D. Berrigan, and R. Ballard-Barbash, "Prevalence of transportation and leisure walking among U.S. adults," *Preventive Medicine*, vol. 47, no. 3, pp. 329–334, 2008.

[17] P. S. Hu and T. R. Reuscher, *Summary of Travel Trends: 2001 National Household Transportation Survey*, US Department of Transportation & Federal Highway Adminstration, Washington, DC, USA, 2004.

[18] D. R. Bassett Jr., J. Pucher, R. Buehler, D. L. Thompson, and S. E. Crouter, "Walking, cycling, and obesity rates in Europe, North America and Australia," *Journal of Physical Activity and Health*, vol. 5, no. 6, pp. 795–814, 2008.

[19] J. F. Sallis, R. B. Cervero, W. Ascher, K. A. Henderson, M. K. Kraft, and J. Kerr, "An ecological approach to creating active living communities," *Annual Review of Public Health*, vol. 27, pp. 297–322, 2006.

[20] K. R. McLeroy, D. Bibeau, A. Steckler, and K. Glanz, "An ecological perspective on health promotion programs," *Health Education Quarterly*, vol. 15, no. 4, pp. 351–377, 1988.

[21] M. Bopp, A. T. Kaczynski, and P. Wittman, "The relationship of eco-friendly attitudes with walking and biking to work," *Journal of Public Health Management and Practice*, vol. 17, no. 5, pp. E9–E17, 2011.

[22] M. Bopp, A. Kaczynski, and P. Wittman, "Active commuting patterns at a large, midwestern college campus," *Journal of American College Health*, vol. 59, no. 7, pp. 605–611, 2011.

[23] J. R. Panter and A. Jones, "Attitudes and the environment as determinants of active travel in adults: what do and don't we know?" *Journal of Physical Activity and Health*, vol. 7, no. 4, pp. 551–561, 2010.

[24] G.-J. de Bruijn, S. P. J. Kremers, A. Singh, B. van den Putte, and W. van Mechelen, "Adult active transportation: adding habit strength to the theory of planned behavior," *American Journal of Preventive Medicine*, vol. 36, no. 3, pp. 189–194, 2009.

[25] M. Bopp, A. T. Kaczynski, and G. Besenyi, "Active commuting influences among adults," *Preventive Medicine*, vol. 54, no. 3-4, pp. 237–241, 2012.

[26] A. T. Kaczynski, M. J. Bopp, and P. Wittman, "Association of workplace supports with active commuting," *Preventing Chronic Disease*, vol. 7, no. 6, article A127, 2010.

[27] J. F. Sallis, M. F. Floyd, D. A. Rodríguez, and B. E. Saelens, "Role of built environments in physical activity, obesity, and cardiovascular disease," *Circulation*, vol. 125, no. 5, pp. 729–737, 2012.

[28] A. Lake and T. Townshend, "Obesogenic environments: exploring the built and food environments," *Journal of the Royal Society for the Promotion of Health*, vol. 126, no. 6, pp. 262–267, 2006.

[29] N. Owen, N. Humpel, E. Leslie, A. Bauman, and J. F. Sallis, "Understanding environmental influences on walking: review and research agenda," *American Journal of Preventive Medicine*, vol. 27, no. 1, pp. 67–76, 2004.

[30] C. L. Craig, R. C. Brownson, S. E. Cragg, and A. L. Dunn, "Exploring the effect of the environment on physical activity: a study examining walking to work," *American Journal of Preventive Medicine*, vol. 23, no. 2, pp. 36–43, 2002.

[31] M. Lemieux and G. Godin, "How well do cognitive and environmental variables predict active commuting?" *International Journal of Behavioral Nutrition and Physical Activity*, vol. 6, article 12, 2009.

[32] National Center for Education Statistics, *Digest of Education Statistics*, U.S. Department of Education, Alexandria, Va, USA, 2010.

[33] L. G. P. M. van Amelsvoort, M. G. Spigt, G. M. H. Swaen, and I. Kant, "Leisure time physical activity and sickness absenteeism; a prospective study," *Occupational Medicine*, vol. 56, no. 3, pp. 210–212, 2006.

[34] M. Bopp, A. T. Kaczynski, and M. E. Campbell, "Social ecological influences on work-related active commuting among adults," *American Journal of Health Behavior*, vol. 37, no. 4, pp. 543–554, 2013.

[35] C. L. Blue, D. G. Marrero, and D. R. Black, "Physical activity belief scales for diabetes risk: development and psychometric testing," *Health Education and Behavior*, vol. 35, no. 3, pp. 316–331, 2008.

[36] V. S. Conn, T. Tripp-Reimer, and M. L. Maas, "Older women and exercise: theory of planned behavior beliefs," *Public Health Nursing*, vol. 20, no. 2, pp. 153–163, 2003.

[37] New York State School Boards Association, *Condition Critical: Can Health Insurance Consortiums Rein in School District Health Care Costs?*, 2009.

[38] M. Olabarria, K. Pérez, E. Santamariña-Rubio, A. M. Novoa, and F. Racioppi, "Health impact of motorised trips that could be replaced by walking," *European Journal of Public Health*, vol. 23, no. 2, p. 217, 2012.

[39] A. Andersen, "The XY perspective for the next decade," *The Perspective*, pp. 3–4, 2000.

[40] M. Bopp and E. Fallon, "Community-based interventions to promote increased physical activity: a primer," *Applied Health Economics and Health Policy*, vol. 6, no. 4, pp. 173–187, 2008.

[41] D. L. Katz, M. O'Connell, M.-C. Yeh et al., "Public health strategies for preventing and controlling overweight and obesity in school and worksite settings: a report on recommendations of the task force on community preventive services," *MMWR Recommendations and Reports*, vol. 54, no. RR-10, pp. 1–12, 2005.

[42] A. Bandura, *Social Foundations of Thought and Action: A Social Cognitive Theory*, Prentice-Hall, Englewood Cliffs, NJ, USA, 1986.

[43] Centers for Disease Control Prevention, "Youth risk behavior surveillance system," 2012, http://www.cdc.gov/HealthyYouth/yrbs/index.htm.

13

An Attempt at Quantifying Factors that Affect Efficiency in the Management of Solid Waste Produced by Commercial Businesses in the City of Tshwane, South Africa

Yohannes Worku[1] and Mammo Muchie[2]

[1] *Department of Civil Engineering, Faculty of Engineering, Tshwane University of Technology, Private Bag X680, Pretoria 0001, South Africa*
[2] *Faculty of Economics and Finance, Institute for Economic Research on Innovation (IERI), Tshwane University of Technology, Private Bag X680, Pretoria 0001, South Africa*

Correspondence should be addressed to Yohannes Worku, Johannes.Worku@gmail.com

Academic Editor: Oladele A. Ogunseitan

Objective. The objective was to investigate factors that affect the efficient management of solid waste produced by commercial businesses operating in the city of Pretoria, South Africa. *Methods.* Data was gathered from 1,034 businesses. Efficiency in solid waste management was assessed by using a structural time-based model designed for evaluating efficiency as a function of the length of time required to manage waste. Data analysis was performed using statistical procedures such as frequency tables, Pearson's chi-square tests of association, and binary logistic regression analysis. Odds ratios estimated from logistic regression analysis were used for identifying key factors that affect efficiency in the proper disposal of waste. *Results.* The study showed that 857 of the 1,034 businesses selected for the study (83%) were found to be efficient enough with regards to the proper collection and disposal of solid waste. Based on odds ratios estimated from binary logistic regression analysis, efficiency in the proper management of solid waste was significantly influenced by 4 predictor variables. These 4 influential predictor variables are lack of adherence to waste management regulations, wrong perception, failure to provide customers with enough trash cans, and operation of businesses by employed managers, in a decreasing order of importance.

1. Introduction

The city of Tshwane is the capital of South Africa. According to Statistics South Africa, the population size of the city of Tshwane in 2011 was roughly equal to 3 million. The city is home to over 5,000 businesses out of which 1,603 businesses operate within the Central Business District of Tshwane, known as Pretoria [1]. According to the annual report issued by the city of Tshwane Metropolitan Municipality for the budget year 2010-2011, about 1,734,295 tons of solid waste are collected each year from businesses operating in the city [2]. The solid waste produced by businesses in the city includes trash or garbage such as wood, product packaging, empty bottles, used tyres and car parts, and cans, garden refuse, furniture, clothing, leftover food, newspapers, wires, grease, appliances, paint, pieces of metal, broken containers, sheet metal, used medicine, and the like. These businesses produce massive volumes of solid and liquid waste on a daily basis. Taxi ranks, bus stations, open flea markets, food outlets, and small businesses located in Pretoria are synonymous with litter, uncontrolled solid and liquid waste, as well as lack of capacity in the efficient management of waste. The annual report released by the city of Tshwane Metropolitan Municipality for the year 2011 shows that massive waste is accumulated during strike action by municipal workers responsible for the removal of waste from households and businesses [2]. The collection, disposal, and processing of waste produced by businesses and households are regulated by legislative policies set out and enforced by the Municipality of Tshwane and the South African National Department of Environmental Affairs and Tourism [2, 3]. The use of an integrated municipal solid waste management system [4–7] has been shown to be essential for improving overall efficiency in municipal waste management in almost all developed nations of the world. In order for an integrated waste management system to perform efficiently, all relevant stakeholders of the waste chain must play a mutually collaborative role in the collection, disposal, processing and management of waste. A review of the relevant literature shows that such a measure is essential for reducing the overall cost of waste management, and for the protection of the environment [8–10]. Overall efficiency in the management of waste depends on adherence to municipal acts on waste disposal and management [11–13]. Research work carried out in several developing nations of the world has shown that health education on environmental sanitation and primary health care [14], socioeconomic incentives [15], as well as a strict enforcement of municipal bylaws [16] are all needed for ensuring overall environmental cleanliness and the efficient management of waste in metropolitan cities such as Tshwane.

The study was conducted against the background of a host of factors that are well known to undermine overall efficiency in the management of solid waste in almost all metropolitan cities of the developing world. These background factors are lack of infrastructural capacity required for the efficient management and processing of solid waste [2, 3, 17, 18], poor awareness about the benefits of proper waste management [19], lack of socioeconomic incentives to stakeholders relevant to the waste management chain [20], failure to adequately utilize modern waste management and processing technology [21, 22], failure to vigorously enforce municipal bylaws [2, 3], and the absence of an integrated waste management system in Tshwane [23, 24]. The study aims to identify and quantify the key predictors of inefficiency in the management of solid waste in the city of Tshwane. With a view to ensure optimal efficiency in the management of solid waste, this research work will assess the degree to which municipal bylaws and regulations that are relevant to solid waste management are adhered to by businesses conducting business in the city of Tshwane. The bylaws and regulations are relevant to all stages of the waste management chain (sorting of waste at source, collection, treatment, disposal, and processing). The model considers 4 categories of solid waste (municipal, organic, plastics, and electronic) and is designed for realizing a sustainable and optimally efficient solid waste management system for the city of Tshwane. The model is accompanied by a comprehensive monitoring and evaluation plan that could be used for assessing the current status-quo, and for assessing and evaluating efficiency in waste management at each stage of the waste management chain. Norms and standards set out by the South African National Department of Environment and Tourism are used for benchmarking [4].

Municipal bylaws that are relevant to waste management are not enforced with full vigour. Although more than 25% of small and medium-sized businesses as well as informal traders operating in the city of Tshwane generate waste in the course of conducting routine business [2, 3, 17], the pace at which such waste is properly collected and disposed of by municipal workers employed by the city of Tshwane is significantly lower than the pace at which waste is generated. This situation is exacerbated at times of civil action carried out by municipal workers responsible for routine waste collection and disposal. Taxi ranks, the various sources of solid and liquid waste and pollution, bus stations, liquor stores, petrol stations, schools, shops, open markets, garages, and so forth are well known contributors for the generation of high volume of solid and liquid waste in the CBD of Pretoria. There is room for improvement of the current level of efficiency in the management of waste produced by the various sources of solid and liquid waste and pollution. In terms of the strategic plan adopted by the South African Department of Environmental Affairs and Tourism (DEAT) to improve efficiency in the management of waste, the various sources of solid and liquid waste and pollution are a major stakeholder, and no progress can be made unless otherwise the various sources of solid and liquid waste and pollution are involved in the implementation of the plan drawn up by the DEAT [4, 17].

There is a significant accumulation of solid waste especially in townships such as Mamelodi and Marabastad, and at the various taxi ranks in and around the city of Pretoria. There is a shortage of essential facilities such as trash cans, seats, shelters, public toilets, and clean tap water at taxi ranks and public gathering arenas. Some of the various sources of solid and liquid waste and pollution do not have properly functioning toilets and washrooms although the proper functioning of such facilities is an essential requirement for business. The various sources of solid and liquid waste and pollution, taxi ranks, and public gathering arenas are often characterized by bad smell and a large accumulation of solid and liquid waste. Such places are conducive for the spread of communicable diseases such as food poisoning and diarrhoea unless they are controlled and managed efficiently by the CTMM. Not enough is known so far about the extent to which efficiency in waste disposal can be improved in view of the fact that there is lack of empirical evidence in this area of research interest. Not enough research has been done in the CBD of Pretoria to assess and identify factors that affect efficiency in proper waste disposal. There is a shortage of empirical evidence based on a properly designed multivariate modelling in areas related to the quantification of factors that contribute to poor environmental sanitation and the accumulation of solid and liquid waste in the CBD of Pretoria. Low level of awareness in areas related to recycling, classification of waste at source and composting plays a major role in compounding the current lack of efficiency in the efficient utilization of resources such as broken bottles, empty cans, used goods, plastic bags, and so forth. Far from being put to economic use, broken bottles are harming pedestrians and school children in addition to polluting the environment and decreasing the beauty of the city in the eyes of visitors and residents. Ratepayers are disgusted with the level of incompetence, inefficiency, and indifference. Some irresponsible inhabitants of the city and visitors who travel to the city from outside do not have adequate respect for environmental sanitation and demonstrate total disregard for cleanliness of the streets of the city. Such irresponsible inhabitants and visitors often throw away rubbish on the streets. Examples of such rubbish are beer bottles, empty cans, and used food packages. Empty bottles break into harmful pieces as they are thrown onto the streets from moving taxis and private cars. There is a need to have irresponsible inhabitants and visitors educated and disciplined so that they show respect for environmental sanitation and cleanliness. Experience drawn from large municipalities in Sweden, the United States, and Kenya shows that these deeply ingrained problems could be addressed adequately by enforcing the relevant municipal bylaws with vigour [18], by promoting health and environmental education, and by providing socioeconomic incentives to stakeholders and role-players in the waste management chain [19].

A review of the literature shows that in cities as big as Tshwane, modern waste treatment technologies such as composting, incineration, landfills, recycling, and window composting should be used for solid waste management [20–23]. Modern solid waste management techniques such as landfills, incineration, recycling, biological processing, energy recovery, radio frequency identification tags, global positioning system tracking integrated software packages, rear vision cameras, and the like are used in cities such as Geneva and Stockholm [18]. Examples of advanced solid waste treatment technologies that are suitable for the city are anaerobic digestion, ethanol production, biodrying, gasification, in-vessel composting, mechanical biological treatment, mechanical heat treatment, plasma arc waste disposal, pyrolysis, sewage treatment, and tunnel composting are also highly appropriate technologies for the city [19, 20]. In the city of Tshwane, the management of solid waste involves collection, transportation, processing or disposal, management, and monitoring of waste materials. The South African Department of Environmental Affairs and Tourism [4] promotes the use of modern technologies and evaluation techniques that are necessary for the efficient management of waste although advanced technologies that are used for waste management and evaluation are poorly utilized in South African cities including the City of Tshwane [2].

Globally, diverse methods have been used for improving efficiency in the collection and disposal of solid waste. The most commonly used methods are designed for ensuring efficiency in solid waste management and are outlined in the UN-Habitat's Third Global Report of 2010 [21]. In the world's cleanest cities, the following methods are used: integrated sustainable waste management, the enforcement of municipal bylaws, the promotion of primary health care services and environmental sanitation, the promotion of health education on proper waste management, financial sustainability, institutional framework, good governance, community based campaigns of awareness, the provision of incentives for good performance in the collection of solid waste, process flow diagrams, as well as monitoring and evaluation programmes designed for the assessment of municipal service delivery programmes [22–25].

In this study, assessment of efficiency in waste management was made by using the classic structural time-based model constructed by Tchobanoglous et al. [26] as well as adherence to municipal bylaws. The city of Tshwane uses the model for assessing overall efficiency in the collection of solid waste by municipal service providers. The model is suitable for assessing efficiency in the collection of solid waste from fixed containers that are used for depositing solid waste by businesses and ordinary residents. The model assesses overall efficiency as a function of time taken for the management of waste.

The aim of this research is to identify and quantify factors that affect overall efficiency in the management of solid waste generated by businesses that operate in the city of Tshwane. Based on data collected from a random sample of $n = 1{,}034$ businesses operating in the city of Tshwane, the research article aims to:

(1) assess the current state of solid waste management with regards to type of wastes and quantities of waste generated,

(2) identify key factors that affect efficiency in the management of solid waste, and

(3) assess the degree to which businesses adhere to norms and standards that are recommended for businesses in terms of solid waste disposal.

2. Methods

2.1. Data. Data was collected in 2010 from a random sample of 1,034 businesses operating in the city of Tshwane. Eligible businesses were identified based on a sampling frame belonging to Statistics South Africa [1]. Managers and owners of the businesses as well as employees were asked a total of 89 questions related to the type of business they were operating, the type and volume of waste generated, how waste was collected, sorted out, disposed of and managed, the extent of cleanliness and sanitation at the workplace, their socioeconomic and demographic characteristics, as well as their personal opinion on the benefits of the proper management of waste.

2.2. Statistical Analyses. Efficiency in solid waste management was assessed by using the model proposed by Tchobanoglous et al. [26] for estimating the median time required for the collection of solid waste from the businesses that took part in the study. The model measures efficiency in the collection of solid waste from fixed locations and containers based on the mathematical expression shown below:

$$E = 1 - A + B. \tag{1}$$

In (1), A denotes an off-route factor, and B is a measure of off-route activity time by individuals collecting waste. In cases where $A = B$, the collection of solid waste becomes perfectly efficient. The larger the difference between A and B, the less efficient becomes the waste collection procedure. The time required per trip is given by the expression shown below:

$$t = \frac{t_1 + t_2 + Y}{1 - A}. \tag{2}$$

In (2), t is the time required for waste collection from a fixed site per trip, t_1 is equal to pick up time of container at the site of collection, t_2 is equal to on-site time per trip, Y denotes the total haul time during waste collection, and X denotes the average round-trip haul distance per trip.

Since the relationship between Y and X follows simple linear regression, we have

$$Y = \beta_0 + \beta X. \tag{3}$$

In (3), β_0 is the constant term in the simple linear regression of Y on X, and β is the regression coefficient in the simple linear regression of Y on X. In cases where waste is collected from fixed sites, the time required to collect waste per trip follows a stationary model, and is expressed by the expression shown below:

$$t_1 = P + Q + R. \tag{4}$$

In (4), P is the time taken to pick up a container that is full of solid waste; Q is the time taken to unload an empty container; R is the time taken for driving from one container to the next container.

The number of trips per day is given by the expression shown below:

$$n = Y(1 - A) - \frac{(t_3 + t_4)}{t}. \tag{5}$$

In (5), variable t is the time required for waste collection from a fixed site per trip; t_3 is the time required to drive from dispatch station to first container location to be served by the day; t_4 is the time required to drive from the last container location to be served by the day to the dispatch station.

The time taken per trip is given by the expression shown below:

$$t_5 = \frac{t_6 - t}{Y}. \tag{6}$$

In (6), variable t_6 is the number of trips made in a week. The number of trips made per week is given by the expression shown below:

$$t_6 = \frac{K}{RQ}. \tag{7}$$

In (7), variable K is a measure of the volume of waste generated in a week in cubic meters per kg; R is the average size of the container in cubic meters per kg; Q is the weighted average container utilization factor.

Since $t = (t_1 + t_2 + Y)/(1 - A)$ as shown above in (2), it follows that

$$t_1 + t_2 + Y = (1 - A)t. \tag{8}$$

Efficiency can thus be measured by the following relationship:

$$\begin{aligned} E &= \frac{Y + t_1 + t_2 + Bt}{t} = \frac{(t_1 + t_2 + Y) + Bt}{t} \\ &= \frac{(1 - A)t + Bt}{t} = 1 - A + B. \end{aligned} \tag{9}$$

Values of E in the expression $E = 1 - A + B$ were calculated for each of the 1,034 businesses that took part in the study. Businesses for which values of E fell below the median were used for identifying businesses in which efficiency in waste management was inadequate. Businesses for which values of E were greater than or equal to the median were used for identifying businesses in which efficiency in waste management was deemed adequate. That is,

$$\text{overall efficiency} = \begin{cases} \text{inadequate if score is below} \\ \text{the median of } E \\ \text{adequate if score is greater than} \\ \text{or equal to the median of } E. \end{cases} \tag{10}$$

Pearson's chi-square tests of association [27] were used for the screening of variables. This was done by performing two-by-two tests of associations between overall efficiency in the management of waste and the various socioeconomic, demographic, sanitary, environmental, and health-related variables on which data was gathered as part of the study. At the 5% level of significance, an association was deemed significant if the P value was below 5%. The dependent variable of study is a measure of overall efficiency in the management of waste. The variable has only 2 possible values (Inadequate, Adequate). Since the dependent variable of study is dichotomous, binary logistic regression analysis [28] was used in order to identify key predictors of inefficiency in the management of waste. Multilevel analysis [29] was used in order to estimate the extent of variation with regards to efficiency in the management of waste by geographical zone and category of business enterprise. Multilevel analysis is a statistical procedure that enables planners and policy makers to allocate resources that are needed for intervention based on the extent of variation observed at various hierarchical levels. In this study, the two hierarchical levels depending on which efficiency in waste management varies are geographical location and category of business.

The degree of adherence to municipal bylaws and guidelines for the disposal of solid waste was measured by using a 2-point scale. The guidelines used for measuring adherence were the ISO 14000 and ISO 14031 guidelines for environmental management and performance monitoring in the management of waste and the environment [30–32]. At each of the 1,034 businesses selected for the study, the degree of adherence to municipal bylaws and procedures recommended for solid waste management by businesses by the city of Tshwane was graded based on ISO 14000 and ISO 14031 guidelines. That is, at each business enterprise, binary grades (Adequate, Not adequate) were allocated as a measure of compliance according to criteria stipulated in ISO 14000 and ISO 14031 guidelines. The binary variable created for assessing degree of adherence to ISO guidelines or municipal bylaws was used as one of the predictor variables of study. Category 1 of the binary variable represented inadequate adherence to ISO guidelines or municipal bylaws. Category 2 of the binary variable represented adequate adherence to ISO guidelines or municipal bylaws.

The purpose of conducting binary logistic regression analysis was to identify influential predictors of inefficiency in the management of waste among businesses operating in the city of Tshwane. The use of binary logistic regression analysis was appropriate as the dependent variable of study had only 2 possible values (1, 0). In binary logistic regression analysis, odds ratios were used as an epidemiological measure of effect. At the 5% level of significance, influential predictors of inefficiency in waste management are characterized by estimated odds ratios that differ from 1 significantly, P-values that are smaller than 0.05, and 95% confidence intervals of odds ratios that do not contain 1. The adequacy of the fitted logistic regression model was assessed by using standard diagnostic procedures such as the classification table, the Hosmer and Lemeshow goodness-of-fit test, receiver operating characteristics (ROC) plots, and sensitivity/specificity plots [28].

3. Results

Table 1 shows a comparison between businesses that were efficient with regards to solid waste management with those that were not. It can be seen from the table that 857 of the 1,034 businesses (83%) were efficient, while the remaining 177 businesses (17%) were inefficient. The table shows that a significant percentage of businesses located in the central and western parts of the city were inefficient, whereas businesses located in the eastern and northern parts of the city were by and large efficient. The table shows that 76% of operators who managed businesses that were efficient with regards to waste management have acquired formal education at college level or better. In general, businesses that are inefficient in the management of waste are relatively younger, poor in personal hygiene and cleanliness of premises, and are by and large commercial. The majority of old businesses (6 years or more) are efficient in waste management. Businesses that are operated by owners are more efficient in comparison with businesses that are operated by employed managers. Utilization of private contractors for waste removal and management, regular inspection of premises by municipal workers, familiarity with the South African White Paper on waste management, source reduction of waste, good perception on the benefits of proper waste management, and adherence to waste management regulations recommended by the municipality are much more common among businesses that are efficient in waste management.

Two-by-two Pearson chi-square tests of associations [27] was used for performing a preliminary screening of influential factors that were significantly associated with inefficient management of waste. Table 2 shows a list of 15 factors that are significantly associated with poor or less than satisfactory waste disposal at the 0.001 level of significance. In each of the tests, the outcome variable of study, Y, was defined as follows:

$$\text{overall efficiency} = \begin{cases} \text{inadequate if score is below} \\ \text{the median of } E \\ \text{adequate if score is greater than} \\ \text{or equal to the median of } E. \end{cases} \tag{11}$$

At the 0.001 level of significance, significant associations are characterized by large observed chi-square values and P-values that are smaller than 0.001. Table 2 provides a list of 15 variables that are significantly associated with inefficient waste management.

At the 0.001 level of significance, all 15 variables shown in Table 2 are significantly associated with overall efficiency in the management of waste. It can be seen from the table that the top 5 significant variables are: lack of adherence to municipal bylaws and regulations, wrong perception on the potential benefits of proper waste management, failure of businesses to provide customers with enough trash cans, the status of the business operator (owner or employee), and the frequency at which business premises are inspected by municipal sanitation and health workers, in a decreasing order of strength.

Results from binary logistic regression analysis are theoretically more reliable than results from Pearson's chi-square tests of association [28]. This is because the measure of effect in binary logistic regression is the odds ratio, and not two-by-two significant associations. Logistic regression analysis allows multivariate analysis involving several variables that are influential over waste disposal. It is also possible to assess the reliability of the fitted logistic regression model based on highly reliable diagnostic tests such as the classification table, the likelihood ratio test, the Hosmer-Lemeshow goodness-of-fit test, as well as receiver operating characteristic (ROC) and sensitivity/specificity plots [28].

At the 0.05 level of significance, influential predictor variables are characterized by estimated odds ratios that differ from 1 significantly, P-values that are smaller than 0.05, and 95% confidence intervals of odds ratios that do not contain 1. Accordingly, it can be seen from Table 3 that all 4 predictor variables are significant at the 0.05 level. The results show that efficiency in the proper management of solid waste is significantly influenced by 4 predictor variables. These 4 influential predictor variables are lack of adherence to municipal bylaws and regulations (OR = 9.17; 95% C.I. = (6.42, 12.54)), wrong perception (OR = 8.81; 95% C.I. = (6.01, 11.35)), failure to provide customers with enough trash cans (OR = 3.15; 95% C.I. = (1.46, 5.87)), and the operation of businesses by employed managers (OR = 2.69; 95% C.I. = (1.66, 4.32)), in a decreasing order of importance.

The adjusted odds ratio of the variable poor adherence is 9.17. This shows that a business that is managed by an operator who fails to adhere to guidelines set out for waste management by the city of Tshwane is 9.17 times as likely to be inefficient in the proper management of solid waste in comparison with a business that is managed by an operator who adheres to recommended guidelines. The adjusted odds ratio of the variable wrong perception is 8.81. This shows that a business operator who has the wrong perception on the benefits of proper management of solid waste is 8.81 times as likely to be inefficient in comparison with another business operator with the correct perception on the benefits of proper waste management. The adjusted odds ratio of the variable failure to provide customers with enough trash cans is 3.15. This shows that a business in which there are not enough trash cans for customers is 3.15 times as

TABLE 1: Comparison with regards to overall efficiency in waste management.

Characteristic	Efficient (n = 857)	Inefficient (n = 177)
Category of business	Agricultural: 1% Commercial: 71% Construction: 6% Industrial: 11% Institutional: 2% Municipal: 6% Manufacturing: 3%	Agricultural: 1% Commercial: 83% Construction: 3% Industrial: 3% Institutional: 3% Municipal: 5% Manufacturing: 2%
Geographical location of business in the city of Tshwane	Central: 31% East: 21% West: 19% North: 17% South: 12%	Central: 41% East: 13% West: 23% North: 13% South: 10%
Age of business in years	Less than a year: 5% 1 to 2 years: 6% 3 to 5 years: 29% 6 years or more: 60%	Less than a year: 34% 1 to 2 years: 35% 3 to 5 years: 15% 6 years or more: 16%
Status of business operator	Owner: 76% Manager: 24%	Owner: 31% Manager: 69%
Level of education of operator	College level or better: 76% High school level or less: 24%	College level or better: 39% High school level or less: 61%
Gender of operator	Male: 76% Female: 24%	Male: 73% Female: 27%
Use of private contractor for waste management	Yes: 23% No: 77%	Yes: 16% No: 84%
Sorting waste	Yes: 76% No: 24%	Yes: 45% No: 55%
Adherence to waste management regulations	Yes: 95% No: 5%	Yes: 52% No: 48%
Personal hygiene	Excellent: 9% Very good: 43% Satisfactory: 37% Less than satisfactory: 10% Poor: 1%	Excellent: 0% Very good: 21% Satisfactory: 41% Less than satisfactory: 33% Poor: 5%
Perception on the benefits of proper waste management	Excellent: 3% Very good: 56% Satisfactory: 35% Less than satisfactory: 5% Poor: 1%	Excellent: 1% Very good: 6% Satisfactory: 29% Less than satisfactory: 55% Poor: 9%
Source reduction of waste	Yes: 80% No: 20%	Yes: 52% No: 48%
Amount of waste generated in 1,000 kg per week	$\leq$0.9 : 25% 1 to 1.9 : 46% 2 to 4.9 : 27% 5 to 9.9 : 2% $\geq$10 : 0%	$\leq$0.9 : 49% 1 to 1.9 : 42% 2 to 4.9 : 8% 5 to 9.9 : 1% $\geq$10 : 0%
Enough trash cans available for customers	Yes: 77% No: 23%	Yes: 46% No: 54%
Regular inspection of premises by municipality	Yes: 84% No: 16%	Yes: 41% No: 59%
Familiarity of operator with White Paper on Waste Management	Yes: 86% No: 14%	Yes: 28% No: 72%

TABLE 2: List of top 15 significant associations from Pearson's chi-square tests of associations with overall efficiency in waste disposal ($P < 0.001$).

Variable of study associated with overall efficiency in waste management	Observed chi-square value	P value
Adherence: degree of adherence to waste management regulations	716.04	0.0000
Perception: perception on the benefits of proper waste management	705.99	0.0000
Trashcan: availability of enough trash cans for customers	701.42	0.0000
Status: status of person operating business (owner or employee)	469.21	0.0000
Frequency: frequency at which business premises are inspected by municipality	299.57	0.0000
Hygiene: personal hygiene of employees at business premises	251.72	0.0000
Maintenance: degree of maintenance of trash bins and their environment in business premises	167.09	0.0000
Cleanliness: degree to which business premises are kept clean	139.88	0.0000
Education: level of education of business operator	127.52	0.0000
Inspection: regular inspection of premises by municipal workers	115.14	0.0000
Volume: volume of waste generated	109.59	0.0000
Contractor: use of private contractors for waste management	104.44	0.0000
White Paper: familiarity with White Paper on waste management	103.87	0.0000
Implement: degree to which a waste management plan is implemented	100.11	0.0000
Sort: sorting waste generated at source	93.12	0.0000

TABLE 3: Odds ratios estimated from binary logistic regression analysis.

Variable	Unadjusted OR and 95% C.I.$^{+}$	P value	Adjusted* OR and 95% C.I.$^{+}$
Poor adherence	9.18 (6.43, 12.55)	0.000	9.17 (6.42, 12.54)
Wrong perception	8.84 (6.02, 11.36)	0.000	8.81 (6.01, 11.35)
Failure to provide customers with enough trash cans	3.17 (1.48, 5.89)	0.000	3.15 (1.46, 5.87)
Status of operator (owner, manager)	2.71 (1.69, 4.35)	0.000	2.69 (1.66, 4.32)

* Adjustment was done for level of education, gender, and location of business.
$^{+}$C.I.: Confidence interval.

likely to be inefficient in the management of solid waste in comparison with a business in which enough trash cans are provided to customers. The adjusted odds ratio of the variable status of operator is 2.69. This shows that an outlet that is operated by someone who does not own the business being operated is 2.69 times as likely to beinefficient in the proper management of solid waste in comparison with an outlet that is operated by someone who actually owns the business. Adjusted odds ratios are more reliable than unadjusted odds ratios in epidemiological studies of this kind. In this study, the estimated odds ratios were adjusted for two potential confounding variables (level of education of business operator and the physical location of business). The adjusted odds ratios did not differ much from the unadjusted odds ratios, thereby showing that none of the variables used for adjustment was a confounding variable. There was no effect modifying variable.

3.1. Goodness-of-Fit Tests. The reliability of the fitted logistic regression model was assessed using standard goodness-of-fit tests suitable for binary logistic regression analysis [28]. The classification table showed that the fitted model had an overall percentage of correct classification of 88.78%, a percentage sensitivity of 57.06%, and a percentage specificity of 95.33%. This shows that the fitted model is highly reliable in accurately classifying observations. The Hosmer-Lemeshow goodness-of-fit test gave a P-value of 0.0701, a figure which is greater than 0.05, thereby showing that there was no reason to doubt the reliability of the fitted logistic regression model. Figure 1 below shows a plot of sensitivity/specificity versus probability cut-off point. The two plots cross each other fairly close to the vertical axis. This shows that the fitted model is adequately sensitive and specific.

Figure 2 below shows a Receiver Operating Characteristic (ROC) plot. The magnitude of the area that lies under the ROC plot is a measure of variation explained by the fitted logistic regression model. In this case, the area under the ROC plot is 88.82%, a figure that is significantly above 75%. The unexplained proportion of variation is equal to 11.18%. The large proportion of explained variation and the small proportion of unexplained variation show that the fitted model is highly reliable in explaining variability in waste disposal as a function of the explanatory variables used for logistic regression analysis.

The likelihood ratio test is used for assessing the collective efficiency of the 8 predictor variables used for performing binary logistic regression analysis. At the 5% level of significance, a P-value that is smaller than 0.05 shows that the 8 predictor variables used for performing binary logistic regression analysis are jointly efficient. In this case, the P-value from the likelihood ratio test is equal to 0.000, a figure that is smaller than 0.05. This small P-value shows that the 8 predictor variables used for binary logistic regression

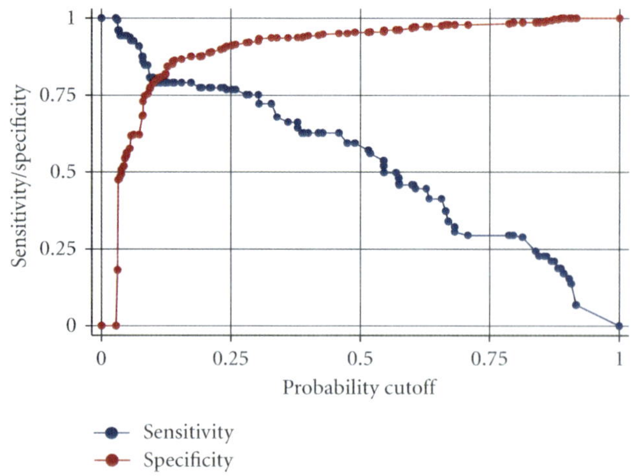

Figure 1: Plot of sensitivity/specificity versus probability cut-off point.

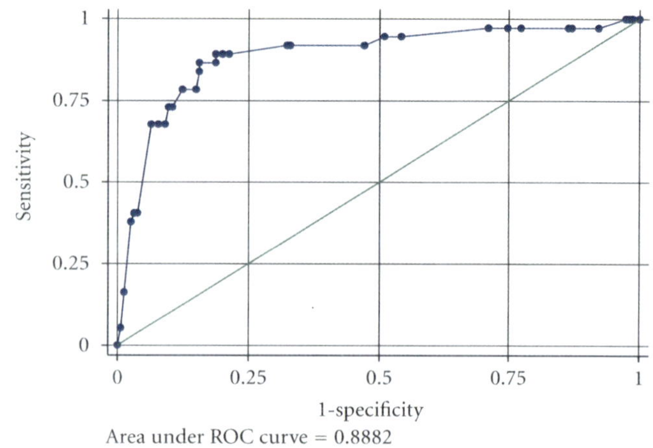

Figure 2: Area under the Receiver Operating Characteristic (ROC) plot.

analysis are collectively efficient in accounting for failure in the proper disposal of waste.

Multilevel analysis [29] was used in order to estimate the extent of variation with regards to efficiency in the management of waste by geographical zone and category of business enterprise. Table 1 provides frequency distributions for each of the 7 categories of business (agricultural, commercial, construction, industrial, institutional, municipal, and processing and manufacturing) as well as 5 geographical locations (central, east, west, north, south) of the city of Tshwane that were considered in performing multilevel analysis. Results obtained from multilevel analysis showed that there were significant differences among the 7 categories of waste. The results showed that 23.05% of the total variation in efficiency is due to differences among the 7 categories of waste produced by business enterprises operating in the city of Tshwane. The results also showed that businesses within the same category of waste and geographical location were equally efficient in the management of solid waste.

4. Discussion

The key objective of research was to identify and quantify factors that affect efficiency in the management of solid waste by businesses that are operated in the city of Tshwane. The study has shown that efficiency in the management of solid waste is significantly influenced by 4 key predictor variables of study. These 4 influential predictor variables are lack of adherence to municipal bylaws and regulations, wrong perception on the potential benefits of proper waste management, failure to provide customers with enough trash cans for waste disposal, and the practice of operating businesses by employed managers, in a decreasing order of importance. In the city of Tshwane, municipal solid waste consists of everyday items such as product packaging, empty bottles and cans, grass clippings, furniture, clothing, left-over food, newspapers, appliances, paint, batteries, pieces of metals, and so forth. Such solid waste is generated by businesses, households, schools, hospitals, and visitors travelling into the city on foot or by other modes of transport such as cars, train, taxi, or bus. The Health Department of the city of Tshwane [2] has a municipal bylaw that stipulates how solid waste should be packaged, sorted, collected, and disposed of by inhabitants of the city. The bylaw encourages inhabitants of the city to practice source reduction of solid waste, recycling, and composting (collecting organic waste such as left-over food and garden refuse, storing these wastes under conditions that are designed to help them break down naturally, and then use the resulting compost as a natural fertilizer). According to the South African National Department of Environmental Affairs and Tourism [4], the disposal and combustion of municipal solid waste is conducted by the use of landfills, the conversion of non-recyclable waste materials into useable heat, electricity, or fuel, combustion, and transfer stations. Although the use of such mechanisms is consistent with the municipal bylaw in the city of Tshwane, the mechanisms have been poorly utilized mostly due to lack of infrastructural development and technical skills.

Findings from this study are not surprising. The results are expected from a typical sub-Saharan African country in which poverty, unemployment, and massive immigration into urban centres prevail. Environmental hazards arising from the decomposition of solid waste under oversaturated conditions [33] and dumping of solid waste in illegal landfills often cause sludge [34]. Such problems are particularly evident in suburbs of Tshwane such as Mamelodi and Marabastad. In this regard, the city of Tshwane can be viewed as a combination of clean white suburbs and dirty black townships. Generally, awareness and regard for environmental sanitation are poor in black suburbs. The other key environmental hazard is caused by arbitrary landfill sites that dot the peripheries of the city of Tshwane. Green waste from landfills produces potentially harmful gasses such as methane and leachates. Such products pollute water reservoirs in the city. The study by Snyman and Vorster [17] has found that composting and the pretreatment of municipal waste before landfilling are viable options for the city of Tshwane. Silva et al. [35] as well as Wiszniowski et al. have found that composting and pretreatment of municipal waste before landfilling significantly reduce the volume of solid waste and contributes for overall environmental sanitation [36]. At the moment, the city of Tshwane does not have adequate capacity for large scale composting, and there is an acute need for addressing this shortcoming.

The study has shown that a combination of technical and administrative solutions is required in order to improve efficiency in the management of solid waste in the city of Tshwane. To separate waste generated at the various businesses, it is necessary to provide businesses with custom-made containers that are suitable. It is equally important to enforce municipal bylaws in order to ensure compliance. The frequency of collecting waste should be balanced with the volume of waste generated by the various businesses. Studies conducted in various parts of the developed world [37] have shown that there are economic benefits in outsourcing the collection and disposal of recyclable waste to the informal sector, and that sanitary landfills should be used for the final disposal of solid waste. In addition to enforcing the law with vigour, it is equally important to provide community based health education on environmental sanitation by collaborating with the Department of Health. Awareness campaigns and socioeconomic incentives could be provided by civic society and nongovernmental organizations that have a vested interest in improving environmental sanitation and cleanliness. Since most of the waste generated in the city of Tshwane is organic, it is recyclable. As such, the provision of incentives and education at the grass-roots level carries a clear socioeconomic merit. Composting is a form of aerobic treatment, and is suitable for treating organic waste in the city of Tshwane. According to Barlaz [38], facilities used for storage and collection of waste must be compatible with each other. Waste disposal and processing sites must be located strategically so that the cost of waste collection, disposal and processing becomes optimal. The city of Tshwane needs to make the necessary initial investment available in order to benefit from composting in the long-run. Extensive waste management research conducted in various parts of China [39] has shown that educating rural as well as urban people on how to produce compost by using low technology has long-term economic benefits to big metropolitan municipalities such as Tshwane. Large scale compost activities require massive infrastructural investment and skills based training. Research conducted in Nigeria [40] has shown that strategic partnerships and collaboration among academic and research institutions and municipalities have the potential for enhancing overall efficiency in waste management, skills development, and the creation of employment opportunities in municipalities such as Tshwane. One particular area of waste that stands to benefit out of such partnership is the management and processing of plastic and e-waste. This is because unprocessed plastic waste has almost no economic benefit. The collection and recycling of plastic waste is characterized by serious challenges and difficulties in the city of Tshwane. The city of Tshwane has no coherent policy on the collection of e-waste. Neither does it provide clear incentives to entrepreneurs who wish to collect, classify, and process e- and plastic waste. Since e-waste could be hazardous, there is a dire need to build capacity in the classification of e-waste into one of two categories (harmful or hazardous), and processing each category of waste by utilizing an appropriate form of technology. There is an acute need for providing incentives, enforcing municipal bylaws, the provision of health and sanitary education, and a comprehensive monitoring and evaluation programme for assessing the progress made in this regard regularly. A well-functioning integrated solid waste management system can only be realized in the city of Tshwane by providing clear incentives for good practice and behaviour, and by severely penalizing irresponsible behaviour in the city. Liu et al. [41] have found that the provision of direct socioeconomic incentives, clear guidelines on the collection, disposal, and processing of e- and plastic waste, as well as a strict enforcement of municipal bylaws is required for improving overall efficiency in the management of e and plastic waste in the city of Tshwane.

The efficient management of solid waste produced by enterprises that conduct business in the various parts of the city of Tshwane has numerous economic, sanitary, and health-related benefits to the inhabitants of the city. Disposing of waste in landfills is much better than using open dumps. Up until recently, emphasis has been placed on waste disposal, and not on management, recycling, and composting. Poor management of waste has an adverse impact on the environment and public health, particularly in townships such as Mamelodi, Marabastad, Soshanguve, and Attridgeville. In these townships, waste is managed poorly, and landfills are inappropriately sited, designed, managed, and operated. Until recently, the management of waste generated by businesses operating in the city has not been given due consideration. The waste management that took place focused mainly on waste disposal and was reactive in that it addressed needs as they occurred. Holistic, integrated waste management planning was poorly done. The low priority that was historically accorded to waste management has resulted in waste impacting detrimentally on the South African environment and on human health. Standards for medical waste incinerators are generally inadequate in comparison with international best practice.

Efficient waste disposal is a process that requires the full collaboration of all stakeholders on a community based collaborative approach. In addition to providing sanitary education and inspection services to the businesses, clear incentives must be provided to ensure maximum success. The enforcement of regulations, the provision of incentives, adequate logistical resources, additional manpower, financial rewards, public-private partnerships, and awareness campaigns are all essential.

The treatment of waste produced by the businesses in the city of Tshwane is similar to waste produced in a typical developing nation in the sense that treatment of this waste involves simply a reduction of its volume by use of methods such as baling or shredding although incineration and composting is practiced at a small scale. The emphasis remains on disposal of general waste by landfill without treatment as the lowest cost disposal option, as landfill airspace is still available in South Africa. The lack of pretreatment of general waste before disposal is therefore currently not regarded as a problem in South Africa. Incineration of general waste and hazardous waste is not acceptable to many stakeholders due to the poor operation of many existing facilities and noncompliance with existing by-laws. Incineration is not economically feasible in South Africa since its warm climate limits the market for the energy derived from the incineration process. The majority of operating incinerators in South Africa are used for the treatment of infectious medical waste.

Increasing general awareness about the benefits of proper waste disposal is a key requirement for success. The number of waste disposal sites is limited, and the disposal of waste is expensive. Since there are not enough of these facilities, hazardous waste is often transported over long distances, resulting in increased risks of accidents and higher transport costs. Some other helpful steps are to undertake an integrated plan in which waste is gathered and disposed of efficiently based on mutual collaboration among stakeholders, strengthening the technical, financial, administrative, and operating capacity of the institutions in the basic environmental sanitation sector, and encouraging health education and community promotion activities, which are basic to the success of waste collection and disposal, especially at taxi ranks and the streets at the central business district of Pretoria, to provide clear incentives to businesses that improve the quality of waste collection and disposal based on generally accepted standards. Technical cooperation among stakeholders must be directed toward the strengthening of institutions in the basic environmental sanitation sector and emphasis should be given to the following activities: operation and maintenance, community promotion, training, administration and management, the preparation of plans and studies helpful for efficient waste disposal, and the application of technologies that are helpful for efficient waste disposal.

The need for inspection becomes acute during rainy seasons and prolonged civil actions. In-depth interviews conducted with some of the managers of the 1,034 businesses that took part in the study have revealed that the businesses suffer enormously during prolonged strike actions. Waste material gets vandalized by scavengers as a result of delay in collection by service providers. It is too risky to leave waste uncollected during rainy seasons as waste could easily be mixed up with excreta that could be washed away by rainwater, ending up in wells and streams. The germs in the excreta could then easily contaminate drinking or washing water. In such situations, diarrhoeal diseases can spread from one person to another. Failure to dispose of waste can have a significant effect on the health of communities. Where refuse is not disposed of properly, it can lead to pollution of surface water, as rain washes refuse into rivers and streams. There may also be a significant risk of groundwater contamination. Refuse disposed of in storm drains may cause blockages and encourage fly and mosquito breeding. It is therefore very important that household waste is disposed of properly. All business premises operating in the city of Tshwane must be inspected for environmental sanitation and cleanliness regularly with a view to encourage and reward good practice, and to penalize irresponsible behaviour. Municipal bylaws on the collection, disposal and management of waste must be enforced with enough vigour and commitment. Failure to do so can easily result in frustration among businesses that obey municipal guidelines and regulations on waste management.

5. Conclusions

The study showed that 17% of the 1,034 businesses were not efficient enough with regards to the proper collection, disposal, and management of solid waste. The study has shown that efficiency in the management of solid waste is adversely affected by lack of adherence to municipal bylaws and regulations on proper waste management, wrong perception on the potential benefits of proper waste disposal, failure to provide customers with enough trash cans at business premises, and the operation of businesses by employed managers, in a decreasing order of importance. Lack of adherence to municipal bylaws and regulations that are essential for proper waste management constitutes a key challenge in the city of Tshwane. The presence of wrong perception on the potential benefits of waste disposal is also a well known hurdle. To rectify this issue, a combination of three interventions is necessary. The first intervention is to enforce municipal bylaws with vigour. The second intervention is to provide incentives to businesses that manage solid waste properly in accordance with guidelines provided by the city of Tshwane. Regulatory and legislative actions must be taken against those who fail to respect municipal bylaws that are related to cleanliness and proper waste management. The efficient disposal of waste generated by businesses operating in the city has direct economic benefits to all inhabitants of the city. Accordingly, waste should be gathered efficiently and disposed of in accordance with the waste collection and management plan produced by the city of Tshwane. Management of waste must start at the lowest level. The third intervention is to actively promote an education campaign in all parts of the city of Tshwane with a view to ensure the full collaboration of businesses conducting business in the city.

Based on findings of this particular study, the following recommendations are made to the city of Tshwane in order to improve overall efficiency in the management of solid waste that is generated by businesses operating in the city.

(i) The city of Tshwane must produce and implement an integrated plan for the management of solid waste in collaboration and partnership with the relevant stakeholders in the city so that each of the role players in the waste management chain can investment adequately in basic environmental sanitation.

(ii) An initial infrastructural investment needs to be made by the city of Tshwane in order to build adequate capacity for commercial composting. This should be done in collaboration with business enterprises so that they can share the financial burden at the initial stage, and benefit from compost-related business opportunities in the long-run.

(iii) The city of Tshwane must strive to increase awareness about the potential benefits of proper waste collection and disposal by promoting health education on environmental sanitation and techniques that are useful for collecting and sorting waste. Incentives must be provided to businesses that do a good job in terms of the proper collection and disposal of solid waste. The city must support community-based health promotion activities undertaken by nongovernmental organizations. The city must also support research initiatives conducted by academic and research institutions in areas that are related to waste management, environmental sanitation, and personal hygiene by funding them partially or fully.

(iv) The city of Tshwane must improve the conditions of employment of municipal workers responsible for waste collection and disposal.

(v) The city of Tshwane and Gauteng Department of Health must provide technical assistance to businesses that do not have their own waste management plans so that such businesses can contribute for overall efficiency in environmental sanitation.

Conflict of Interests

The authors have no conflict of interests to disclose.

Acknowledgments

The authors would like to acknowledge the various businesses that willingly took part in the study, the Health Department of the city of Tshwane for providing technical and administrative assistance during planning and data collection, and Statistics South Africa for providing the authors with the sampling frame and GIS map of business enterprises operating in the city of Tshwane.

References

[1] Statistics South Africa (SSA), Income and expenditure survey 2010/2011, 2012, http://www.statssa.gov.za/ies/welcome.asp.

[2] City of Tshwane Metropolitan Municipality (CTMM), State of the environment report on Pretoria, 2012, http://www.ceroi.net/reports/pretoria/issues/qual_env/state.htm.

[3] City of Tshwane Metropolitan Municipality(CTMM), Municipal information and services, 2012, http://www.tshwane.gov.za/Services/Pages/default.aspx.

[4] South African National Department of Environmental Affairs and Tourism (SANDEAT), National policy on waste management, 2012, http://www.sciencedirect.com/Science.

[5] L. O. Mbeng, P. S. Phillips, and R. Fairweather, "Developing sustainable waste management practice: application of Q methodology to construct new strategy component in Limbe-Cameroon," *The Open Waste Management Journal*, vol. 2, no. 1, pp. 27–36, 2009.

[6] D. C. Wilson and A. Scheinberg, "What is good practice in solid waste management?" *Waste Management and Research*, vol. 28, no. 12, pp. 1055–1056, 2010.

[7] M. Grosso, A. Motta, and L. Rigamonti, "Efficiency of energy recovery from waste incineration, in the light of the new Waste Framework Directive," *Waste Management*, vol. 30, no. 7, pp. 1238–1243, 2010.

[8] S. T. Wagland, F. Veltre, and P. J. Longhurst, "Development of an image-based analysis method to determine the physical composition of a mixed waste material," *Waste Management*, vol. 32, no. 2, pp. 245–248, 2012.

[9] G. J. Oh, "International comparative study of 3R and waste management policy developments," *Material Cycles and Waste Management*, vol. 13, no. 1, pp. 86–102, 2011.

[10] M. Read, M. K. Gregory, and P. S. Phillips, "Driving the waste prevention agenda—an evaluation of weighing kerbside household waste arisings methodology, in Dorset, UK," *Journal of Solid Waste Technology and Management*, vol. 34, no. 3, pp. 161–176, 2008.

[11] N. Matsueda and Y. Nagase, "Economic instruments and resource use in a recyclable product market," *Economics Bulletin*, vol. 17, no. 21, pp. 1–10, 2011.

[12] A. Bernstad, J. Jansen, and H. Aspegren, "Local strategies for efficient management of solid household waste—the full-scale Augustenborg experiment," *Waste Management v Research*, vol. 30, no. 2, pp. 200–212, 2012.

[13] S. I. Sakai, H. Yoshida, Y. Hirai et al., "International comparative study of 3R and waste management policy developments," *Journal of Material Cycles and Waste Management*, vol. 13, no. 2, pp. 86–102, 2011.

[14] E. Dijkgraaf and R. H. J. M. Gradus, "Cost savings in unit-based pricing of household waste. The case of the Netherlands," *Resource and Energy Economics*, vol. 26, no. 4, pp. 353–371, 2004.

[15] D. Laner and H. Rechberger, "Quantitative evaluation of waste prevention on the level of small and medium sized enterprises (SMEs)," *Waste Management*, vol. 29, no. 2, pp. 606–613, 2009.

[16] C. Berglund, "The assessment of households' recycling costs: the role of personal motives," *Ecological Economics*, vol. 56, no. 4, pp. 560–569, 2006.

[17] J. Snyman and K. Vorster, "Sustainability of composting as an alternative waste management option for developing countries: a case study of the City of Tshwane," *Waste Management & Research*, vol. 29, pp. 1222–1231, 2011.

[18] A. J. Caplan, T. C. Grijalva, and P. M. Jakus, "Waste not or want not? A contingent ranking analysis of curbside waste disposal options," *Ecological Economics*, vol. 43, no. 2-3, pp. 185–197, 2002.

[19] P. Suman, E. Thys, A. Mfoukou-Ntsakala et al., "Methodology for assessing determinants of manure use in urban areas of Africa," *Waste Management and Research*, vol. 28, no. 12, pp. 1076–1086, 2010.

[20] A. Scheinberg, D. C. Wilson, and L. Rodic, *Solid Waste Management in the World's Cities: Third edition in UN-Habitat's State of Water and Sanitation in the World's Cities Series*, Earthscan for UN-Habitat, New York, NY, USA, 2010.

[21] P. Vicente and E. Reis, "Factors influencing households' participation in recycling," *Waste Management and Research*, vol. 26, no. 2, pp. 140–146, 2008.

[22] M. Bates, L. O. Mbeng, and P. S. Phillips, "Managing E-waste—a reuse strategy for UK computers to facilitate developments in third sector organization composting in Cameroon," *Journal of Solid Waste Technology and Management*, vol. 34, no. 4, pp. 204–212, 2008.

[23] United States Environmental Protection Agency (USEPA). Municipal solid waste in the United States: 2005 facts and figures, executive summary, United States Environmental Protection Agency, Office of Solid Waste, Washington, DC, USA, 2006.

[24] O. Hage, P. Söderholm, and C. Berglund, "Norms and economic motivation in household recycling: empirical evidence from Sweden," *Resources, Conservation and Recycling*, vol. 53, no. 3, pp. 155–165, 2009.

[25] A. Bernstad, J. Jansen, and H. Aspegren, "Property-close source separation of hazardous waste and waste electrical and electronic equipment—a Swedish case study," *Waste Management*, vol. 31, no. 3, pp. 536–543, 2011.

[26] G. Tchobanoglous, H. Theisen, and S. A. Vigil, *Integrated Solid Waste Management Engineering Principles and Management Issues*, McGraw Hill, New York, NY, USA, 1993.

[27] B. K. Dawson and R. G. Trapp, *Basic Clinical Biostatistics*, McGraw-Hill, New York, NY, USA, 2nd edition, 2004.

[28] D. W. Hosmer and S. Lemeshow, *Applied Logistic Regression*, John Wiley & Sons, New York, NY, USA, 2nd edition, 2000.

[29] A. H. Leyland and H. Goldstein, *Multilevel Modelling of Health Statistics*, John Wiley & Sons, Chichester, UK, 2011.

[30] Canadian Standards Association, ISO/TC207/SC4/JWG. ISO, 14031, 1999(E)—Environmental Performance Evaluation—Guidelines, Canadian Standards Association, Toronto, Canada, 1999.

[31] Canadian Standards Association, ISO/TC207/SC4/JWG. ISO/TR, 14032: 1999-Examples of Environmental Performance Evaluation (EPE), Canadian Standards Association, Toronto, Canada, 1999.

[32] W. L. Kuhre and ISO, *14031-Environmental Performance Evaluation (EPE): Practical Tools for Conducting an Environmental Performance Evaluation*, Prentice Hall, Upper Saddle River, NJ, USA, 1998.

[33] Y. J. Hao, W. X. Wu, S. W. Wu, H. Sun, and Y. X. Chen, "Municipal solid waste decomposition under oversaturated condition in comparison with leachate recirculation," *Process Biochemistry*, vol. 43, no. 1, pp. 108–112, 2008.

[34] B. Mertoglu, B. Calli, B. Inanc, and I. Ozturk, "Evaluation of in situ ammonia removal in an aerated landfill bioreactor," *Process Biochemistry*, vol. 41, no. 12, pp. 2359–2366, 2006.

[35] A. C. Silva, M. Dezotti, and G. L. Sant'Anna, "Treatment and detoxification of a sanitary landfill leachate," *Chemosphere*, vol. 55, no. 2, pp. 207–214, 2004.

[36] J. Wiszniowski, J. Surmacz-Górska, D. Robert, and J. V. Weber, "The effect of landfill leachate composition on organics and nitrogen removal in an activated sludge system with bentonite additive," *Journal of Environmental Management*, vol. 85, no. 1, pp. 59–68, 2007.

[37] X. Liu, J. Shi, X. Qian, Y. Hu, and G. Peng, "One-dimensional model for municipal solid waste (MSW) settlement considering coupled mechanical-hydraulic-gaseous effect and concise calculation," *Waste Management*, vol. 31, no. 12, pp. 2473–2483, 2011.

[38] M. A. Barlaz, "Forest products decomposition in municipal solid waste landfills," *Waste Management*, vol. 26, no. 4, pp. 321–333, 2006.

[39] Y. Chen, Y. Xie, and L. Zhan, "One-dimensional consolidation model for landfills considering solid-liquid-gas interaction," *Chinese Journal of Geotechnical Engineering*, vol. 28, no. 2, pp. 184–190, 2011.

[40] T. Nzeadibe and C. Ajero, "Development impact of advocacy initiatives in solid waste management in Nigeria," *Environment, Development and Sustainability*, vol. 13, pp. 163–177.

[41] X. Liu, J. Shi, X. Qian, Y. Hu, and G. Peng, "One-dimensional model for municipal solid waste (MSW) settlement considering coupled mechanical-hydraulic-gaseous effect and concise calculation," *Waste Management*, vol. 31, no. 12, pp. 2473–2483, 2011.

14

Cadmium Exposure and Pancreatic Cancer in South Louisiana

Brian G. Luckett,[1,2] L. Joseph Su,[1,3] Jennifer C. Rood,[4] and Elizabeth T. H. Fontham[1]

[1] *Epidemiology Program, School of Public Health, Louisiana State University Health Sciences Center, 2020 Gravier Street, 3rd Floor, New Orleans, LA 70112, USA*
[2] *Department of Global Community Health and Behavioral Sciences, School of Public Health and Tropical Medicine, Tulane University, 1440 Canal Street, Suite 2300, New Orleans, LA 70112, USA*
[3] *Epidemiology and Genomics Research Program, Division of Cancer Control and Population Sciences, National Cancer Institute, 6130 Executive Boulevard, Room 5140, MSC 7393, Bethesda, MD 20892, USA*
[4] *Clinical Chemistry Core, Pennington Biomedical Research Center, 6400 Perkins Road, Baton Rouge, LA 70808, USA*

Correspondence should be addressed to Brian G. Luckett, bluckett@tulane.edu

Academic Editor: Habibul Ahsan

Cadmium has been hypothesized to be a pancreatic carcinogen. We test the hypothesis that cadmium exposure is a risk factor for pancreatic cancer with a population-based case-control study sampled from a population with persistently high rates of pancreatic cancer (south Louisiana). We tested potential dietary and nondietary sources of cadmium for their association with urinary cadmium concentrations which reflect long-term exposure to cadmium due to the accumulation of cadmium in the kidney cortex. Increasing urinary cadmium concentrations were significantly associated with an increasing risk of pancreatic cancer (2nd quartile OR = 3.34, 3rd = 5.58, 4th = 7.70; test for trend $P \leq 0.0001$). Potential sources of cadmium exposure, as documented in the scientific literature, found to be statistically significantly associated with increased risk of pancreatic cancer included working as a plumber, pipefitter or welder (OR = 5.88) and high consumption levels of red meat (4th quartile OR = 6.18) and grains (4th quartile OR = 3.38). Current cigarette smoking, at least 80 pack years of smoking, occupational exposure to cadmium and paints, working in a shipyard, and high consumption of grains were found to be statistically significantly associated with increased concentrations of urinary cadmium. This study provides epidemiologic evidence that cadmium is a potential human pancreatic carcinogen.

1. Introduction

South Louisiana has experienced persistently high mortality rates of pancreatic cancer since at least the 1950s [1], and mapping of mortality from pancreatic cancer in the United States has found significantly elevated rates in southern Louisiana [2]. From 2000 to 2004, south-central Louisiana, the Acadiana region, had the highest incidence rate in the state with 15.9 cases per 100,000 residents [3].

Cadmium is a known human carcinogen [4] and has been hypothesized as a cause of human pancreatic cancer [5]. There is animal model evidence to suggest that it is a plausible pancreatic carcinogen [6]. Cadmium induces trans-differentiation of pancreatic cells [5] and increases synthesis of DNA in the pancreas, possibly through increased synthesis of metallothionein [7]. Metallothioneins are cysteine-rich, low-molecular-weight proteins that bind to xenobiotic heavy metals such as cadmium in the detoxification process [8].

Pancreatic cancer patients were found to have significantly higher serum cadmium levels than noncancer patients in Egypt [9]. However, serum concentration of cadmium may not reflect chronic exposure, typical of many environmental carcinogenic processes, since the half-life of cadmium in blood is only 2 to 3 months [10]. Urinary cadmium concentrations have been found to be a better indicator of long-term cadmium exposure than blood levels due to accumulation of cadmium in the kidney cortex [11, 12].

Higher urinary cadmium concentrations have been found to be associated with increased risk of certain cancers. Menke et al. [13] found that higher creatinine-adjusted urinary cadmium levels were associated with increased cancer mortality among men in the NHANES III Mortality Study. Nawrot et al. [14] found that higher urinary cadmium concentrations were associated with significantly increased incidence of all cancers and lung cancer specifically in a Belgian population-based cohort, while Arisawa et al. [15] found a similar effect among a Japanese cohort. Increased urinary cadmium levels have also been found to be associated with increased risk of breast cancer [16, 17] and bladder cancer [18]. Increased cadmium exposure has been shown to be associated with increased risk of renal cancers [19], endometrial cancer [20], and prostate cancer [21], but these studies did not use urinary cadmium excretion as a biomarker.

Cigarette smoke is a known source of cadmium due to the ability of the *Nicotiana* species to concentrate cadmium. Cadmium oxide released during the burning of a cigarette is highly bioavailable with smokers demonstrating 2 to 3 times the amount of cadmium in their kidneys as nonsmokers [22]. Cigarette smoking is an established risk factor for pancreatic cancer [23–25] with a recent meta-analysis finding about a 75% increase in risk [26]. Although the specific tobacco carcinogens that are linked to pancreatic cancer are not well established [27], cadmium is one possibility. Each cigarette contains 1 to 2 micrograms of cadmium [28].

Phosphate fertilizers and sewage sludge used as fertilizer contain cadmium [29]. Cadmium chloride is used in the production of some pesticides [30]. Continued applications of fertilizers and pesticides have raised cadmium concentrations in Swedish top soil by approximately 30 percent in the period from 1918 to 1980 [31]. Grain dust may contain residual cadmium from fertilizers or pesticides and may contain fungicides using cadmium carbonate [30]. However, cadmium from fertilizer and pesticide applications may not remain isolated. A study of metals in household dust conducted in southern Louisiana found higher mean cadmium concentrations in both indoor and outdoor dust samples in rural households than in urban households [32]. Cadmium from natural sources or from anthropogenic contamination may make its way into well water [33].

Cadmium acetate is used in the refining process to remove mercaptans from crude oil and gasoline [34]. Cadmium has been found in automotive lubricating oils and in diesel oil [35]. Fossil fuel combustion releases cadmium into the air [30].

Cadmium sulfide is used in the manufacture of certain paints to resist blackening by hydrogen sulfide [30]. In addition to the application of cadmium paints, removal of cadmium paints by scraping or blasting may also expose workers [36].

Other metals may contain some cadmium impurities that are released when the metal is smelted, cast, welded, or soldered. Cadmium alloys are used for soldering aluminum [30]. Welders and pipefitters may be occupationally exposed to cadmium through welding fumes [36]. Persons employed in ship yards may also be occupationally exposed [36].

Portland cement contains cadmium [37], and cadmium may also be used as an anticorrosive coating or present as an impurity in galvanized coatings on rebar used in reinforced concrete.

For nonsmokers, food is the primary source of cadmium exposure [22]. Approximately two-thirds of dietary cadmium intake is from plant sources with the remaining one-third coming from animal products [22]. Previous research has found an increased risk of pancreatic cancer among persons residing in south Louisiana consuming large quantities of rice, grains, and pork [23].

Rice and seafood are staples of the south Louisiana diet and may increase exposure to cadmium in this population. Cadmium bioaccumulates in grains and shellfish through uptake of naturally occurring cadmium and cadmium introduced to the environment through industrial emissions, fossil fuel combustion, pesticides, and chemical fertilizers [11]. Cadmium has been detected in high levels in rice in many parts of the world [38, 39]. Shimbo et al. [40] and Watanabe [41] found a correlation between cadmium intake and urinary cadmium concentrations among Japanese women with high consumption levels of rice.

High concentrations of cadmium in mollusks and crustaceans have been demonstrated [41–43]. Elevated cadmium levels have been found in oysters, shrimp, crabs, and crawfish [42, 44, 45] and in rice from south Louisiana (unpublished data).

We test the hypothesis that chronic cadmium exposure is positively associated with pancreatic cancer risk. To address this hypothesis, we regressed disease status on urinary cadmium levels and potential sources of cadmium exposure in a case-control study in south-central Louisiana. We also examined the association between potential sources of cadmium exposure and urinary cadmium concentration to address whether the risk factors we found for pancreatic cancer could be due to cadmium.

2. Materials and Methods

We limited eligibility for cases and controls to noninstitutionalized individuals older than 20 years of age and resident in one of eight south Louisiana parishes (counties) at the time of diagnosis for cases or ascertainment for controls. This human subjects research was reviewed and approved by the Louisiana State University Health Sciences Center: New Orleans, Institutional Review Board. We asked attending physicians for permission before contacting their patients, and every interviewee gave us informed consent.

In collaboration with the Louisiana Tumor Registry, we rapidly ascertained incident cases of pancreatic cancer diagnosed between March 1, 2001, and May 31, 2005, from south Louisiana hospitals. Although we ascertained most cases within one month of diagnosis, 60 percent were already deceased or too ill to participate by the time we attempted to contact them. Seventy-eight percent of cases that were able to participate did so. Since biologic specimens were necessary, no proxy interviews were conducted.

We randomly selected a population-based control group from driver's license and state-issued identification card files for subjects under 65 years of age and from Medicare rolls for subjects 65 years of age or older. Fifty-four percent of the eligible controls we identified participated. Control subjects were frequency matched on age, race (but not ethnicity), and gender in a 2 to 1 ratio to cases. We did not individually match controls to cases on parish of residence to avoid overmatching on environmental exposures; but all controls were residents of the same 8-parish catchment area from which we ascertained cases.

We administered a standardized and previously validated questionnaire to both cases and controls and asked them to provide a one-time blood and urine sample at the time of interview. The questionnaire included demographic data, residential and occupational histories, personal and family medical histories, tobacco and alcohol use, and other relevant information. Also included was a food frequency questionnaire developed at the National Cancer Institute (NCI) which we modified for use in this particular population by adding foods that are common to the south Louisiana diet [46]. The modified Block-NCI questionnaire was used because it employs both frequency and serving size data (ascertained with a visual guide) in the computation of average food consumption. We asked respondents to report their usual diet one year prior to interview to account for dietary changes associated with pancreatic cancer.

The spot urine samples were analyzed at the Pennington Biomedical Research Center on a Perkin Elmer atomic absorption spectrophotometer equipped with a graphite furnace. We measured creatinine in the urine samples using a Beckman-Coulter DXC 600 Pro. Cadmium concentrations are reported here as micrograms per gram of creatinine (μg cadmium/g creatinine).

Cajun ethnicity has previously been demonstrated to be associated with an increased risk of pancreatic cancer in this population [23]. We defined "Cajun" for the purposes of this study as respondents who self-identified themselves as ethnically Cajun and reported that the French language was spoken in their home when they were children. This definition eliminated those persons who identify themselves as Cajun due to cultural affinity. We considered both African-Americans and Whites who met these criteria to be Cajun.

We adjusted for cigarette smoking in the regression models using two measures: pack years (included as a continuous variable) and whether a subject was a current smoker (defined as having smoked cigarettes within three years of interview). Thus, former smokers were defined as quitting at least three years prior to interview. We chose these variable definitions of current and former smoker to capture the expected effect of relatively recent tobacco exposure on urinary excretion of cadmium.

In addition to matching and smoking variables, our models of disease status also included variables for completion of high school, the typical number of alcoholic drinks consumed per day, and whether the subject had any first-degree relatives (parent, sibling, or child) who had been diagnosed with pancreatic cancer. To evaluate whether there is an association between potential cadmium exposures and urinary concentrations of cadmium, we regressed urinary cadmium concentrations on potential sources of cadmium separately with adjustment for matching parameters, pack years, current smoking status, and body weight and height.

We used unconditional logistic regression to calculate odds ratios and confidence intervals for disease risk adjusting for established risk factors for pancreatic cancer and frequency matching variables. We used linear regression to estimate the contribution of potential cadmium sources to urinary cadmium concentrations. We found that the distribution of urinary cadmium concentrations was skewed to the right, but we were able to normalize them using a natural log transformation. We present here the exponentials of the means and coefficients for the natural log transformed values in order to make them comparable to the untransformed values also presented. Our tests for trend were performed by regressing the outcome of interest on the categorical medians instead of categorical dummy variables and including all of the same covariates as previously. All statistical analyses were done using the SAS 9.1 software [47].

3. Results

Table 1 presents the distribution of characteristics of cases and controls included in the study. Cases and controls did not vary significantly by those factors on which the control series was frequency matched: age at interview, race, and gender. Since pancreatic cancer has very poor survival, cases were interviewed within weeks of diagnosis. Therefore, age at interview is practically the same as age at diagnosis.

Of the characteristics listed in Table 1, educational attainment and any first-degree relative with pancreatic cancer were significantly associated with disease status when controlling for matching variables only. Controls were significantly more likely to have completed their high school diploma or a general equivalency diploma (GED) than cases. While 77 percent of controls had a high school diploma or GED, only 62 percent of cases had one. Lack of a high school education more than doubled the risk of pancreatic cancer in this sample (OR = 2.12, 95% CI = 1.09–4.12, not shown in table). Only three percent of controls reported a first-degree relative with pancreatic cancer compared to 10 percent of cases (OR = 3.59, 95% CI = 1.09–11.85, not shown in table).

3.1. Potential Nondietary Sources of Cadmium. Table 2(a) presents odds ratios for disease status with 95 percent confidence intervals for potential sources of nondietary cadmium exposure. Levels of urinary cadmium were categorized into incremental quartiles of 0.5 micrograms of cadmium per gram creatinine with the top quartile capturing any values greater than 1.5 μg/g creatinine. The odds ratios indicate a clear monotonic increase in risk of pancreatic cancer with increasing urinary cadmium concentrations (test for trend $P \leq 0.0001$, not shown in table). Using the group with the lowest concentrations as the referent, the next concentration level group had an odds ratio of 3.34 (95% CI: 1.38–8.07), followed by an odds ratio of 5.58 (95% CI: 2.03–15.34) for the third quartile and 7.70 (95% CI: 3.06–19.34) for the highest levels of urinary cadmium concentration. Urinary cadmium data were not available for all subjects either because the subject did not provide a sample ($n = 16$) or did not provide a sufficient quantity for analysis ($n = 5$). The urinary cadmium datum for one control subject was

Table 1: Demographic characteristics of the study population.

Factor	Level	Cases		Controls	
		n	%	n	%
Gender	Male	35	50.7	78	49.4
	Female	34	49.3	80	50.6
Age	<60	19	27.5	46	29.1
	60–69	17	24.6	41	26.0
	70+	33	47.8	71	44.9
Race	White	54	78.3	125	79.1
	African-American	15	21.7	29	18.4
	Other	0	0.0	4	2.5
Cajun	No	18	26.1	51	32.3
	Yes	51	73.9	107	67.7
Education	< High school	26	37.7	37	23.4
	High school +	43	62.3	121	76.6
Any first-degree relative with pancreatic cancer	No	62	89.9	153	96.8
	Yes	7	10.1	5	3.2

excluded from analysis after being identified as an outlier using the studentized residuals approach.

Current smokers showed an elevated risk of pancreatic cancer, but it was not statistically significant (OR = 1.52, 95% CI: 0.59–3.94). Being a former smoker (quitting at least three years prior to interview) was associated with a nonsignificant increased risk of pancreatic cancer in this sample. Pack years smoked were categorized into 40 pack year intervals with 80 or more pack years the highest category (OR = 2.82, 95% CI: 0.82–9.66). No category of pack years was found to confer a statistically significant risk for pancreatic cancer nor was the test for trend across categories statistically significant ($P = 0.34$). Consumption of alcoholic beverages was not associated with increased risk of pancreatic cancer either measured as current alcohol consumption per day or peak lifetime per day consumption and regardless of adjustment for smoking.

Body mass index and prior diagnosis of diabetes, stomach ulcer, or pancreatitis were not significantly associated with pancreatic cancer in this sample. Subjects reporting any first-degree relative that had been diagnosed with any cancer were found to be at increased, although nonsignificant, risk of pancreatic cancer (OR = 3.04, 95% CI: 0.88–10.50). Being Cajun was associated with a nonsignificant increase in risk for pancreatic cancer (OR = 1.52, 95% CI: 0.76–3.03).

A history of living in a residence in which the primary source of drinking water was from a private well showed an elevated risk for pancreatic cancer but was not significant. Having ever lived on any type of farm was not associated with pancreatic cancer, nor was a history of living on a rice farm or a cotton farm. However, a history of living on a sugar cane farm was found to be a significant risk factor for pancreatic cancer (OR = 3.17, 95%: 1.44–6.97).

A self-reported history of residing within one mile of a petroleum refinery elevated the risk of pancreatic cancer in this sample but was not statistically significant (OR = 1.48, 95% CI: 0.50–4.43).

Self-reported occupational exposures to pesticides (whether on a farm or in any setting), paints, heavy metals, and automotive and diesel exhaust were not associated with an increased risk of pancreatic cancer. Occupational exposure to grain dust, cadmium, aluminum, concrete dust, and petroleum products elevated the risk of pancreatic cancer but were not statistically significant. An occupational history of working as a welder, pipefitter, or plumber was associated with an increased risk of pancreatic cancer in this sample (OR = 5.88, 95% CI: 1.33–26.01). An occupational history of working in a shipyard was not associated with significantly elevated risk (OR = 3.13, 95% CI: 0.70–13.96), nor was a history of working in a refinery (OR = 1.87, 95% CI: 0.27–13.19).

The estimated contributions to urinary cadmium concentration associated with potential nondietary sources of cadmium exposure are presented in Table 3(a). Current cigarette smoking was associated with a significant elevation in urinary cadmium concentration compared to never smokers, while being a former smoker was not associated with increased urinary cadmium concentrations. Compared to lifetime nonsmokers, urinary cadmium concentration increased with increasing pack years with a significant test for trend across pack year categories ($P < 0.0001$). However, only the top category of pack years, at least 80, was statistically significantly associated with elevated urinary cadmium concentration.

Living in a residence in which the primary source of drinking water was from a private well was not significantly associated with an increase in urinary cadmium concentration, nor was ever having lived on any type of farm or ever having lived on a rice farm, cotton farm, or sugar cane farm. Occupational use of pesticides, whether on a farm or in some other setting, was not significantly associated with increased urinary cadmium concentrations. Exposure to grain dust was not associated with increased urinary cadmium concentrations.

Table 2: (a) Distributions and risk estimates for potential cadmium exposures. (b) Distributions and risk estimates for potential dietary cadmium exposures.

(a)

Exposure	Level	Cases n	Cases %	Controls n	Controls %	OR[a]	95% CI
Urinary cadmium	<0.5 μg/g creatinine	10	14.5	71	44.9	ref	
	0.5 to <1 μg/g creatinine	16	23.2	33	20.9	3.34	(1.38, 8.07)
	1 to <1.5 μg/g creatinine	13	18.8	18	11.4	5.58	(2.03, 15.34)
	1.5+ μg/g creatinine	24	34.8	19	12	7.70	(3.06, 19.34)
	Missing/outlier	6	8.7	17	10.8	n/a	
Tobacco							
Cigarette smoking	Never	24	34.8	69	43.7	ref	
	Former	19	27.5	58	36.7	0.75	(0.32, 1.77)
	Current	26	37.7	31	19.6	1.52	(0.59, 3.94)
Pack years	0	24	34.8	69	43.7	ref	
	>0–<40	27	39.1	57	36.1	1.23	(0.60, 2.51)
	≥40–<80	11	15.9	26	16.5	0.80	(0.32, 2.03)
	≥80	7	10.1	6	3.8	2.82	(0.82, 9.66)
Residential							
Well water	No	45	65.2	123	77.9	ref	
	Yes	24	34.8	35	22.2	1.51	(0.77, 2.97)
Ever lived on any farm	No	24	34.8	73	46.2	ref	
	Yes	45	65.2	85	53.8	1.56	(0.81, 3.01)
Resided w/in 1 mile of refinery	No	63	91.3	148	93.7	ref	
	Yes	6	8.7	10	6.3	1.48	(0.50, 4.43)
Occupational							
Occupational any pesticides	No	63	91.3	135	85.4	ref	
	Yes	6	8.7	23	14.6	0.47	(0.17, 1.31)
Occupational paints	No	51	73.9	109	69	ref	
	Yes	18	26.1	49	31	0.73	(0.34, 1.60)
Occupational cadmium	No	68	98.6	156	98.7	ref	
	Yes	1	1.5	2	1.3	1.69	(0.14, 20.39)
Worked as pipefitter/plumber/welder	No	62	89.9	155	98.1	ref	
	Yes	7	10.1	3	1.9	5.88	(1.33, 26.01)
Worked in shipyard	No	65	94.2	154	97.5	ref	
	Yes	4	5.8	4	2.5	3.13	(0.70, 13.96)
Worked in refinery	No	67	97.1	155	98.1	ref	
	Yes	2	2.9	3	1.9	1.87	(0.27, 13.19)

(b)

Food	Weekly servings	Cases n	Cases %	Controls n	Controls %	OR[a]	95% CI	Test for trend
All shellfish	<0.5	8	11.6	36	22.8	ref		
	≥0.5–<1	9	13	21	13.3	2.01	(0.63, 6.40)	
	≥1–<2	15	21.7	37	23.4	2.18	(0.78, 6.07)	
	≥2	37	53.6	64	40.5	2.61	(1.02, 6.69)	0.0898

(b) Continued.

Food	Weekly servings	Cases		Controls		OR[a]	95% CI	Test for trend
		n	%	n	%			
All seafood	<0.5	4	5.8	16	10.1	ref		
	≥0.5–<1	5	7.3	23	14.6	1.10	(0.24, 5.13)	
	≥1–<3	25	36.2	61	38.6	2.15	(0.60, 7.71)	
	≥3	35	50.7	58	36.7	2.87	(0.79, 10.47)	0.0562
Beef	<1	12	17.4	34	21.5	ref		
	≥1–<3	21	30.4	56	35.4	1.03	(0.43, 2.48)	
	≥3–<6	19	24.5	46	29.1	1.21	(0.49, 2.98)	
	≥6	17	24.6	22	13.9	2.36	(0.86, 6.49)	0.0579
Pork	<2	10	14.5	52	32.9	ref		
	≥2–<5	26	37.7	56	35.4	2.21	(0.94, 5.21)	
	≥5–<8	13	18.8	29	18.4	2.14	(0.78, 5.84)	
	≥8	20	29	21	13.3	4.44	(1.66, 11.89)	0.0058
All red meat	<4	10	14.5	51	32.3	ref		
	≥4–<8	25	36.2	48	30.4	2.53	(1.05, 6.07)	
	≥8–<12	10	14.5	37	23.4	1.27	(0.45, 3.56)	
	≥12	24	34.8	22	13.9	6.18	(2.28, 16.76)	0.0009
Rice	<1	7	10.1	31	19.6	ref		
	≥1–<5	25	36.2	70	44.3	1.52	(0.57, 4.01)	
	≥5–<10	16	23.2	33	20.9	1.64	(0.55, 4.87)	
	≥10	21	30.4	24	15.2	3.58	(1.17, 10.91)	0.0203
Wheat	<5	15	21.7	47	29.8	ref		
	≥5–<10	21	30.4	54	34.2	1.42	(0.63, 3.20)	
	≥10–<15	16	23.2	22	13.9	2.43	(0.96, 6.14)	
	≥15	17	24.6	35	22.2	1.87	(0.78, 4.48)	0.1282
All grains	<10	6	8.7	24	15.2	ref		
	≥10–<20	20	29	63	39.9	1.48	(0.50, 4.42)	
	≥20–<30	20	29	38	24.1	2.50	(0.83, 7.57)	
	≥30	23	33.3	33	20.9	3.38	(1.10, 10.36)	0.0112

[a]Models include: age at interview, race, gender, pack years, current smoking, alcoholic drinks per day, family history of pancreatic cancer, and completing high school.

Occupational exposures to cadmium and paints were each significantly associated with increases in urinary cadmium concentration as were exposures to aluminum and concrete dust (not shown). Self-reported occupational exposure to cadmium was estimated to elevate urinary cadmium concentration by 4.8 μg cadmium per gram of creatinine ($P < 0.05$), while exposure to aluminum was estimated to elevate urinary cadmium concentrations by 0.8 μg cadmium/g creatinine ($P \leq 0.01$). Exposure to heavy metals such as lead, chromium, and nickel was not significantly associated with an increase in urinary cadmium concentration.

Occupational exposure to automotive or diesel exhaust was not significantly associated with increased urinary cadmium concentration. However, a history of ever having lived within one mile of a petroleum refinery did significantly predict urinary cadmium concentration with an estimated increase of 2.5 μg cadmium/g creatinine.

An occupational history of ever working in a shipyard was significantly associated with an increase in urinary cadmium concentration, but a history of ever having worked in a refinery or as a pipefitter, welder, or plumber was not.

3.2. Potential Dietary Sources of Cadmium. Table 2(b) reports odds ratios by quartiles of weekly servings for various foods commonly consumed in south Louisiana and for which there is evidence that the food may be a source of dietary cadmium.

Crab and crawfish consumption was not individually associated with pancreatic cancer risk. There was a significantly elevated risk associated with the third highest category of shrimp consumption (OR = 2.69, 95% CI 1.24–5.84), but the test of trend was not statistically significant. Consumption of all shellfish combined (shrimp, crabs, and crawfish) was significantly associated with increased risk of pancreatic cancer among subjects consuming at least two servings of shellfish per day compared to those subjects consuming less than one-half serving per day (OR = 2.61, 95% CI: 1.02–6.69) although the test of trend was not significant ($P = 0.09$). Consumption of fish showed elevated risks for

TABLE 3: (a) Means, estimates, and significance levels for potential cadmium exposures on urinary cadmium concentrations. (b) Means, estimates, and significance levels for potential dietary cadmium sources on urinary cadmium concentrations.

(a)

Exposure	Weekly servings	Creatinine-adjusted urinary cadmium (μg/g creatinine) Mean	Coefficient[a]	P value
Tobacco use				
Cigarette smoking	Never	0.4764	ref	
	Former	0.5599	0.9923	0.9705
	Current	1.1647	2.1871	0.0013
Pack years	0	0.4764	ref	
	>0–<40	0.5892	1.0813	0.6806
	≥40–<80	1.1207	1.4802	0.1229
	≥80	1.2859	2.1231	0.0242
Residential				
Drank well water	No	0.6686	ref	
	Yes	0.5620	0.7603	0.1138
Ever lived on any farm	No	0.5901	ref	
	Yes	0.6769	1.1257	0.4449
Resided w/in 1 mile of refinery	No	0.6099	ref	
	Yes	1.3879	2.5056	0.0052
Occupational				
Any pesticides	No	0.6211	ref	
	Yes	0.7567	1.2395	0.3424
Cadmium	No	0.6291	ref	
	Yes	1.5530	4.7979	0.0117
Paints	No	0.6064	ref	
	Yes	0.7131	1.6692	0.0057
Worked in shipyard	No	0.6234	ref	
	Yes	1.1034	2.2175	0.0403
Worked in refinery	No	0.6315	ref	
	Yes	0.9328	1.7401	0.2584
Pipefitter, plumber or welder	No	0.6342	ref	
	Yes	0.7069	1.3642	0.3775

(b)

Food	Weekly servings	Creatinine-adjusted urinary cadmium (μg/g creatinine) Mean	Coefficient[a]	P value	Test for trend
All shellfish	<0.5	0.5910	ref		
	≥0.5–<1	0.7460	1.2048	0.4957	
	≥1–<2	0.6335	1.1813	0.4751	
	≥2	0.6304	1.1845	0.4311	0.6251
All seafood	<0.5	0.8146	ref		
	≥0.5–<1	0.5582	0.7748	0.4658	
	≥1–<3	0.6317	0.9090	0.7416	
	≥3	0.6347	0.9514	0.8648	0.6586

(b) Continued.

Food	Weekly servings	Creatinine-adjusted urinary cadmium (μg/g creatinine)			
		Mean	Coefficient[a]	P value	Test for trend
Beef	<1	0.6552	ref		
	≥1–<3	0.5571	0.8778	0.5393	
	≥3–<6	0.6778	1.0781	0.7274	
	≥6	0.7094	1.2335	0.4129	0.2175
Pork	<2	0.5437	ref		
	≥2–<5	0.6688	1.1852	0.3826	
	≥5–<8	0.5010	0.8883	0.6092	
	≥8	0.9080	1.5445	0.0620	0.1490
All red meat	<4	0.5488	ref		
	≥4–<8	0.6807	1.1506	0.4871	
	≥8–<12	0.5678	0.9704	0.8926	
	≥12	0.7709	1.5221	0.0688	0.0867
Rice	<1	0.5055	ref		
	≥1–<5	0.6323	1.1886	0.4283	
	≥5–<10	0.7591	1.1673	0.5356	
	≥10	0.6518	1.2893	0.3280	0.4723
Wheat	<5	0.5381	ref		
	≥5–<10	0.5402	1.0538	0.7833	
	≥10–<15	0.7042	1.1326	0.5897	
	≥15	0.9044	1.7108	0.0105	0.0066
All grains	<10	0.5516	ref		
	≥10–<20	0.5297	1.6985	0.6299	
	≥20–<30	0.6407	1.8978	0.2120	
	≥30	0.8960	2.4498	0.0089	0.0012

[a]Models include age at interview, race, gender, body weight, height, pack years, and current smoking status.

increased consumption but was not significantly associated with disease status nor was the test for trend statistically significant. Consumption of all seafood combined (crabs, crawfish, shrimp, oysters, and fish) showed an increasing risk with increasing consumption, but the test for trend was only marginally significant ($P = 0.06$).

Increasing levels of beef consumption were associated with increasing risk of pancreatic cancer although none of the odds ratios were significant and the test for trend was only marginally significant ($P = 0.06$). Increasing levels of pork consumption were associated with disease status (OR 2nd: 2.21, 95% CI: 0.94–5.21, OR 3rd: 2.14, 95% CI: 0.78–5.84 and OR 4th: 4.44, 95% CI: 1.66–11.89) with a significant test for trend ($P \leq 0.01$). Increasing levels of consumption of red meat (beef and pork) were significantly associated with increased risk of pancreatic cancer (test for trend $P \leq 0.01$). Consumption of at least 12 servings per week of red meat was found to increase the risk of pancreatic cancer in this sample by more than five hundred percent compared to subjects eating less than four servings per week (OR 4th: 6.18, 95% CI 2.28–16.76). Consumption of chicken and turkey was not found to be associated with pancreatic cancer in this sample.

Rice consumption shows increasing risk by quartile (OR 2nd: 1.52, OR 3rd: 1.64, and OR 4th: 3.58) with a significant test for trend ($P = 0.02$), although only the highest category of consumption, at least 10 servings per week, was statistically significant. Wheat products showed increased risk of pancreatic cancer at higher consumption levels but none were statistically significant nor was the test for trend significant. All grain products combined show significantly increasing risk with levels of consumption (test for trend P value = 0.01), although only the odds ratio for the top category of consumption, at least 30 servings per week, was statistically significant (OR = 3.38, 95% CI: 1.10–10.36).

Table 3(b) presents the results from the predictive model of urinary cadmium concentrations. The top category of consumption of wheat products (at least 15 servings per week) predicted an increase of 1.7 μg cadmium/g creatinine compared to subjects who consumed less than five servings of wheat products per week and was statistically significant at the 0.05 level as was the test for trend. All grains combined (wheat, rice, corn, rye, and oats) showed monotonically increasing estimates of contribution to urinary cadmium concentrations, but only the top category of at least 30 servings per week was statistically significant. The test for trend across categories of consumption of all grains was statistically significant.

Pork consumption was not significantly associated with increased urinary cadmium concentrations, although the top category (at least 8 servings per week) approached significance ($P = 0.06$). Consumption of red meat (beef and pork combined) was not significantly associated with urinary cadmium concentrations although the top category (at least 12 servings per week) approached significance ($P = 0.07$).

Consumption of rice, legumes, fruits and juices, or vegetables was not found to significantly contribute to urinary cadmium concentrations in this sample, nor was consumption of shellfish, fish, beef, or poultry (not shown).

4. Discussion

This study is the first to our knowledge to establish an increased risk of pancreatic cancer with increased urinary cadmium concentrations: the measure considered to be most indicative of long-term cadmium exposure. The monotonically increasing risk of disease with incremental quartiles of 0.5 micrograms of cadmium per gram creatinine is evidence of an etiologic link between cadmium exposure and pancreatic cancer. Given the history of excess incidence of pancreatic cancer among the population of south Louisiana, cadmium exposure should be considered as a potential environmental carcinogen driving these rates.

Our results confirmed some findings from an earlier study of pancreatic cancer done between 1979 and 1983 in south Louisiana [48] using hospital-based controls. That study found that consumption of at least 31 servings of pork per month increased risk by 44%, at least 30 servings of rice per month increased risk by 55%, and at least 60 servings of bread and cereals per month increased risk by 64%. Falk et al. [48] found a significantly elevated risk associated with Cajun ethnicity and moderate, and heavy cigarette smoking was nonsignificantly associated with pancreatic cancer risk. This earlier study also found a significant protective effect for the consumption of fruits and juices among persons consuming at least 64 servings per month that was not found here. It should be noted though that the earlier study employed a much larger sample size made possible through next-of-kin interviews.

Both studies of this population found that sugar cane farming was statistically significantly associated with increased risk of pancreatic cancer. No specific exposure that might explain this observed association that is related to sugar cane farming but not rice or other crops is known at this time. A significant association was found between residential proximity to an oil refinery and urinary concentrations of cadmium, but since proximity was self-reported recall bias cannot be ruled out for this result. We find it surprising that cigarette smoking was not found to be a significant risk factor for pancreatic cancer in this sample despite being a significant contributor to urinary cadmium concentrations. This may be related to the small sample size and limited statistical power.

This study had limited statistical power to detect weak associations; however, the elevated risk of pancreatic cancer associated with urinary concentration of cadmium found in this study provides support for the hypothesis that cadmium plays a role in its etiology. Further, this study provides some evidence that previous findings of increased risk associated with high consumption levels of red meat and grains may be related to their cadmium content. Pork may have higher cadmium content than beef due to being exclusively grain-fed, whereas cattle are generally grazed until six months before moving to feed lots to be finished with grain.

Increased synthesis of metallothionein may represent a mechanism through which cadmium acts in pancreatic carcinogenesis [7]. Ohshio et al. [49] found that positive staining for metallothionein in pancreatic carcinomas was more often associated with liver metastases, worse histological grade of the tumors, and shorter survival in a sample of 75 pancreatic duct cell carcinomas from Japan. Therefore, it is possible that the cases that were deceased at the time of contact or were too ill to participate had higher cadmium exposures than those found in participating cases. If so, that would bias our risk estimates associated with urinary cadmium concentrations and potential sources of cadmium exposure toward the null.

The lack of clear correlation between consumption levels of potential dietary sources of cadmium and urinary cadmium concentrations may be explained by previous findings that dietary cadmium intake and urinary excretion are poorly correlated at low levels of cadmium intake but improve at higher levels [50, 51]. Individual uptake of dietary cadmium may vary by other dietary characteristics such as fiber content as well as individual physiology such as blood iron stores [22, 51, 52].

The Cajun population and especially the older age cohort that we examined here consume large amounts of seafood, rice, and pork which could increase their exposure to cadmium. Additional research into sources of cadmium exposure and the carcinogenic effects of cadmium in the pancreas is warranted.

Acknowledgments

This research was made possible by a grant from the Louisiana State Board of Regents. We are grateful to the dedicated staff of the Region 4 Louisiana Tumor Registry for the identification of incident cases. We are especially indebted to everyone who volunteered personal information for this study; particularly the pancreatic cancer patients who trusted us enough to allow us into their homes during a very difficult time in their lives.

References

[1] T. J. Mason, F. W. McKay, R. Hoover, W. J. Blot, and J. F. Fraumeni Jr., "Atlas of cancer mortality for US counties 1950–1969," DHEW Publication NIH 75-780, United States Government Printing Office, Washington, DC, USA, 1975.

[2] W. J. Blot, J. F. Fraumeni Jr., and B. J. Stone, "Geographic correlates of pancreas cancer in the United States," *Cancer*, vol. 42, no. 1, pp. 373–380, 1978.

[3] E. S. Peters, B. A. Schmidt, P. A. Andrews et al., *Cancer in Louisiana, 2000–2004*, vol. 22, Louisiana Tumor Registry, New Orleans, La, USA, 2007.

[4] International Agency for Research on Cancer, "IARC Monographs on the evaluation of carcinogenic risk to humans: Cadmium and cadmium compounds," Vol. 100C, 2011,

http://monographs.iarc.fr/ENG/Classification/Classifications GroupOrder.pdf.

[5] G. G. Schwartz and I. M. Reis, "Is cadmium a cause of human pancreatic cancer?" *Cancer Epidemiology Biomarkers and Prevention*, vol. 9, no. 2, pp. 139–145, 2000.

[6] M. P. Waalkes, M. G. Cherian, J. M. Ward, and R. A. Goyer, "Immunohistochemical evidence of high concentrations of metallothionein in pancreatic hepatocytes induced by cadmium in rats," *Toxicologic Pathology*, vol. 20, no. 3 I, pp. 323–326, 1993.

[7] G. K. Andrews, K. Page, P. Palmiter-Thomas, and M. P. Sarras, "Metal ions induce expression of metallothionein in pancreatic exocrine and endocrine cells," *Pancreas*, vol. 5, no. 5, pp. 548–554, 1990.

[8] J. H. R. Kägi and A. Schäffer, "Biochemistry of metallothionein," *Biochemistry*, vol. 27, no. 23, pp. 8509–8515, 1988.

[9] A. M. Kriegel, A. S. Soliman, Q. Zhang et al., "Serum cadmium levels in pancreatic cancer patients from the East Nile Delta region of Egypt," *Environmental Health Perspectives*, vol. 114, no. 1, pp. 113–119, 2006.

[10] H. Welinder, S. Skerfving, and O. Henriksen, "Cadmium metabolism in man," *British Journal of Industrial Medicine*, vol. 34, no. 3, pp. 221–228, 1977.

[11] G. F. Nordberg, R. F. M. Herber, and L. Alessio, Eds., *Cadmium in the Human Environment: Toxicity and Carcinogenicity*, International Agency for Research on Cancer, Lyon, France, 1992, IARC Scientific Publ. No. 118.

[12] Centers for Disease Control and Prevention, "Third national report on human exposure to environmental chemicals," Tech. Rep., US Department of Health and Human Services, Public Health Services, www.cdc.gov/exposurereport, 2005.

[13] A. Menke, P. Muntner, E. K. Silbergeld, E. A. Platz, and E. Guallar, "Cadmium levels in urine and mortality among U.S. adults," *Environmental Health Perspectives*, vol. 117, no. 2, pp. 190–196, 2009.

[14] T. Nawrot, M. Plusquin, J. Hogervorst et al., "Environmental exposure to cadmium and risk of cancer: a prospective population-based study," *Lancet Oncology*, vol. 7, no. 2, pp. 119–126, 2006.

[15] K. Arisawa, H. Uemura, M. Hiyoshi et al., "Cause-specific mortality and cancer incidence rates in relation to urinary β2-microglobulin: 23-Year follow-up study in a cadmium-polluted area," *Toxicology Letters*, vol. 173, no. 3, pp. 168–174, 2007.

[16] J. A. McElroy, M. M. Shafer, A. Trentham-Dietz, J. M. Hampton, and P. A. Newcomb, "Cadmium exposure and breast cancer risk," *Journal of the National Cancer Institute*, vol. 98, no. 12, pp. 869–873, 2006.

[17] C. M. Gallagher, J. J. Chen, and J. S. Kovach, "Environmental cadmium and breast cancer risk," *Aging*, vol. 2, no. 11, pp. 804–814, 2010.

[18] E. Kellen, M. P. Zeegers, E. D. Hond, and F. Buntinx, "Blood cadmium may be associated with bladder carcinogenesis: the Belgian case-control study on bladder cancer," *Cancer Detection and Prevention*, vol. 31, no. 1, pp. 77–82, 2007.

[19] D. Il'yasova and G. G. Schwartz, "Cadmium and renal cancer," *Toxicology and Applied Pharmacology*, vol. 207, no. 2, pp. 179–186, 2005.

[20] A. Akesson, B. Julin, and A. Wolk, "Long-term dietary cadmium intake and postmenopausal endometrial cancer incidence: a population-based prospective cohort study," *Cancer Research*, vol. 68, no. 15, pp. 6435–6441, 2008.

[21] M. Vinceti, M. Venturelli, C. Sighinolfi et al., "Case-control study of toenail cadmium and prostate cancer risk in Italy," *Science of the Total Environment*, vol. 373, no. 1, pp. 77–81, 2007.

[22] S. Satarug and M. R. Moore, "Adverse health effects of chronic exposure to low-level cadmium in foodstuffs and cigarette smoke," *Environmental Health Perspectives*, vol. 112, no. 10, pp. 1099–1103, 2004.

[23] R. T. Falk, L. W. Pickle, E. T. Fontham, P. Correa, and J. F. Fraumeni, "Life-style risk factors for pancreatic cancer in Louisiana: a case-control study," *American Journal of Epidemiology*, vol. 128, no. 2, pp. 324–336, 1988.

[24] P. Maisonneuve, A. B. Lowenfels, H. B. Bueno-de-Mesquita et al., "Past medical history and pancreatic cancer risk: results from a multicenter case-control study," *Annals of Epidemiology*, vol. 20, no. 2, pp. 92–98, 2010.

[25] E. L. Wynder, K. Mabuchi, N. Maruchi, and J. G. Fortner, "A case control study of cancer of the pancreas," *Cancer*, vol. 31, no. 3, pp. 641–648, 1973.

[26] S. Iodice, S. Gandini, P. Maisonneuve, and A. B. Lowenfels, "Tobacco and the risk of pancreatic cancer: a review and meta-analysis," *Langenbeck's Archives of Surgery*, vol. 393, no. 4, pp. 535–545, 2008.

[27] E. T. H. Fontham and P. Correa, "Epidemiology of pancreatic cancer," *Surgical Clinics of North America*, vol. 69, no. 3, pp. 551–567, 1989.

[28] R. A. Goyer, "Toxic effects of metals," in *Casarett and Doull's Toxicology: The Basic Science of Poisons*, C. D. Klaassen, Ed., pp. 691–736, McGraw Hill, New York, NY, USA, 1996.

[29] M. J. McLaughlin and B. R. Singh, "Cadmium in soils and plants," in *Developments in Plant and Soil Sciences*, M. J. McLaughlin and B. R. Singh, Eds., vol. 85, pp. 1–7, Kluwer Academic, Dordrecht, The Netherlands, 1999.

[30] International Agency for Research on Cancer, *IARC Monographs on the Evaluation of Carcinogenic Risk of Chemicals to Man: Cadmium, Nickel, Some Epoxides, Miscellaneous Industrial Chemicals and General Considerations on Volatile Anaesthetics*, vol. 11, International Agency for Research on Cancer, Lyon , France, 1976.

[31] A. Anderson, "Trace elements in agricultural soils—fluxes, balances and background values," Tech. Rep. 4077, Swedish Environmental Protection Agency, Stockholm, Sweden, 1992.

[32] R. Lemus, A. A. Abdelghani, T. G. Akers, and W. E. Horner, "Health risks from exposure to metals in household dusts," *Reviews on Environmental Health*, vol. 11, no. 4, pp. 179–189, 1996.

[33] J. A. Staessen, R. R. Lauwerys, G. Ide, H. A. Roels, G. Vyncke, and A. Amery, "Renal function and historical environmental cadmium pollution from zinc smelters," *The Lancet*, vol. 343, no. 8912, pp. 1523–1527, 1994.

[34] G. V. Greene, "Cadmium compounds," in *Encyclopedia of Chemical Technology*, R. E. Kirk and D. F. Othmer, Eds., vol. 3, pp. 889–911, John Wiley & Sons, New York, NY, USA, 2nd edition, 1974.

[35] J. V. Lagerwerff and A. W. Specht, "Contamination of roadside soil and vegetation with cadmium, nickel, lead, and zinc," *Environmental Science and Technology*, vol. 4, no. 7, pp. 583–586, 1970.

[36] United States Department of Labor: Occupational Safety and Health Administration, "Safety and Health Topics: Cadmium," http://www.osha.gov/SLTC/cadmium, 2009.

[37] T. Sugiyama, S. Takahashi, M. Honda, and E. Sakai, "Current state of the JSCE standard on test method for leaching of trace elements from hardened concrete," in *Proceedings of the International Conference on Sustainable Construction Materials and*

Technologies, R. N. Kraus, T. R. Naik, P. Claisse, and Sadeghi-Pouya, Eds., pp. 197–203, UW Milwaukee CBU, Milwaukee, Wis, USA, June 2007, Coventry, Special papers proceedings.

[38] M. Ikeda, "Biological monitoring of the general population for cadmium," in *Cadmium in the Environment: Toxicity and Carcinogenecity*, G. F. Nordberg, R. F. M. Herber, and A. L. Lyon, Eds., pp. 65–72, International Agency for Research on Cancer, Lyon, France, 1992.

[39] S. W. Al-Rmalli, R. O. Jenkins, and P. I. Haris, "Dietary intake of cadmium from Bangladeshi foods," *Journal of Food Science*, vol. 77, pp. 26–33, 2012.

[40] S. Shimbo, Z. W. Zhang, C. S. Moon et al., "Correlation between urine and blood concentrations, and dietary intake of cadmium and lead among women in the general population of Japan," *International Archives of Occupational and Environmental Health*, vol. 73, no. 3, pp. 163–170, 2000.

[41] T. Watanabe, Z. W. Zhang, C. S. Moon et al., "Cadmium exposure of women in general populations in Japan during 1991–1997 compared with 1977–1981," *International Archives of Occupational and Environmental Health*, vol. 73, no. 1, pp. 26–34, 2000.

[42] L. Jorhem, J. Engman, B. Sundstrom, and A. M. Thim, "Trace elements in crayfish: regional differences and changes induced by cooking," *Archives of Environmental Contamination and Toxicology*, vol. 26, no. 2, pp. 137–142, 1994.

[43] G. M. Kruzynski, "Cadmium in oysters and scallops: the BC experience," *Toxicology Letters*, vol. 148, no. 3, pp. 159–169, 2004.

[44] S. M. Naqvi, R. D. Howell, and M. Sholas, "Cadmium and lead residues in field-collected red swamp crayfish (Procambarus clarkii) and uptake by alligator weed, Alternanthera philoxiroides," *Journal of Environmental Science and Health B*, vol. 28, no. 4, pp. 473–485, 1993.

[45] P. B. Tchounwou, A. A. Abdelghani, Y. V. Pramar, L. R. Heyer, and C. M. Steward, "Assessment of potential health risks associated with ingesting heavy metals in fish collected from a hazardous-waste contaminated wetland in Louisiana, USA," *Reviews on Environmental Health*, vol. 11, no. 4, pp. 191–203, 1996.

[46] "HHHQ-Dietsys Analysis Software Version 4.02," National Cancer Institute, 1999.

[47] SAS Institute, Inc., SAS 9. 1. 3. 2002. Cary, N.C.

[48] R. T. Falk, L. W. Pickle, E. T. Fontham et al., "Occupation and pancreatic cancer risk in Louisiana," *American Journal of Industrial Medicine*, vol. 18, no. 5, pp. 565–576, 1990.

[49] G. Ohshio, T. Imamura, N. Okada et al., "Immunohistochemical study of metallothionein in pancreatic carcinomas," *Journal of Cancer Research and Clinical Oncology*, vol. 122, no. 6, pp. 351–355, 1996.

[50] M. Berglund, A. Akesson, B. Nermell, and M. Vahter, "Intestinal absorption of dietary cadmium in women depends on body iron stores and fiber intake," *Environmental Health Perspectives*, vol. 102, no. 12, pp. 1058–1066, 1994.

[51] I. M. Olsson, I. Bensryd, T. Lundh, H. Ottosson, S. Skerfving, and A. Oskarsson, "Cadmium in blood and urine—impact of sex, age, dietary intake, iron status, and former smoking—association of renal effects," *Environmental Health Perspectives*, vol. 110, no. 12, pp. 1185–1190, 2002.

[52] S. Satarug, S. H. Garrett, M. A. Sens, and D. A. Sens, "Cadmium, environmental exposure, and health outcomes," *Environmental Health Perspectives*, vol. 118, no. 2, pp. 182–190, 2010.

Arsenic, Cadmium, Lead, and Mercury in Sweat: A Systematic Review

Margaret E. Sears,[1, 2] Kathleen J. Kerr,[3, 4] and Riina I. Bray[3, 4]

[1] *Children's Hospital of Eastern Ontario Research Institute, Ottawa, ON, Canada K1H 8L1*
[2] *Clinical Epidemiology, Ottawa Hospital Research Institute, Ottawa, ON, Canada K1Y 4E9*
[3] *Environmental Health Clinic, Women's College Hospital, Toronto, ON, Canada M5S 1B2*
[4] *Department of Family and Community Medicine, University of Toronto, Toronto, ON, Canada M5T 1W7*

Correspondence should be addressed to Margaret E. Sears, megsears@ncf.ca

Academic Editor: Gerry Schwalfenberg

Arsenic, cadmium, lead, and mercury exposures are ubiquitous. These toxic elements have no physiological benefits, engendering interest in minimizing body burden. The physiological process of sweating has long been regarded as "cleansing" and of low risk. Reports of toxicant levels in sweat were sought in Medline, Embase, Toxline, Biosis, and AMED as well as reference lists and grey literature, from inception to March 22, 2011. Of 122 records identified, 24 were included in evidence synthesis. Populations, and sweat collection methods and concentrations varied widely. In individuals with higher exposure or body burden, sweat generally exceeded plasma or urine concentrations, and dermal could match or surpass urinary daily excretion. Arsenic dermal excretion was severalfold higher in arsenic-exposed individuals than in unexposed controls. Cadmium was more concentrated in sweat than in blood plasma. Sweat lead was associated with high-molecular-weight molecules, and in an interventional study, levels were higher with endurance compared with intensive exercise. Mercury levels normalized with repeated saunas in a case report. Sweating deserves consideration for toxic element detoxification. Research including appropriately sized trials is needed to establish safe, effective therapeutic protocols.

1. Introduction

No person is without some level of toxic metals in their bodies, circulating and accumulating with acute and chronic lifetime exposures. An individual may take numerous measures to minimize exposures and to optimize metabolism and excretion of toxic elements in the stool and urine with diet, supplements, and chelation therapy [1, 2]; however, an often overlooked route of excretion of toxicants is via the process of sweating [3].

Sweating with heat and/or exercise has been viewed throughout the ages, by groups worldwide, as "cleansing." As part of a scoping review regarding arsenic, cadmium, lead, and mercury, we reviewed the scientific literature pertaining to toxicant excretion in sweat.

1.1. Arsenic, Cadmium, Lead, and Mercury: Background. While many chemical elements are essential for life, arsenic, cadmium, lead, and mercury have no known beneficial effect in humans. On the contrary, all four elements are confirmed or probable carcinogens, and they exhibit wide-ranging toxic effects on many bodily systems, including the nervous, endocrine, renal, musculoskeletal, immunological, and cardiovascular systems [4–7].

Children and the fetus are most at risk of harm, with early exposures potentially predisposing the youngster over his/her lifetime to multisystem ailments, as well as lower IQ and dysfunctional behavior. In older populations there is increased likelihood of early cognitive decline, as well as a range of conditions including kidney and cardiovascular disease, diabetes, and osteoporosis [4–7].

Some populations are exposed to elevated levels of toxic elements by virtue of geochemistry, resulting in groundwater or foods with elevated levels of toxic elements (e.g., elevated arsenic in groundwater, most famously in parts of Asia such as Bangladesh but also elsewhere; cadmium that accumulates in foods grown in particular locations with high levels in soils or from fertilizers, including shellfish [8], grains [9], and brassicas [10]; and mercury in fish and seafoods). Tobacco avidly accumulates cadmium and lead from soil, making smoking a major source of exposure. In addition, valuable and unique properties of arsenic, cadmium, lead, and mercury have made them integral in many products, including electronics, batteries, and alloys. Modern environmental exposures arise from mining, refining, and industrial processes (e.g., arsenic from precious metal mining and refining, mercury from chloralkali production, or lead and cadmium from mining, refining, and recycling these and other metals such as zinc); the vestiges of older products (e.g., pesticides, leaded gasoline, paint and plumbing, mercury-containing switches and thermometers, and arsenical wood preservatives); ongoing uses (e.g., arsenical veterinary drugs, and mercury-containing dental amalgams, preservatives, and lamps); as well as emissions from burning coal and other incineration (including cremation).

With toxic elements ubiquitous in our air, water, food, and the physical environment, as well as in many consumer products, prudent avoidance is not always possible. Although signs and symptoms of chronic disease are consistent with effects of arsenic, cadmium, lead, and/or mercury, physicians commonly have a low index of clinical suspicion, and therefore levels of toxic elements are seldom investigated. Diagnosis may be challenging because multiple chemicals may contribute to subtle effects in chronic illnesses of an individual, and the effects may be synergistic. A recent review called for mercury assessment in all patients presenting with hypertension or any vascular disease [11], but other toxic elements such as lead [12] may also be implicated at levels commonly observed in the population. "Interaction Profiles" [13] compiled by the US Agency for Toxic Substances and Disease Registry report that renal toxicities of mixtures of lead plus mercury are greater than would be predicted knowing the toxicity dose response of the individual elements. Similarly, neurological toxicities of mixtures of lead plus arsenic, lead plus methylmercury, and lead plus cadmium are supra-additive [13].

1.2. Sweating: Background. Increasing the thermal load on the body activates heat loss mechanisms including increased circulation throughout the skin and sweating [14], with blood flow to the skin increasing from a baseline of 5–10%, to 60–70% of the cardiac output [15]. Maximal sweating occurs within 15 minutes and the fluid loss may be as high as 2 L/h in an "acclimatized" person who regularly sweats [16].

Eccrine sweat is produced in tubular coil glands under the skin surface in response to heat and, or work stress. Capillaries as well as adjacent adipose tissue may contribute to secretions from sebaceous and apocrine glands, as has been seen in research using sweat patches to detect drugs of abuse [17]. Sweat arises from the blood supply to the sweat gland, but is not simply an ultrafiltrate of blood plasma; sodium and chloride are lower in sweat than in serum, as salt loss is restricted by reabsorption in the gland [18]. Both the concentration and total loss of salt (sodium chloride) in sweat vary widely among individuals [19], as well as with acclimatization to exercise and heat [20]. In an early study, Robinson et al. demonstrated that with serum salt depletion the kidneys responded within hours by restricting excretion into the urine, while the sweat glands responded only after days with decreased concentrations in the sweat [21]. Potassium, urea, ammonia, and lactic acid concentrations are higher in sweat than in plasma, although these levels are also regulated to some extent by reabsorption in the ductal tubule of the sweat gland [22]. In one study of successive exercise sessions with cool-down breaks, over the short-term sodium, potassium, calcium, and magnesium excretion in sweat remained constant, while zinc excretion fell [23]. It is unclear whether reabsorption or depletion of plasma supply resulted in diminishing zinc losses.

Children, with greater surface area in comparison to body mass, have been observed in research studies to sweat less than adults, with sweating increasing through puberty [24]. Although some research has indicated that children's thermoregulation and heat tolerance may be less robust than adults, these findings may be at least in part an artifact of study designs and models for interpretation [25]. In research involving exercise and heat, it may be a challenge to maintain ongoing, consistent motivation among children.

2. Methods

2.1. Search Strategy. Medline, Embase, Toxline, Biosis, and AMED were searched, with no restriction on date or language, to March 22, 2011. These records were supplemented with searches for other research by key authors, searches of citations and reference lists of key reports, and "related articles."

Neither sweating nor toxic elements are exclusively modern topics of research, so in order to search older literature for all chemical forms, the online version of the Chemical Rubber Company Handbook was searched for all arsenic, cadmium, lead, and mercury compounds, and lists of keywords were extracted from these lists. Searches using these keywords yielded records that were not identified in searches using the four chemical abstracts service (CAS) numbers or the medical subject headings (MeSHs) for arsenic, cadmium, lead, and mercury. CAS numbers and MeSHs are intended for specific individual chemicals or records referring to unspecified compounds—the tool cannot simultaneously be both specific and general. Toxic element records were searched for terms related to sweating, perspiration, sauna, steam baths, exercise, depuration, and secretion or excretion from skin. Bibliographic records were imported, duplicates were removed, and reports were screened using Zotero 2.03 (http://www.zotero.org/).

2.2. Report Screening and Inclusion. Titles and abstracts were screened by one investigator (MS), for primary reports with data on one or more of the toxic elements in sweat, with at least a substantial abstract in English. Reviews were included at this level, to search reference lists. Two investigators (MS and KK) independently screened studies

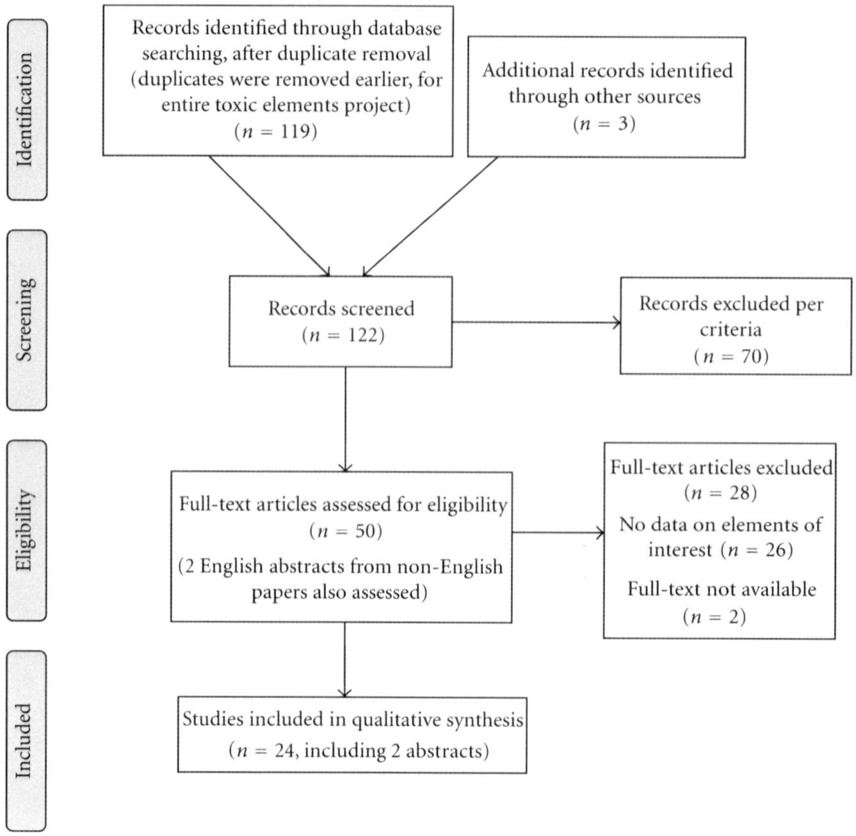

FIGURE 1: PRISMA flow diagram of evidence searches and inclusion.

for inclusion, and extracted and verified data. All studies presenting quantitative human data on levels of arsenic, cadmium, lead, and/or mercury were included, regardless of experimental design, or methods of sweat collection or chemical analysis.

3. Results

Of 122 bibliographic records identified, 70 did not meet inclusion criteria at first screening, 52 full-text articles were sought for full-text screening, and 50 were obtained and screened. Data from the extended abstract of a report in German [26] and the conclusion from the abstract of one report in Russian [27] that were not obtained in full text were noted. Twenty-four reports of 22 or 23 trials or studies (it is unclear if two studies from one institution reported results twice for a subset of participants [22, 28]) were included in evidence synthesis. Searching, screening, and study inclusion are summarized in the modified PRISMA flow diagram, Figure 1.

3.1. Excretion of Toxic Elements in Sweat. Along with essential minerals, sweat is an acknowledged excretory route for toxic metals. For instance, it is recommended to sample hair close to the scalp because content of toxic elements may be elevated along the shaft, from either environmental contamination or excreted toxins in sweat and sebum [32, 42]. The minerals generally arise from blood serum [28], with contribution from dermally absorbed occupational exposures, which might not be reflected in blood or urine [35, 37]. Sweating was induced by sauna, exercise, or pilocarpine iontophoresis to measure the concentration of the heavy metals in the sweat, while sauna and exercise were used for therapy. Study participants included workers with occupational exposures and individuals with no occupational exposures who were well or experiencing chronic ill health, and in two studies participants were intentionally dosed with lead [34, 37]. Studies that have examined the presence of toxic metals in sweat are summarized in Tables 1, 2, 3, and 4, for arsenic, cadmium, lead, and mercury, respectively.

Arsenic accumulates highly in the skin, and causes characteristic skin lesions, but little information is available on levels in sweat. Yousuf et al. recently found that excretion of arsenic was greatest from the skin of patients with skin lesions, slightly but not statistically significantly lower from arsenic-exposed controls, and severalfold lower from nonexposed controls [29]. Genuis et al. measured numerous toxic elements in blood plasma, urine, and sweat of 20 study subjects (10 healthy and 10 with chronic health problems) [3]. The maximum sweat arsenic concentration was 22 μg/L. On average, arsenic was 1.5-fold (in males) to 3-fold (in females) higher in sweat than in blood plasma; however,

TABLE 1: Studies of excretion of arsenic in sweat.

Study	Country, participants	Study design and intervention	Key findings (concentrations of μg/L unless otherwise indicated)
Yousuf et al. 2011 [29]	Bangladesh 20 arsenicosis patients with melanosis and leucomelanosis 20 controls with As in drinking water 20 unexposed controls	Secretions from chest, back, and abdomen collected for 24 h, on gauze pads (8-fold; 2 × 3 inches) attached to fitted T-shirt	As secretion severalfold greater for As-exposed groups No significant difference between patients and As-exposed controls 2 zinc atoms excreted per As atom Vitamin E excreted with As
Genuis et al. 2010 [3]	Canada 10 with chronic conditions 10 healthy	Simultaneous measurement of As in blood plasma, urine, and sweat Sweating induced by exercise or sauna, collected directly into bottle	17 participants with As detected in all samples Blood plasma mean: 2.5 (range 0.9–13) (n = 17) Urine mean: 37 (range 4.8–200) (n = 20) Sweat mean: 3.1 (range 3.7–22) (n = 20)

TABLE 2: Studies of cadmium excretion in sweat.

Study	Country, participants	Study design and intervention	Key findings (concentrations μg/L unless otherwise indicated)
Genuis et al., 2010 [3]	Canada 10 with chronic conditions 10 healthy	Simultaneous measurement of toxic trace elements in blood plasma, urine, and sweat Exercise or sauna Sweat collected directly into bottle	3 participants with cadmium detected in all samples Blood plasma mean: 0.03 (range 0.02–0.07) (n = 11) Urine mean: 0.28 (0.18–0.39) (n = 3) Sweat mean: 5.7 (0.36–36) (n = 18)
Omokhodion and Howard, 1994 [30]	UK 15 healthy participants	Sweat collected using modified arm bag (hand excluded) Participants exercised at room temperature	Cadmium detected in 13 sweat samples Mean 1.9 Range 1.1–3.1
Stauber and Florence, 1988 [28]	Australia 24 males 13 females taking oral contraceptives 26 females not taking oral contraceptives	Forearm sweat induced by pilocarpine iontophoresis and collected on a membrane filter	Males mean sweat cadmium 1.4 (range <0.5–10) Females not taking contraceptives 2.6 (<0.5–18) Females taking contraceptives 2.4 (<0.5–5.5)
Stauber and Florence, 1987 [22]	Australia 9 males 7 females taking oral contraceptives 6 not taking oral contraceptives (unclear overlap with 1988 participants)	Forearm sweat induced by pilocarpine iontophoresis and collected on a membrane filter	Cadmium not detected in sweat (0.5 detection limit) Mean blood cadmium 0.8
Robinson and Weiss, 1980 [31]	USA 28 males (university faculty members)	Exercise and shower preceded sauna for sweat collection. Sweat collected as drips from forehead or nose	Sweat cadmium (range 11–200) Urine cadmium (range ND–67) Sweat/urine ratio (range 1.0–16) No correlation between the concentrations in urine and sweat
Robinson and Weiss, 1980 [32] (companion to previous)	USA 2 males (university faculty members)	As previous, cadmium also measured in hair segments.	Daily excretion of cadmium estimated as follows: (i) 30 μg/day in urine (ii) 120 μg/day in sweat (iii) 0.2 μg/day in hair Cadmium concentrations in hair and sweat were lower in one participant than the other
Cohn and Emmett, 1978 [33]	USA 6 males 3 females	Total body washdown and arm bag techniques	Mean concentration of cadmium in sweat > urine Arm bags yielded lower levels than whole body measurements

Table 3: Studies of lead excretion in sweat.

Study	Country, participants	Study design and intervention	Key findings (concentrations μg/L unless otherwise indicated)
Genuis et al., 2010 [3]	Canada 10 with chronic health conditions 10 healthy	Analyses of blood plasma, urine, and sweat Sweating induced by exercise or sauna, collected directly into bottle	Sweat mean 31 (range 1.5–94) ($n = 20$) Blood plasma mean 0.12 (0.39–1.7) ($n = 20$) Urine mean 1.8 (0.91–7.5) ($n = 20$)
Omokhodion and Crockford, 1991 [34]	UK 2 participants	Blood, urine, and sweat lead measured before and following ingestion of lead chloride: 1 or 2 doses of lead chloride (20 mg $PbCl_2$ total, in 1 or 2 divided doses).	Blood lead peaked at 4 h Sweat concentrations did not increase significantly (range 0–11) Blood concentration range 6–51 Urine concentration range 10–97 Arm sweat collections varied by more than 2-fold between arms at the same time on the same person
Omokhodion and Howard, 1991 [35]	Unidentified "tropics" 19 workers in a lead battery factory 8 controls (medical students)	Measured lead in sweat, blood, and urine simultaneously Sweating induced by exercising at room temperature. Sweat collected in arm bags.	Workers: (i) blood lead 13–36 (ii) urine lead 28–290 μg/g creatinine (iii) sweat lead 72–260 Controls: (i) blood lead 90–120 (ii) urine lead 9–20 μg/g creatinine (iii) sweat lead 9–30
Omokhodion and Crockford, 1991 [36]	UK 24 normal, healthy subjects	Measured lead in sweat, urine, blood, and saliva Sweat collected in arm bags, sitting in a hot chamber	(i) Blood lead 86 (range 60–140) (ii) Urine lead 18 μg/g creatinine (range 7.7–44 μg/g creatinine) (iii) Mean sweat lead 5.2 (2.5–13) (iv) Saliva lead 4.8 (2.5–10)
Parpaleĭ et al., 1991 [27] (in Russian—English abstract only)	Russia NR in abstract	NR in abstract	"... sauna increased excretion with sweat fluid of toxic substances [lead] that penetrated the body during work. Sauna is recommended."
Lilley et al., 1988 [37]	Australia 9 lead workers volunteers had lead applied to skin	Lead dust 6 h/day for 4 days 20 mg Pb dust on L arm of volunteer $PbNO_3$ 24 h of 60 mg $PbNO_3$ on L arm of volunteer.	Sweat lead in workers: 71–18,000 Following exposure, sweat lead from R arm increased approximately by 10x, returning to baseline after approximately by 2–4 days. Saliva increased approximately 5-6x. Urine and blood levels were unchanged
Stauber and Florence, 1988 [28]	Australia 24 males 13 females taking oral contraceptives 26 not taking oral contraceptives	Sweating induced on the forearms by pilocarpine iontophoresis and collected on a membrane filter	Mean sweat lead: (i) males: 41 (range 6–87) (ii) females not taking contraceptives: 24 (<5–66) (difference with males $P < 0.01$) (iii) females taking contraceptives: 36 (<5–70)
Stauber and Florence, 1987 [22]	Australia 9 males 7 females taking oral contraceptives 6 not taking oral contraceptives (unclear overlap with 1988 participants)	Sweating induced in the forearms by pilocarpine iontophoresis and collected on a membrane filter	No significant differences among groups Mean blood lead 200 Mean blood plasma lead 10 Mean sweat lead 15

TABLE 3: Continued.

Study	Country, participants	Study design and intervention	Key findings (concentrations μg/L unless otherwise indicated)
Haber et al., 1985 [26] (in German-used extended abstract)	Germany 4 groups of 8 males 2 groups with occupational lead exposure 2 control groups	Comparison of precisely defined physical work (intensive cycling and extended rowing in a pool), examining lead excretion in persons with elevated blood levels compared with nonexposed controls	Aerobic endurance training (rowing) caused a significant drop in the blood lead level in the occupationally exposed group (mean 430 (range 320–580) decreased to 370 (240–450)) ($P < 0.05$) Endurance training was more effective than shorter, more intensive training (cycling) Urine lead levels were not significantly affected by training
Cohn and Emmett, 1978 [33]	USA 6 males 3 females	Total body washdown and arm bag techniques	The mean concentration of lead in sweat was similar to that in urine (1) Total body sweat lead mean: (i) males: 24 (SD 16) (ii) females: 53 (range 40–60) (2) Body minus 1 arm/arm bag sweat lead 60 (SD 16) (40–120)/83 (86) (20–250)
Hohnandel et al., 1973 [38]	33 healthy males 15 females	15 min of arm bag collection	Mean sweat lead: (i) males: 51 (range 8–180) (ii) females: 120 (SD 72) (49–280)

TABLE 4: Studies of mercury excretion in sweat.

Study	Country, participants	Study design and intervention	Key findings (concentrations μg/L unless otherwise indicated)
Genuis et al., 2010 [3]	Canada 10 with chronic conditions 10 healthy	Sweating induced by exercise or sauna, collected directly into bottle	16 participants had mercury detected in all samples Blood plasma mercury mean 0.61 (range 0.26–1.6) ($n = 16$) Urine mean 0.65 (range 0.32–1.3) ($n = 16$) Sweat mean 0.86 (range 0.48–1.5) ($n = 20$)
Robinson and Skelly, 1983 [39]	USA 21 males at university 7 sampled more than once	Mercury in sweat dripping from forehead or nose, compared with urine	Sweat mean 0.5 (range 0.1–1.4)
Sunderman 1978 [40]	USA 1 case with mercury intoxication	Case report of chelating agents to treat mercury intoxication, followed by a regimen of daily sweat and physiotherapy for a protracted period of several months	Appreciable quantities of mercury were excreted in sweat. With the sweating regimen mercury, levels in sweat decreased to within the normal range
Lovejoy et al., 1973 [41]	USA 3 mercury-exposed workers 3 nonexposed workers 1 control	Participants wore rubber chest waders from 7 : 30 to 9 : 00 am Sweat accumulated in the feet was collected, as well as a 16-hour urine sample	Exposed workers: 1.5 h sweat: 120–350 ng mercury 16 h urine: 160–190 ng mercury Unexposed workers: 1.5 h sweat: 5–8 ng mercury 16 h urine: 5–7 ng mercury Internal controls: 1.5 h sweat: 43–70 ng mercury 16 h urine: 30–46 ng mercury Mercury concentrations in sweat > urine for exposed workers; similar for controls

arsenic was excreted at lower concentrations in sweat than in urine [3].

Cadmium in sweat was examined in six studies [3, 22, 28, 30–33], with concentrations in sweat ranging from <0.5–10 μg/L [28] to 0.36–35.8 μg/L [3]. Stauber and Florence concluded that sweat may be an important route for excretion of cadmium when an individual is exposed to high levels [22, 28], a finding that was confirmed by observing that the total daily excretion of cadmium was greater in sweat than in urine [3, 32]. The maximum cadmium concentration observed in sweat was 35.8 μg/L [3].

Lead was examined in eleven studies [3, 22, 26–28, 33–38]. In 1973, Hohnadel et al. suggested that "sauna bathing might provide a therapeutic method to increase elimination of toxic trace metals" [38]. In two males, 36% and 50% of sweat lead was of molecular weight > 30,000, as measured by ultrafiltration, suggesting excretion of organic complexes rather than simple ions [22]. Lead excretion was lower in females taking birth control medications compared with females not taking medications, or males [28]. Haber et al. found that prolonged endurance workouts (rowing) ameliorated elevated blood lead levels in exposed workers but did not alter levels in control subjects and did not affect urine levels [26]. They suggested that the elimination route was not urine, but potentially sweat or/and bile. Omokhodion and Crockford carried out several studies of trace elements in sweat, including a study of lead ingestion by two human participants [34]. Sweat lead levels did not increase immediately with elevated blood lead, although the authors make reference to an older study with longer followup wherein lead in underarm pads doubled in the five days following ingestion. Omokhodion and Howard also reported higher lead in sweat of exposed workers compared with unexposed controls [35], and in another study that sweat and blood lead levels were the only two variables that correlated among blood, urine, sweat, and saliva [36]. The English abstract of a 1991 case report in Russian indicated that sauna increased excretion of toxic elements and resulted in clinical improvements [27]. Sweat lead levels up to 283 μg/L have been observed in nonoccupationally exposed subjects [38] and up to 17,700 μg/L in workers [37], where it is noted that lead in sweat may partially originate from material absorbed within the skin that was not removed by pretest cleaning protocols [35]. Indeed, although dermal application of lead via hair follicles, sweat ducts, and diffusion does not result in immediate increases in blood or urine lead concentrations, dermal absorption was demonstrated using the Pb-204 isotope [43], lead powder, and salt [37].

Mercury. In 1973, Lovejoy et al. noted that exposure to mercury does not always correlate with urine mercury levels and that elimination by other routes such as sweat may be an explanation [41]. They suggested, "sweating should be the initial and preferred treatment of patients with elevated mercury urine levels." In a 1978 case report, a severely poisoned worker was rescued with chelation therapy, followed by a regimen of daily sweat and physiotherapy over several months during which the sweat mercury level returned to normal and the patient recovered [40]. Robinson measured mercury in sweat repeatedly in two volunteers, observing sweat to urine concentration ratios ranging from less than 0.1 to greater than 5. Sweat mercury concentrations varied widely from day to day, and there was no correlation with urine levels. Sweat mercury levels of 1.5 μg/L were observed by Genuis et al. [3] and 1.4 μg/L by Robinson and Skelly [39].

4. Discussion

Arsenic, cadmium, lead, and mercury may be excreted in appreciable quantities through the skin, and rates of excretion were reported to match or even exceed urinary excretion in a 24-hour period. This is of particular interest should renal compromise limit urinary excretion of toxic elements.

Most of the research identified was over 20 years old, and collection methods varied widely. Although authors described thorough precleaning methods, sweat concentrations measured in research settings are not well validated and varied according to the location on the body, collection method, and from day to day according to other variables such as hydration. Sweat contains metals not only from the blood plasma, but also evidently originating from dermal layers (particularly with significant dermal exposures, as for workers in welding, smelting, or battery manufacturing). It would appear that large variabilities in measured concentrations, apart from collection methods as mentioned above, were likely the result of differences in excretion amongst widely varying individuals with ranges of body burdens, genetic polymorphisms affecting detoxification efficiency, and physiological states, coupled with necessarily crude if simple experimental techniques. These variations were very much greater than would be expected due to limitations of analytical methods. Although analytical methods have improved over the years, analysis of these metals was commonplace at the time of the studies. Authors generally reported analytical methods rigorously or provided references to thorough descriptions and included internal standards and some indication of sensitivity.

The observation that between a third and a half of lead in sweat may be associated with high-molecular-weight molecules [22] merits replication, including examination of additional toxic elements and characterization of the associated molecules previously observed. Excretion of these large molecules also suggests that sweating may be a means of excretion of metals complexed with natural or synthetic chelating agents.

Yousuf et al.'s recent study demonstrating a 2 : 1 molar ratio of zinc : arsenic and increased vitamin E in skin secretions suggests potential therapeutic supplementation to accommodate these biochemical requirements. Vitamin E, zinc, and other nutrients are required for methylation and detoxification of arsenic within the body, and vitamin E supplementation improves the skin manifestations in arsenicosis [29].

From an occupational health perspective, lead, and presumably other toxic elements, may be absorbed via the skin, which supports showering at work and further suggests the possibility of purging workers' skin by washing with a chelating agent (e.g., EDTA rinses extracted lead from workers' skin in methods validation experimentation [38]). It is unknown if sweating during the workday may affect dermal absorption, or if forced sweating at the end of the workday would be beneficial. It is also unknown if increased blood flow to the skin could possibly enhance absorption into the bloodstream, or if worker health could be optimized by a combination of workplace skin cleaning and sweating interventions.

Sweating has long been perceived to promote health, not only accompanying exercise but also with heat. Worldwide traditions and customs include Roman baths, Aboriginal sweat lodges, Scandinavian saunas (dry heat; relative humidity from 40% to 60%), and Turkish baths (with steam). Infrared saunas heat exposed tissues with infrared radiation, while air temperatures remain cooler than in other saunas.

Sweating is a long-standing, if recently forgotten, aspect of mercury detoxification. Various strategies used to maintain the mercury mining workforce have been explored over the centuries. In Spain and colonies, long the western world's primary sources of mercury, sending ill workers to warmer climes away from the exposure to drink weak beer (the hydrogen peroxide catalase oxidation of elemental mercury to ionic mercury is competitively inhibited by alcohol, increasing mercury in exhaled breath [44]) and to work in the heat (presumably to sweat out the "vapors") was a common and effective strategy centuries ago; tremors, salivation, and mouth ulcers resolved generally within a few weeks [45].

With acclimatization and regular use, the sauna is generally well tolerated by all ages [46], though medical supervision may be recommended during initial sessions for children, the elderly, or those with compromised health. Varying qualities of evidence indicate potential short- and long-term improvements for cardiovascular, rheumatological and respiratory conditions; contraindications include unstable angina pectoris, recent myocardial infarction, severe aortic stenosis, and high-risk pregnancy [15, 46]. Sweating is not only observed to enhance excretion of the toxic elements of interest in this paper, but also may increase excretion of diverse toxicants, as observed in New York rescue workers [47], or in particular persistent flame retardants [48] and bisphenol-A [49].

Optimizing the potential of sweating as a therapeutic excretory mechanism merits further research. To date, the large body of research into homeostasis of the most common metals (sodium, potassium, and to a lesser extent, magnesium, calcium, and zinc) and conditioning or adaptation to regular sweating by athletes has not been matched with studies of excretion of trace elements. Limited research suggests indirectly that conditioning may not restrict excretion of nonessential elements. Combination therapies, such as administration of *n*-acetyl cysteine, vitamin C, a chelating agent, or low doses of ethanol (for mercury), to name a few possibilities, along with sauna and/or exercise therapy to induce sweating, may be fruitful avenues of investigation.

It has been noted that among people whose health is compromised by toxicants, heat regulatory mechanisms of the autonomic nervous system are often affected, resulting in a failure to sweat readily [3]. In these cases, along with diet and nutritional supplementation to remediate biochemical imbalances, interventions to consider include brushing the skin, niacin to assist with vasodilation, and exercise prior to sauna use [50]. Clinical experience is that with persistence and ample hydration patients do eventually start to sweat. This is often a sign that the autonomic nervous system function is beginning to improve. With enhanced ability to sweat, detoxification is facilitated, which can ultimately result in clinical improvement.

For biomonitoring and research purposes, modern validated methods are desirable to collect and measure elements in sweat, so this means of excretion may be considered in the context of other measures such as urine, blood, feces, and hair concentrations. Considerations for dry and wet collection methods were recently discussed in the context of essential solutes [51, 52].

Undoubtedly further research in this area would improve understanding, but the available evidence suggests that physicians could consider recommending sweating as tolerated via exercise (preferred) and/or use of a sauna as a low-risk, potentially beneficial treatment for individuals who may be experiencing effects of toxic elements, or for individuals with regular exposure to or accretion of toxicants.

5. Conclusions

Sweating offers potential and deserves consideration, to assist with removal of toxic elements from the body. As toxic elements are implicated in many serious chronic conditions, research is needed in patients with select conditions to evaluate the body burden and to test the efficacy of source removal, dietary choices and supplements, interventions that induce sweating, and treatments with drugs, all to enhance excretion of toxic elements with the goal of clinical improvement. There is a clear need for robust trials, appropriately sized to assess clinical outcomes, from which therapeutic protocols can be derived. Both biochemical and clinical outcomes should be examined in order to develop and monitor clinical interventions that are both safe and effective.

Conflicts of Interests

The authors declare that they have no conflicts of interests.

Acknowledgments

The scoping review from which this work is derived was generously supported by a grant from the Canadian Institutes of Health Research, and the Social Sciences and Humanities Research Council of Canada. There are no conflicts of interest.

References

[1] Institute for Functional Medicine, *Textbook of Functional Medicine*, Gig Harbor, Wash, USA, 3rd edition, 2010.

[2] M. E. Sears and S. J. Genuis, "Environmental determinants of chronic disease, and medical approaches: recognition, avoidance, supportive therapy and detoxification," *Journal of Environmental and Public Health*, 2012.

[3] S. J. Genuis, D. Birkholz, I. Rodushkin, and S. Beesoon, "Blood, urine, and sweat (BUS) study: monitoring and elimination of bioaccumulated toxic elements," *Archives of Environmental Contamination and Toxicology*, vol. 61, no. 2, pp. 344–357, 2011.

[4] Agency for Toxic Substances and Disease Registry. Toxicological Profile: Arsenic, 2007, http://www.atsdr.cdc.gov/ToxProfiles/TP.asp?id=22&tid=3.

[5] Agency for Toxic Substances and Disease Registry. Toxicological Profile: Cadmium, 2008, http://www.atsdr.cdc.gov/toxprofiles/tp.asp?id=48&tid=15.

[6] Agency for Toxic Substances and Disease Registry. Toxicological Profile: Lead, 2007, http://www.atsdr.cdc.gov/ToxProfiles/tp.asp?id=96&tid=22.

[7] Agency for Toxic Substances and Disease Registry. Toxicological Profile: Mercury. US Department of Health and Human Services. Public Health Service, 1999, http://www.atsdr.cdc.gov/ToxProfiles/TP.asp?id=115&tid=24.

[8] R. Copes, N. A. Clark, K. Rideout, J. Palaty, and K. Teschke, "Uptake of cadmium from Pacific oysters (*Crassostrea gigas*) in British Columbia oyster growers," *Environmental Research*, vol. 107, no. 2, pp. 160–169, 2008.

[9] P. Perilli, L. G. Mitchell, C. A. Grant, and M. Pisantea, "Cadmium concentration in durum wheat grain (*Triticum turgidum*) as influenced by nitrogen rate, seeding date and soil type," *Journal of the Science of Food and Agriculture*, vol. 90, no. 5, pp. 813–822, 2010.

[10] W. Liu, Q. Zhou, J. An, Y. Sun, and R. Liu, "Variations in cadmium accumulation among Chinese cabbage cultivars and screening for Cd-safe cultivars," *Journal of Hazardous Materials*, vol. 173, no. 1–3, pp. 737–743, 2010.

[11] M. C. Houston, "Role of mercury toxicity in hypertension, cardiovascular disease, and stroke," *Journal of Clinical Hypertension*, vol. 13, no. 8, pp. 621–627, 2011.

[12] Health Canada. Government of Canada. Draft Human Health State of the Science Report on Lead—2011 Health Canada Consultation Document, 2011, http://www.hc-sc.gc.ca/ewh-semt/pubs/contaminants/dhhssrl-rpecscepsh/index-eng.php.

[13] Agency for Toxic Substances and Disease Registry. Interaction Profiles Home Page, http://www.atsdr.cdc.gov/interactionprofiles/index.asp.

[14] J. Leppaluoto, "Human thermoregulation in sauna," *Annals of Clinical Research*, vol. 20, no. 4, pp. 240–243, 1988.

[15] M. L. Hannuksela and S. Ellahham, "Benefits and risks of sauna bathing," *American Journal of Medicine*, vol. 110, no. 2, pp. 118–126, 2001.

[16] A. Eisalo and O. J. Luurila, "The Finnish sauna and cardiovascular diseases," *Annals of Clinical Research*, vol. 20, no. 4, pp. 267–270, 1988.

[17] J. A. Levisky, D. L. Bowerman, W. W. Jenkins, and S. B. Karch, "Drug deposition in adipose tissue and skin: evidence for an alternative source of positive sweat patch tests," *Forensic Science International*, vol. 110, no. 1, pp. 35–46, 2000.

[18] G. W. Cage and R. L. Dobson, "Sodium secretion and reabsorption in the human eccrine sweat gland," *Journal of Clinical Investigation*, vol. 44, no. 7, pp. 1270–1276, 1965.

[19] D. B. Dill, F. G. Hall, and W. van Beaumont, "Sweat chloride concentration: sweat rate, metabolic rate, skin temperature, and age," *Journal of Applied Physiology*, vol. 21, no. 1, pp. 96–106, 1966.

[20] D. B. Dill, F. G. Hall, and H. T. Edwards, "Changes in composition of sweat during acclimatization to heat," *American Journal of Physiology*, vol. 123, no. 2, p. 412, 1938.

[21] S. Robinson, J. R. Nicholas, J. H. Smith, W. J. Daly, and M. Pearcy, "Time relation of renal and sweat gland adjustments to salt deficiency in men," *Journal of Applied Physiology*, vol. 8, no. 2, pp. 159–165, 1955.

[22] J. L. Stauber and T. M. Florence, "The determination of trace metals in sweat by anodic stripping voltammetry," *Science of the Total Environment*, vol. 60, pp. 263–271, 1987.

[23] S. J. Montain, S. N. Cheuvront, and H. C. Lukaski, "Sweat mineral-element responses during 7 h of exercise-heat stress," *International Journal of Sport Nutrition and Exercise Metabolism*, vol. 17, no. 6, pp. 574–582, 2007.

[24] B. Falk, O. Bar-Or, R. Calvert, and J. D. MacDougall, "Sweat gland response to exercise in the heat among pre-, mid-, and late- pubertal boys," *Medicine and Science in Sports and Exercise*, vol. 24, no. 3, pp. 313–319, 1992.

[25] B. Falk and R. Dotan, "Children's thermoregulation during exercise in the heat—a revisit," *Applied Physiology, Nutrition and Metabolism*, vol. 33, no. 2, pp. 420–427, 2008.

[26] P. Haber, F. Ring, O. Jahn, and V. Meisinger, "Influence of intensive and extensive aerobic circulatory stress on blood lead levels," *Zentralblatt für Arbeitsmedizin, Arbeitsschutz, Prophylaxe und Ergonomie*, vol. 35, no. 10, pp. 303–306, 1985 (German).

[27] I. A. Parpaleĭ, L. G. Prokof'eva, and V. G. Obertas, "The use of the sauna for disease prevention in the workers of enterprises with chemical and physical occupational hazards," *Vracebnoe Delo Kiev*, no. 5, pp. 93–95, 1991, English abstract.

[28] J. L. Stauber and T. M. Florence, "A comparative study of copper, lead, cadmium and zinc in human sweat and blood," *Science of the Total Environment*, vol. 74, pp. 235–247, 1988.

[29] A. K. M. Yousuf, M. Misbahuddin, and M. S. Rahman, "Secretion of arsenic, cholesterol, vitamin E, and zinc from the site of arsenical melanosis and leucomelanosis in skin," *Clinical Toxicology*, vol. 49, no. 5, pp. 374–378, 2011.

[30] F. O. Omokhodion and J. M. Howard, "Trace elements in the sweat of acclimatized persons," *Clinica Chimica Acta*, vol. 231, no. 1, pp. 23–28, 1994.

[31] J. W. Robinson and S. Weiss, "The direct determination of cadmium in urine and perspiration using a carbon bed atomizer for atomic absorption spectroscopy," *Journal of Environmental Science and Health, Part A*, vol. 15, no. 6, pp. 635–662, 1980.

[32] J. W. Robinson and S. Weiss, "The direct determination of cadmium in hair using carbon bed atomic absorption spectroscopy. Daily rate of loss of cadmium in hair, urine and sweat," *Journal of Environmental Science and Health, Part A*, vol. 15, no. 6, pp. 663–697, 1980.

[33] J. R. Cohn and E. A. Emmett, "The excretion of trace metals in human sweat," *Annals of Clinical and Laboratory Science*, vol. 8, no. 4, pp. 270–275, 1978, (only abstract available online).

[34] F. O. Omokhodion and G. W. Crockford, "Sweat lead levels in persons with high blood lead levels: experimental elevation of blood lead by ingestion of lead chloride," *Science of the Total Environment*, vol. 108, no. 3, pp. 235–242, 1991.

[35] F. O. Omokhodion and J. M. Howard, "Sweat lead levels in persons with high blood lead levels: lead in sweat of lead

workers in the tropics," *Science of the Total Environment*, vol. 103, no. 2-3, pp. 123–128, 1991.
[36] F. O. Omokhodion and G. W. Crockford, "Lead in sweat and its relationship to salivary and urinary levels in normal healthy subjects," *Science of the Total Environment*, vol. 103, no. 2-3, pp. 113–122, 1991.
[37] S. G. Lilley, T. M. Florence, and J. L. Stauber, "The use of sweat to monitor lead absorption through the skin," *Science of the Total Environment*, vol. 76, no. 2-3, pp. 267–278, 1988.
[38] D. C. Hohnadel, F. W. Sunderman, M. W. Nechay, and M. D. McNeely, "Atomic absorption spectrometry of nickel, copper, zinc, and lead in sweat collected from healthy subjects during sauna bathing," *Clinical Chemistry*, vol. 19, no. 11, pp. 1288–1292, 1973.
[39] J. W. Robinson and E. M. Skelly, "The direct determination of mercury in sweat," *Spectroscopy Letters*, vol. 16, no. 2, p. 133, 1983.
[40] F. W. Sunderman, "Clinical response to therapeutic agents in poisoning from mercury vapor," *Annals of Clinical and Laboratory Science*, vol. 8, no. 4, pp. 259–269, 1978.
[41] H. B. Lovejoy, Z. G. Bell, and T. R. Vizena, "Mercury exposure evaluations and their correlation with urine mercury excretions. 4. Elimination of mercury by sweating," *Journal of Occupational Medicine*, vol. 15, no. 7, pp. 590–591, 1973.
[42] D. Airey, "Mercury in human hair due to environment and diet: a review," *Environmental Health Perspectives*, vol. 52, pp. 303–316, 1983.
[43] J. L. Stauber, T. M. Florence, B. L. Gulson, and L. S. Dale, "Percutaneous absorption of inorganic lead compounds," *Science of the Total Environment*, vol. 145, no. 1-2, pp. 55–70, 1994.
[44] G. Sällsten, S. Kreku, and H. Unosson, "A small dose of ethanol increases the exhalation of mercury in low-level-exposed humans," *Journal of Toxicology and Environmental Health, Part A*, vol. 60, no. 2, pp. 89–100, 2000.
[45] K. W. Brown, "Workers' health and colonial mercury mining at Huancavelica, Peru," *The Americas*, vol. 57, no. 4, pp. 467–496, 2001.
[46] K. Kukkonen-Harjula and K. Kauppinen, "Health effects and risks of sauna bathing," *International Journal of Circumpolar Health*, vol. 65, no. 3, pp. 195–205, 2006.
[47] J. Dahlgren, M. Cecchini, H. Takhar, and O. Paepke, "Persistent organic pollutants in 9/11 world trade center rescue workers: reduction following detoxification," *Chemosphere*, vol. 69, no. 8, pp. 1320–1325, 2007.
[48] S. J. Genuis, D. Birkholz, M. Ralitsch, and N. Thibault, "Human detoxification of perfluorinated compounds," *Public Health*, vol. 124, no. 7, pp. 367–375, 2010.
[49] S. J. Genuis, S. Beesoon, D. Birkholz, and R. A. Lobo, "Human excretion of bisphenol-A: blood, urine and sweat (BUS) study," *Journal of Environmental and Public Health*, 2012.
[50] G. H. Ross and M. C. Sternquist, "Methamphetamine exposure and chronic illness in police officers: significant improvement with sauna-based detoxification therapy," *Toxicology and Industrial Health*. In press.
[51] L. B. Weschler, "Sweat electrolyte concentrations obtained from within occlusive coverings are falsely high because sweat itself leaches skin electrolytes," *Journal of Applied Physiology*, vol. 105, no. 4, pp. 1376–1377, 2008.
[52] L. E. Armstrong, "Commentary on viewpoint: sweat electrolyte concentrations obtained from within occlusive coverings are falsely high because sweat itself leaches skin electrolytes," *Journal of Applied Physiology*, vol. 105, no. 4, p. 1378, 2008.

16

Human Excretion of Bisphenol A: Blood, Urine, and Sweat (BUS) Study

Stephen J. Genuis,[1] Sanjay Beesoon,[2] Detlef Birkholz,[3] and Rebecca A. Lobo[4]

[1] *Faculty of Medicine, University of Alberta, 2935-66 Street, Edmonton, AB, Canada T6K 4C1*
[2] *Department of Laboratory Medicine, University of Alberta, Edmonton, AB, Canada T6G 2B7*
[3] *Environmental Division, ALS Laboratory Group, Edmonton AB, Canada T6E 5C1*
[4] *Department of Family Medicine, University of Alberta, Edmonton, AB, Canada T6G 2C8*

Correspondence should be addressed to Stephen J. Genuis, sgenuis@ualberta.ca

Academic Editor: Robin Bernhoft

Background. Bisphenol A (BPA) is an ubiquitous chemical contaminant that has recently been associated with adverse effects on human health. There is incomplete understanding of BPA toxicokinetics, and there are no established interventions to eliminate this compound from the human body. Using 20 study participants, this study was designed to assess the relative concentration of BPA in three body fluids—blood, urine, and sweat—and to determine whether induced sweating may be a therapeutic intervention with potential to facilitate elimination of this compound. *Methods.* Blood, urine, and sweat were collected from 20 individuals (10 healthy participants and 10 participants with assorted health problems) and analyzed for various environmental toxicants including BPA. *Results.* BPA was found to differing degrees in each of blood, urine, and sweat. In 16 of 20 participants, BPA was identified in sweat, even in some individuals with no BPA detected in their serum or urine samples. *Conclusions.* Biomonitoring of BPA through blood and/or urine testing may underestimate the total body burden of this potential toxicant. Sweat analysis should be considered as an additional method for monitoring bioaccumulation of BPA in humans. Induced sweating appears to be a potential method for elimination of BPA.

1. Introduction

First synthesized in 1891 and with current production estimated at 4 billion kilograms each year globally [1], bisphenol A (BPA) is a multipurpose compound that is widely used in the modern industrial world. BPA was initially investigated for its potentially therapeutic estrogenic properties in the 1930s; when diethylstilbestrol (DES) was found to be more potent, however, BPA was temporarily cast aside. Its commercial value was reassessed in the 1950s with the introduction of BPA as a fundamental component in the manufacturing of some plastics. As its primary use currently, BPA is a key monomer in the production of the most common form of clear and shatter-proof polycarbonate plastic, but it has also been incorporated into a variety of everyday goods.

Questions regarding the safety and side effects of BPA began to emerge in the late 1990s when BPA was found to leech out of plastics and into experimental animal subjects, resulting in an increased incidence of chromosomal anomalies in offspring [2]. There has since been ongoing discussion in both scientific and political spheres about the potential for harm resulting from human BPA exposure and potential bioaccumulation. An overview of the literature regarding the effects of BPA on human health is provided, followed by a presentation of data from 20 subjects whose blood, urine, and sweat were tested for BPA. Results and discussion regarding BPA bioaccumulation and elimination are presented for consideration.

2. Background

Currently, BPA is most commonly found as a component in polycarbonates (~74% of total BPA produced) and in the production of epoxy resins (~20%). As well as being found in a myriad of products including plastic food and beverage containers (including baby and water bottles), BPA is also commonly found in various household appliances, electronics, sports safety equipment, adhesives, cash register receipts, medical devices, eyeglass lenses, water supply pipes, and many other products. It is also frequently used as an adjunct in the production of brominated flame retardants and brake fluid [1]. Moreover, BPA derivatives, such as bisphenol A-glycidyl methacrylate and bisphenol A-dimethacrylate, have recently been incorporated into the dental industry and used in dental fillings and sealants. The widespread use of this compound is receiving increasing scrutiny as concerns about BPA effects on human health have recently emerged.

The main mechanism by which the population is exposed to BPA is through leaching from plastic products. This results from either the release of unpolymerized monomers or the slow decay of polymer bonds in polycarbonates leading to monomer release into proximal foods and liquids. Occupational exposures are also present where plastics are burned and manufactured, and thus BPA may be inhaled by workers [3, 4]. An analysis of Chinese employees in factories where BPA and epoxy resins are produced, for example, revealed that over 90% of exposed workers have notable levels of BPA in their serum and urine [5].

A plethora of recent studies affirms that the majority of the population (91–99%) does indeed have detectable levels of BPA, but the level and the toxicological relevance of current exposure levels is a subject of intense academic and public health debate [6–13]. An extensive review conducted in 2007 concluded that BPA levels in human blood and/or urine are within the range shown to be dangerous in animals and are therefore likely to be biologically active in humans [6]. (As will be discussed, however, blood and urine testing may underestimate the full extent of exposure and bioaccumulation.) Conversely, an industry-sponsored literature review from 2008 declared that daily human consumption was far below dangerous levels and is therefore of minimal concern [7].

Sources of BPA ingestion may vary. In infants and children, baby and beverage bottles used by most individuals in the pediatric population provide ongoing daily sources of BPA [14–22]. Le et al. found that at room temperature, leaching of BPA occurred into the contained fluid, which increased 55-fold if boiling water was added [14]. Another study found that exposure levels increased not only with temperature, but also with repeated use of a container [15].

Other common sources of ingestion include foods stored in food cans, which are lined with BPA epoxy resin films to prevent corrosion [23–28], thermal printing paper commonly used in cash register receipts [29–31], and BPA containing dental composites and sealants [32–34]. Medical equipment is also raising concerns about BPA levels as a study of newborns found that those who regularly spent time in a neonatal intensive care unit had significantly higher serum BPA levels than the general population—thought to be due to exposure to plastics in medical devices [35]. Likewise, dialysis patients appear to have higher rates of exposure, which may be attributable to circulating solvents which expedite the leaching of BPA from polycarbonate hemodialysis equipment [36, 37].

When ingested, unconjugated BPA—the biologically active form of BPA—has historically been thought to be rapidly conjugated in the liver and then excreted through bile or urine, with a half life of approximately 5.3 hours [38–40]. This rapid excretion has been the basis of reassuring safety evaluations and declarations given by some public health authorities worldwide. However, within many tissues, particularly the lungs, livers and kidneys in rats, and the placenta of animals and humans, β-glucuronidase enzyme is present at detectable concentration. This enzyme is able to deconjugate BPA and thus release its active form again [41]. This is of great significance, as it is plausible that, in pregnancy, the conjugated form of BPA will circulate through the placenta, undergo deconjugation, and cause subsequent fetal exposure in utero. This may also result in bioaccumulation of some portion of BPA after exposure. In fact, recent evidence suggests that at low concentrations, while most plasma BPA (about 95%) is bound to serum proteins, BPA has lipophilic affinity with a fat: blood coefficient of 3.3 [42]. Furthermore, BPA appears to have a disproportionate affinity to fat in comparison to other tissues such as kidney, muscle, and other sites; "in fat, the accumulation of BPA was about three times higher than in other tissues" [42]. With evidence of potential bioaccumulation, BPA has the prospect of exerting ongoing metabolic effects.

2.1. Potential Implications of BPA Exposure. BPA is thought to wield its effects through endocrine disruption, epigenetic modification, cytokine release, and oxidative stress. When first discovered, BPA was investigated for its estrogenic properties, as it is thought to alter the synthesis of estradiol and testosterone and interfere with receptor binding [43, 44]. Consequently, exposure to BPA has been linked with a number of developmental and reproductive pathologies in both animal models and human subjects. These include abnormalities in reproductive organ function (irregular cycles, multiple ovarian cysts, reduction in primordial follicles [45–49]), placental dysfunction [50], increased incidence of miscarriage and neonatal mortality [50, 51], precocious puberty [52], and sexual dysfunction such as erectile dysfunction, decreased libido, and ejaculation difficulties [53–55]. Moreover, interference with the production and signaling of sex hormones has led to neurological impairment [56–60]. Synapse formation during development is regulated by estrogen and androgens; however with exposure to BPA, a recent study found that levels deemed safe by the US Environment Protection Agency, completely abolish the response of synapses to estrogen in the prefrontal cortex and hippocampus [61].

Epigenetic effects of BPA have been associated with an increased risk of cancer, particularly breast and prostate malignancies [62–69]. The exposure of breast epithelial cells to BPA was found to alter gene expression of 170 genes and increase their vulnerability to other carcinogens [62, 63]. Additionally, there was silencing of lysosomal-associated membrane protein 3, as occurs in ERα-positive breast cancer [62]. Similar effects have been seen with respect to prostatic disease, as exposure to BPA has been repeatedly shown to modify methylation of implicated genes [64–66].

Low dose BPA exposure at weaning during the perinatal period has also been found to increase adipogenesis in female animals [70]. As it is hypothesized that adult body weight may be programmed during early life, these results are noteworthy with regards to the childhood obesity pandemic and the action of endocrine disruptors as determinants of obesity [70]. BPA exposure appears to have widespread impact as it has also been linked by various researchers and studies throughout the world with a whole host of other health problems, including metabolic syndrome, obesity, non-insulin-dependent diabetes mellitus, allergies and asthma, ADHD, autism, cognitive decline, memory impairment, depression, and anxiety [71–92]. With the rise of sensitivity-related illness, there is also concern that BPA may be a determinant of this recently recognized causative mechanism of disease and source etiology of assorted clinical conditions [93] by stimulating the release of proinflammatory adipokines such as interleukin-6 (IL-6) and tumor necrosis factor alpha (TNF-alpha) from human adipose tissue [71].

As a result of all the emerging attention in the scientific literature, various governments have also embarked on research and policy decisions relating to BPA. In 2010, for example, the Minister of Health for the Canadian Government declared the results of a four-year study indicating, "The Government of Canada is a world leader in chemicals management. Our science indicated that Bisphenol A may be harmful to both human health and the environment" [94]. With emerging information of concern about BPA, the Canadian government became the first to prohibit the sale of BPA-containing polycarbonate baby bottles. France, Denmark and several American states have since implemented similar regulations.

2.2. Limitations of Toxicant Biomonitoring. It is often assumed that after exposure, BPA is rapidly metabolized to a hormonally inactive metabolite and efficiently excreted in toto from the body [95–97]. As a result, there has been little concern about bioaccumulation. The question arises, however, that if the compound is rapidly excreted without any accrual, why is there increasing evidence that BPA exposure is anything but innocuous and is able to cause potentially serious problems in animal and human organisms? While some believe that only unremitting ongoing exposure to BPA generates risk, concern has been raised that unrecognized bioaccumulation of some fraction of BPA may occur in some exposed individuals. How does one monitor to determine if toxicant compounds bioaccumulate and thus remain within the human organism?

Throughout the world, blood and urine sampling are the general modalities used to biomonitor levels of most toxicant compounds including toxic elements, synthetic compounds, petrochemical compounds, biologic toxicants such as mycotoxins, and xenobiotics sometimes produced as byproducts from processing of parent compounds [98]. There is increasing evidence, however, that relying on blood and urine measurements as indicators of bioaccumulation can be very flawed [99]. Many compounds sequester in tissues and do not remain in blood; testing of whole blood or serum may miss toxicants which have exited the blood compartment and are being stored primarily in tissues such as bone, muscle, or adipose compartments. Levels of toxicant compounds can also rapidly fluctuate with changes in immediate status such as caloric restriction, level of hydration, underlying nutrient status, thermal changes, or exercise [98, 100].

Reliance on blood or urine testing for assessment of the body burden of many toxicants may thus be less than reliable clinically or for public health purposes. As a result, attempts to biomonitor toxicant levels by sampling other tissues and bodily excretions have been explored, including hair sampling, salivary testing, stool sampling, perspiration testing, breath analysis, provocation testing, and biopsies of adipose tissue through needle aspiration into fat pads under the skin. It is evident, however, that there are limitations with each of these approaches. Hair samples, for example may only reflect what has been in the blood stream for the last few weeks, while stool samples only assess what is being eliminated though fecal waste—these do not measure the body burden. As detailed toxicokinetics for many xenobiotic compounds are not fully understood, it is difficult to know which proportion of parent compounds and their metabolites accrue within various bodily compartments.

Some researchers have recently commenced doing fat biopsies as a tool to biomonitor toxicant levels—this technique involves taking a sample of fat, usually from the abdominal or gluteal area and sending the sample for analysis. Recent evidence, however, confirms that toxicants sequester differently even within specific compartments such as adipose tissue; one adipose tissue site may display toxicant concentrations that are totally different than concentrations at another site [101]. So the toxicant concentration in brain adipose tissue, for example, may be very different than that found in breast or abdominal wall adipose tissue.

In review, attempts to biomonitor the levels of toxicant compounds, including BPA, in humans using a single modality such as blood or urine are inadequate at best. This is a challenging realization as most population studies on toxicant compounds reported in the scientific literature as well as most ongoing biomonitoring research is based on blood or urine testing.

2.3. Study Objective. BPA exposure is generally assessed by measuring urine levels of this compound. In this research, we endeavor to determine the relative concentrations of BPA in blood, urine, and sweat. By assessing BPA levels in these three compartments, the possibility of identifying retained BPA will be explored as well as the potential for induced perspiration as a means to eradicate this compound.

3. Methods

3.1. Participant Recruitment. 9 males and 11 females with mean ages 44.5 ± 14.4 years and 45.6 ± 10.3 years, respectively, were recruited to participate in the study after appropriate ethical approval from the Health Research Ethics Board of the University of Alberta. 10 participants were patients with various clinical conditions and 10 were otherwise healthy adults. Participants with health issues were recruited from the first author's clinical practice by invitation. Each

Table 1: Participant results for BPA in three body compartments: serum, urine, and sweat.

Participant	Gender	Age	Clinical diagnosis	Serum conc.	Urine conc.	Sweat conc.	Sweat/urine ratio	Technique used for sweat collection
1	M	61	Diabetes, obesity, hypertension	0	4	82	20.5	Exercise
2	F	40	Rheumatoid arthritis	0	22	24	1.1	Steam sauna
3	M	38	Addiction disorder	0	20	22	1.1	Steam sauna
4	F	25	Bipolar disorder	0	40	22	0.6	Steam sauna
5	F	47	Lymphoma	0	10	24	2.4	Steam sauna
6	F	43	Fibromyalgia	0	32	0	n/a	Steam sauna
7	F	48	Depression	0	0	16	n/a	Steam sauna
8	F	40	Chronic fatigue	0	0	22	n/a	Infrared sauna
9	F	68	Diabetes, fatigue, obesity	0	0	10	n/a	Steam sauna
10	M	49	Chronic pain, cognitive decline	0	8	10	1.3	Exercise
11	M	53	Healthy	10	32	20	0.6	Exercise
12	M	23	Healthy	0	30	46	1.5	Infrared sauna
13	M	21	Healthy	30	4	10	2.5	Infrared sauna
14	F	47	Healthy	0	8	12	1.5	Infrared sauna
15	M	53	Healthy	0	4	35	8.8	Infrared sauna
16	F	43	Healthy	0	0	12	n/a	Infrared sauna
17	F	51	Healthy	0	0	0	n/a	Infrared sauna
18	M	46	Healthy	0	42	0	n/a	Infrared sauna
19	M	57	Healthy	0	0	0	n/a	Infrared sauna
20	F	50	Healthy	0	8	22	2.8	Infrared sauna

participant in the study provided informed consent and volunteered to give one 200 mL random sample of blood, one sample of first morning urine, and one 100 mL sample of sweat. Demographic and clinical characteristics of all research participants are provided in Table 1.

3.2. Samples Collection. All blood samples were collected at one Dynalife laboratory site in Edmonton, Alberta, Canada through vacutainer blood collection equipment (BD Vacutainer, Franklin Lakes, NJ, 07417, USA) using 21 gauge stainless steel needles which were screwed into the "BD Vacutainer One-Use Holder" (REF 364815). The 10 mL glass vacutainer was directly inserted into the holder and into the back end of the needle. This process and the use of glass were used to preclude contamination. Blood was collected directly into plain 10 mL glass vacutainer tubes, allowed to clot, and spun down 30 minutes later. After serum was separated off, samples were picked up by ALS Laboratories (about 3 kilometres from the blood collection site) for storage pending analysis. When received at ALS, serum samples were transferred to 4-mL glass vials and stored in a freezer at −20°C, pending transfer to the analytical laboratory. We chose to analyze BPA in serum rather than in whole blood, based on the fact that matrix effect of serum is much lower than whole blood.

For urine collection, participants were instructed to collect a first morning urine sample directly into a provided 500 mL glass jar container with Teflon-lined lid on the same day that blood samples were collected. Urine samples were delivered by the participants directly to Edmonton ALS Laboratories. Samples were transferred to 4-mL glass vials and stored in a freezer at −20°C, pending transfer.

For sweat collection, participants were instructed to collect perspiration from any site on their body directly into the provided 500 mL glass jar container with Teflon-lined lid—by placing the jar against their prewashed skin when actively sweating or by using a stainless steel spatula against their skin to transfer perspiration directly into the glass jar. (Stainless steel—made up primarily of iron, chromium, and nickel—was chosen as it is the same material as the needles used in standard blood collections and is reported not to off-gas or leach at room or body temperature.) Excess of 100 mL of sweat was provided in all but one case. Each of the glass bottles used for sampling in this study was provided by ALS laboratories and had undergone extensive cleaning and rinsing. The containers were deemed appropriate for sweat collection with negligible risk of contamination: laboratory-grade phosphate-free detergent wash; acid rinse; multiple hot and cold deionized water rinses; oven-dried; capping and packing in quality controlled conditions. Sweat was collected within 1 week before or after doing the blood work. No specifications were given as to how long sweating had commenced before collection. 10 participants collected sweat

TABLE 2: Comparison of urine BPA levels across published studies.

Urine levels of BPA (ng/mL)-comparison across studies							
Study	Location	Detection method	DL (ng/mL)	Participants	Detection(%)	AM/GM/Median	Range
This study	Canada	LC-MS	0.2	20 adults	70	AM:13 Median 8	0–42
Bushnik et al. [10]	Canada	GC-MS	0.2	5462 (age 6–79)	90.7	GM 1.16 (1.08–1.24)	N/A
Calafat et al. [9]	USA	LC-MS	0.4	950 adults	N/A	GM 2.4	N/A
Calafat et al. [8]	USA	GC-MS	0.1	394 adults	95	GM 1.33 Median 1.28	0.1–5.18 (*95th Centile*)
Moors et al. [108]	Germany	GC-MS	3	15 adults	60		ND-55
Mendiola et al. [107]	USA	LC-MS	0.4	375 males	90	GM 1.50	<0.4–6.5 (*95th Centile*)

DL: detection limit; AM: arithmetic mean; GM: geometric mean; ND: non detect; N/A: not available.
LC-MS: liquid chromatography-mass spectrometry.
GC-MS: gas chromatography-mass spectrometry.

inside an infrared sauna; 7 collected inside a regular steam sauna, and 3 collected during and immediately after exercise—no specific instruction was given regarding the type or location of exercise. Sweat was delivered by the participants directly to ALS laboratories. Samples were transferred to 4 mL glass vials and stored in a freezer at −20°C, pending analysis. No preservatives were used in the jars provided for sweat and urine collection, nor in the serum storage vials.

3.3. Analytical Methods. Human serum was analyzed for levels of bisphenol A (BPA) at ALS Canada following the general procedures presented by the Centres for Disease Control and Prevention [8, 102]. Briefly, samples were fortified with 12.5 nanograms of isotopically labelled phthalate metabolites, 50 nanograms of labeled bisphenol-A, 250 nanograms of 4-methylumbelliferone glucuronide, 300 microliters of ammonium acetate buffer (pH 6.5), and 10 microliters of β-glucuronidase (Escherichia coli K12, Roche Biomedical). The samples were mixed and incubated at 37°C overnight to allow for the deglucuronidation.

Following enzymatic hydrolysis, a 20 uL aliquot of the sample is added to 70 uL of HPLC-grade water and 10 ng of labelled 4-methylumbelliferone to determine deglucuronidation efficiency (done once every 100 samples). The remaining sample is loaded onto a Zymark Rapid Trace Station for automated solid phase extraction (SPE). The 60 milligram/3 mL Oasis-HLB cartridges were conditioned with HPLC-grade methanol (2 mL) and 0.1 M formic acid (2 mL). The samples were diluted with 5 mL of 0.1 M formic acid and loaded onto the SPE cartridge at a rate of 1.0 mL/min. The cartridge was washed with water (1 mL) and 10% methanol in water (2 mL) at a flow rate of 1 mL/min. The samples were eluted with 1.0 mL of acetonitrile at a flow rate of 0.5 mL/min. The eluate was evaporated to dryness under a stream of dry nitrogen and the residue was resuspended in 85% methanol in water (200 microliters) and transferred to glass autosampler vials.

Quality control of the analysis was maintained by analysing a method blank (calf serum) and two spiked calf serum samples (20 ng/mL, all analytes) along with every 17 samples. The detection limit (0.2 ng/mL) was based upon our lower calibration standard (0.5 ng/mL) which gave an instrument signal to noise response of 3 : 1. Analysis was performed using an API 4000 liquid chromatograph/tandem mass spectrometer.

4. Results and Discussion

Demographic characteristics as well as results for each individual participant are summarized in Table 1. All concentrations are in nanograms per milliliter.

The fact that some subjects showed undetectable levels confirms that generalized contamination of these samples is not likely. Furthermore, the levels of BPA were similar to those recently published in studies from Italy and Greece [103] and are comparable with the serum levels found (0.79–7.12 ng/mL) in a recent study by Cobellis et al. in 2009 [104]. The rather low percentage detection among the serum samples in North America is hard to compare as (to our knowledge) there is only one study in the literature that documents BPA levels in blood of North Americans [105]. In that study, using the same extraction method as the methodology used in this study, the authors reported BPA levels in the range of <0.5 (detection limit) to 22.3 ng/mL in the blood plasma of 40 pregnant American women in the state of Michigan. However, the authors did not report in how many of these 40 women that BPA was detected above their current limit of detection of 0.5 ng/mL. In general, there is major variability in the range of concentrations of BPA detected in blood, and this may be explained by the fact that detection methods vary widely and the specific populations studied also vary considerably [106].

For the urine samples, the percentage detection in the current study (70%) is lower than that of the large scale Canadian biomonitoring study (90.7%) also known as the Canadian Health Measures Survey as reported by Bushnik et al. [10]. However, the geometric mean level of urine BPA in this study is generally higher than those in other biomonitoring studies in North America. Comparative levels for urine BPA as found in the literature are presented in Table 2. For example, Bushnik et al. reported a geometric

A	Serum+	Serum−
Urine+	2	12
Urine−	0	6

B	Serum+	Serum−
Sweat+	2	14
Sweat−	0	4

C	Urine+	Urine−
Sweat+	12	4
Sweat−	2	2

FIGURE 1: 2×2 tables indicating the presence of BPA in specific body compartments. Each cell represents number of study participants.

mean of 1.15 ng/mL urine BPA in Canada for a sample size of 5462 [10], Calafat et al. found a value of 2.4 ng/mL for urine BPA among 950 American adults aged between 20 and 59 [9] and more recently Mendolia et al. reported on 375 American males with a geometric mean value of 1.50 ng/mL of urine BPA [107]. As far as sweat data is concerned, comparison across studies is impossible as to our knowledge this is the first study which attempts to quantify BPA in sweat.

One obvious qualitative interpretation of the data from the cohort of 20 study participants is that BPA is rarely detected in blood, and this is probably why most large scale biomonitoring studies, such as the NHANES (National Health and Nutrition Examination Survey) and CHMS (Canadian Health Measures Survey), use urine as the human sample of choice to determine exposure levels in populations. In an attempt to summarize the findings on the distribution of BPA in the 3 different body fluids, we give three 2×2 tables in Figure 1. As discussed earlier, the 2 discordant pairs urine+/serum− and sweat+/serum−, with 12 and 14 in their respective grids show clearly that serum is not the appropriate body fluid to test if BPA biomonitoring in humans is to be characterised. Although there seems to be high correlation between urine and sweat in terms of the presence/absence of BPA in these media, with 12 individuals in the urine+/sweat+ concordant pair, what is more surprising is that there are 4 individuals for which BPA was detected in sweat but undetectable in urine (Figure 1C).

In an attempt to compare the excretion efficiencies of urine and sweat for BPA, we calculated the ratio of BPA concentration in sweat versus urine for those 12 individuals who are in the urine+/sweat+ concordant pair. As shown in Table 1, with the exception of 2 individuals (participants 4 and 11) where urine concentration of BPA is slightly higher than in sweat, in general the ratio is higher than 1, suggesting that induced sweating may be an efficient method for eliminating BPA from the body. This is not surprising in the light of the findings of Csanády et al. whereby they found a preferential partitioning of BPA in adipose tissue compared to blood with a ratio of 3.3 [42]. This suggests that the BPA in blood which is then conjugated and excreted in the urine may only represent about one-third of the body burden of BPA. It is not surprising therefore that induced sweating in saunas can mobilise BPA in adipose tissue thus leading to enhanced excretion in sweat. Given that BPA in body fat is mostly unconjugated, further studies looking at the ratio of free BPA to conjugated BPA in sweat will help to confirm whether the BPA excreted in sweat comes from adipose tissue. Given that in normal circumstances the daily volume of urine is much higher than sweat, urine remains an important mode of elimination of BPA from the human body.

An important consideration in response to the results is why there are two participants with evidence of BPA in their urine with no positive level in their sweat. Presumably, the sweat level may be reflective of accrued toxicants in tissue, whereas urine may reflect in part at least recent exposure which the body is endeavoring to eliminate. It may be that BPA begins to bioaccumulate only after a threshold of exposure is reached or once the detoxification mechanisms of the organism are unable to completely eliminate the BPA load that presents after exposure. Further research is required in order to clarify, but this result may indicate that the two individuals have had some recent exposure, but no significant level of stockpiled toxicant. Similarly, the marked variation in the range of the sweat/urine ratio may once again be reflective of different phenomenon: the sweat results may represent transcutaneous excretion of accured BPA toxicant, while the urine results are perhaps reflecting recent BPA exposure in addition to some release of accrued BPA that the body is able to eliminate through renal mechanisms. It is also noteworthy that there was no statistically significant difference (P-value >0.05) in sweat BPA levels depending on the method of sweat collection whether through exercise, infrared sauna, or regular sauna.

Although this study sheds light on the importance of sweat as a pathway of elimination for BPA from the body, it has some limitations. First, given the small study size (n = 20) it is not possible to extrapolate the findings to the general population. Secondly, samples were analysed for total BPA, instead of unconjugated BPA and conjugated BPA separately. Thirdly, other rare forms of BPA such as chlorinated and sulfated BPA were not analysed for.

5. Conclusion

As a result of increased scrutiny of health sequelae associated with human BPA exposure, it is apparent that this endocrine-disrupting compound has potentially negative consequences for the human organism. With new evidence for the possibility of BPA accrual within the body, interventions to facilitate elimination of this toxic compound have clinical relevance with regards to the prevention and treatment of adverse outcomes associated with BPA bioaccumulation. The results of this study suggest that: (i) Sweat testing may be an additional tool for BPA bio-monitoring; and (ii) Induced sweating appears to be a clinically useful tool to facilitate the release of BPA through the skin in order to eliminate this toxicant from the human body.

Notable findings and implications of data from this study
(i) BPA is excreted in sweat
(ii) Sweat BPA concentrations are consistently much higher than urine
(iii) Only 2/20 participants had BPA in serum, while 16/20 had BPA in sweat
(iv) The data suggests that BPA likely bioaccumulates to some degree in humans
(v) The data suggests that BPA retained in tissues (likely adipose) excretes via sweat
(vi) The finding in some individuals that little or no BPA is excreted in urine while considerable levels are found in sweat suggests that current biomonitoring via serum (as done in Europe) or urine (as done in North America) may not provide a reliable indication of the BPA toxicant burden
(vii) With the recognition that BPA has the potential for hormonal dysregulation, the significance of accrued BPA remains to be conclusively elucidated

Conflict of Interests

There is no conflict of interests. No funding has been received for any part of this work.

Acknowledgment

The authors thank Jarrod Roberts for his technical work and assistance with analysis of samples.

References

[1] Environment Canada, Consultation Document Bisphenol A—Phenol, 4,4′-(1-Methylethylidene) bis-(Bisphenol A), 2009, http://www.ec.gc.ca/lcpe-cepa/79A93C66-1EE0-4F72-89C1-114DFD7B7292/pba-eng.pdf.

[2] P. A. Hunt, K. E. Koehler, M. Susiarjo et al., "Bisphenol a exposure causes meiotic aneuploidy in the female mouse," *Current Biology*, vol. 13, no. 7, pp. 546–553, 2003.

[3] N. K. Wilson, J. C. Chuang, M. K. Morgan, R. A. Lordo, and L. S. Sheldon, "An observational study of the potential exposures of preschool children to pentachlorophenol, bisphenol-A, and nonylphenol at home and daycare," *Environmental Research*, vol. 103, no. 1, pp. 9–20, 2007.

[4] L. N. Vandenberg, M. V. Maffini, C. Sonnenschein, B. S. Rubin, and A. M. Soto, "Bisphenol-a and the great divide: a review of controversies in the field of endocrine disruption," *Endocrine Reviews*, vol. 30, no. 1, pp. 75–95, 2009.

[5] Y. He, M. Miao, C. Wu et al., "Occupational exposure levels of Bisphenol a among Chinese workers," *Journal of Occupational Health*, vol. 51, no. 5, pp. 432–436, 2009.

[6] L. N. Vandenberg, R. Hauser, M. Marcus, N. Olea, and W. V. Welshons, "Human exposure to bisphenol A (BPA)," *Reproductive Toxicology*, vol. 24, no. 2, pp. 139–177, 2007.

[7] W. Dekant and W. Völkel, "Human exposure to bisphenol A by biomonitoring: methods, results and assessment of environmental exposures," *Toxicology and Applied Pharmacology*, vol. 228, no. 1, pp. 114–134, 2008.

[8] A. M. Calafat, Z. Kuklenyik, J. A. Reidy, S. P. Caudill, J. Ekong, and L. L. Needham, "Urinary concentrations of bisphenol A and 4-Nonylphenol in a human reference population," *Environmental Health Perspectives*, vol. 113, no. 4, pp. 391–395, 2005.

[9] A. M. Calafat, X. Ye, L. Y. Wong, J. A. Reidy, and L. L. Needham, "Exposure of the U.S. population to bisphenol A and 4-tertiary-octylphenol: 2003-2004," *Environmental Health Perspectives*, vol. 116, no. 1, pp. 39–44, 2008.

[10] T. Bushnik, D. Haines, P. Levallois, J. Levesque, J. Van Oostdam, and C. Viau, "Lead and bisphenol A concentrations in the Canadian population," *Health Reports*, vol. 21, no. 3, pp. 7–18, 2010.

[11] H. Mielke and U. Gundert-Remy, "Bisphenol A levels in blood depend on age and exposure," *Toxicology Letters*, vol. 190, no. 1, pp. 32–40, 2009.

[12] K. Becker, T. Güen, M. Seiwert et al., "GerES IV: phthalate metabolites and bisphenol A in urine of German children," *International Journal of Hygiene and Environmental Health*, vol. 212, no. 6, pp. 685–692, 2009.

[13] J. H. Kang, F. Kondo, and Y. Katayama, "Human exposure to bisphenol A," *Toxicology*, vol. 226, no. 2-3, pp. 79–89, 2006.

[14] H. H. Le, E. M. Carlson, J. P. Chua, and S. M. Belcher, "Bisphenol A is released from polycarbonate drinking bottles and mimics the neurotoxic actions of estrogen in developing cerebellar neurons," *Toxicology Letters*, vol. 176, no. 2, pp. 149–156, 2008.

[15] S. H. Nam, Y. M. Seo, and M. G. Kim, "Bisphenol A migration from polycarbonate baby bottle with repeated use," *Chemosphere*, vol. 79, no. 9, pp. 949–952, 2010.

[16] J. L. Carwile, H. T. Luu, L. S. Bassett et al., "Polycarbonate bottle use and urinary bisphenol A concentrations," *Environmental Health Perspectives*, vol. 117, no. 9, pp. 1368–1372, 2009.

[17] Health C, "Survey of bisphenol A in bottled water products," 2009, http://www.hc-sc.gc.ca/fn-an/alt_formats/hpfb-dgpsa/pdf/securit/bpa_survey-enquete-bot-bou-eng.pdf.

[18] K. A. Ehlert, C. W. E. Beumer, and M. C. E. Groot, "Migration of bisphenol A into water from polycarbonate baby bottles during microwave heating," *Food Additives and Contaminants—Part A*, vol. 25, no. 7, pp. 904–910, 2008.

[19] N. De Coensel, F. David, and P. Sandra, "Study on the migration of bisphenol-A from baby bottles by stir bar sorptive extractionthermal desorption-capillary GC-MS," *Journal of Separation Science*, vol. 32, no. 21, pp. 3829–3836, 2009.

[20] C. Kubwabo, I. Kosarac, B. Stewart, B. R. Gauthier, K. Lalonde, and P. J. Lalonde, "Migration of bisphenol A from plastic baby bottles, baby bottle liners and reusable polycarbonate drinking bottles," *Food Additives and Contaminants—Part A*, vol. 26, no. 6, pp. 928–937, 2009.

[21] X. L. Cao and J. Corriveau, "Migration of bisphenol A from polycarbonate baby and water bottles into water under severe conditions," *Journal of Agricultural and Food Chemistry*, vol. 56, no. 15, pp. 6378–6381, 2008.

[22] N. C. Maragou, A. A. Makri, E. Lampi, N. S. Thomaidis, and M. A. Koupparis, "Migration of bisphenol A from polycarbonate baby bottles under real use conditions," *Food Additives and Contaminants—Part A*, vol. 25, no. 3, pp. 373–383, 2008.

[23] J. Sajiki, F. Miyamoto, H. Fukata, C. Mori, J. Yonekubo, and K. Hayakawa, "Bisphenol A (BPA) and its source in foods in Japanese markets," *Food Additives and Contaminants*, vol. 24, no. 1, pp. 103–112, 2007.

[24] R. Braunrath, D. Podlipna, S. Padlesak, and M. Cichna-Markl, "Determination of bisphenol A in canned foods by immunoaffinity chromatography, HPLC, and fluorescence detection," *Journal of Agricultural and Food Chemistry*, vol. 53, no. 23, pp. 8911–8917, 2005.

[25] L. Grumetto, D. Montesano, S. Seccia, S. Albrizio, and F. Barbato, "Determination of bisphenol A and bisphenol B residues in canned peeled tomatoes by reversed-phase liquid chromatography," *Journal of Agricultural and Food Chemistry*, vol. 56, no. 22, pp. 10633–10637, 2008.

[26] X. L. Cao, J. Corriveau, S. Popovic, G. Clement, F. Beraldin, and G. Dufresne, "Bisphenol A in baby food products in glass jars with metal lids from canadian markets," *Journal of Agricultural and Food Chemistry*, vol. 57, no. 12, pp. 5345–5351, 2009.

[27] X. L. Cao, J. Corriveau, and S. Popovic, "Bisphenol a in canned food products from canadian markets," *Journal of Food Protection*, vol. 73, no. 6, pp. 1085–1089, 2010.

[28] X. L. Cao, J. Corriveau, and S. Popovic, "Levels of bisphenol a in canned soft drink products in Canadian markets," *Journal of Agricultural and Food Chemistry*, vol. 57, no. 4, pp. 1307–1311, 2009.

[29] S. Biedermann, P. Tschudin, and K. Grob, "Transfer of bisphenol A from thermal printer paper to the skin," *Analytical and Bioanalytical Chemistry*, vol. 398, no. 1, pp. 571–576, 2010.

[30] S. Lunder, D. Andrews, and J. Houlihan, "Synthetic estrogen BPA coats cash register receipts," 2010, http://www.ewg.org/bpa-in-store-receipts.

[31] T. Mendum, E. V. Stoler, and J. Warner, "Concentration of bisphenol A in thermal paper," 2010, http://advancinggreenchemistry.org/?p=1176.

[32] N. Olea, R. Pulgar, P. Pérez et al., "Estrogenicity of resin-based composites and sealants used in dentistry," *Environmental Health Perspectives*, vol. 104, no. 3, pp. 298–305, 1996.

[33] D. Arenholt-Bindslev, V. Breinholt, A. Preiss, and G. Schmalz, "Time-related bisphenol-A content and estrogenic activity in saliva samples collected in relation to placement of fissure sealants," *Clinical Oral Investigations*, vol. 3, no. 3, pp. 120–125, 1999.

[34] J. M. Zimmerman-Downs, D. Shuman, S. C. Stull, and R. E. Ratzlaff, "Bisphenol A blood and saliva levels prior to and after dental sealant placement in adults," *Journal of Dental Hygiene*, vol. 84, no. 3, pp. 145–150, 2010.

[35] A. M. Calafat, J. Weuve, X. Ye et al., "Exposure to bisphenol A and other phenols in neonatal intensive care unit premature infants," *Environmental Health Perspectives*, vol. 117, no. 4, pp. 639–644, 2009.

[36] Y. Kanno, H. Okada, T. Kobayashi, T. Takenaka, and H. Suzuki, "Effects of endocrine disrupting substance on estrogen receptor gene transcription in dialysis patients," *Therapeutic Apheresis and Dialysis*, vol. 11, no. 4, pp. 262–265, 2007.

[37] K. Murakami, A. Ohashi, H. Hori et al., "Accumulation of bisphenol A in hemodialysis patients," *Blood Purification*, vol. 25, no. 3, pp. 290–294, 2007.

[38] W. Völkel, T. Colnot, G. A. Csanády, J. G. Filser, and W. Dekant, "Metabolism and kinetics of bisphenol a in humans at low doses following oral administration," *Chemical Research in Toxicology*, vol. 15, no. 10, pp. 1281–1287, 2002.

[39] H. Inoue, G. Yuki, H. Yokota, and S. Kato, "Bisphenol A glucuronidation and absorption in rat intestine," *Drug Metabolism and Disposition*, vol. 31, no. 1, pp. 140–144, 2003.

[40] H. Yokota, H. Iwano, M. Endo et al., "Glucuronidation of the environmental oestrogen bisphenol A by an isoform of UDP-glucuronosyltransferase, UGT2B1, in the rat liver," *Biochemical Journal*, vol. 340, no. 2, pp. 405–409, 1999.

[41] G. Ginsberg and D. C. Rice, "Does rapid metabolism ensure negligible risk from bisphenol A?" *Environmental Health Perspectives*, vol. 117, no. 11, pp. 1639–1643, 2009.

[42] G. Csanády, H. Oberste-Frielinghaus, B. Semder, C. Baur, K. Schneider, and J. Filser, "Distribution and unspecific protein binding of the xenoestrogens bisphenol A and daidzein," *Archives of Toxicology*, vol. 76, no. 5-6, pp. 299–305, 2002.

[43] T. Galloway, R. Cipelli, J. Guralnik et al., "Daily bisphenol a excretion and associations with sex hormone concentrations: results from the InCHIANTI adult population study," *Environmental Health Perspectives*, vol. 118, no. 11, pp. 1603–1608, 2010.

[44] S. Arase, K. Ishii, K. Igarashi et al., "Endocrine disrupter bisphenol a increases in situ estrogen production in the mouse urogenital sinus," *Biology of Reproduction*, vol. 84, no. 4, pp. 734–742, 2011.

[45] H. Kato, T. Ota, T. Furuhashi, Y. Ohta, and T. Iguchi, "Changes in reproductive organs of female rats treated with bisphenol A during the neonatal period," *Reproductive Toxicology*, vol. 17, no. 3, pp. 283–288, 2003.

[46] S. Honma, A. Suzuki, D. L. Buchanan, Y. Katsu, H. Watanabe, and T. Iguchi, "Low dose effect of in utero exposure to bisphenol A and diethylstilbestrol on female mouse reproduction," *Reproductive Toxicology*, vol. 16, no. 2, pp. 117–122, 2002.

[47] R. R. Newbold, W. N. Jefferson, and E. Padilla-Banks, "Prenatal Exposure to Bisphenol A at environmentally relevant doses adversely affects the murine female reproductive tract later in life," *Environmental Health Perspectives*, vol. 117, no. 6, pp. 879–885, 2009.

[48] C. Lawson, M. Gieske, B. Murdoch et al., "Gene expression in the fetal mouse ovary is altered by exposure to low doses of bisphenol A," *Biology of Reproduction*, vol. 84, no. 1, pp. 79–86, 2011.

[49] H. A. Rodríguez, N. Santambrosio, C. G. Santamaría, M. Muñoz-de-Toro, and E. H. Luque, "Neonatal exposure to bisphenol A reduces the pool of primordial follicles in the rat ovary," *Reproductive Toxicology*, vol. 30, no. 4, pp. 550–557, 2010.

[50] T. Tachibana, Y. Wakimoto, N. Nakamuta et al., "Effects of bisphenol A (BPA) on placentation and survival of the neonates in mice," *Journal of Reproduction and Development*, vol. 53, no. 3, pp. 509–514, 2007.

[51] M. Sugiura-Ogasawara, Y. Ozaki, S. I. Sonta, T. Makino, and K. Suzumori, "Exposure to bisphenol A is associated with recurrent miscarriage," *Human Reproduction*, vol. 20, no. 8, pp. 2325–2329, 2005.

[52] K. L. Howdeshell, A. K. Hotchkiss, K. A. Thayer, J. G. Vandenbergh, and F. S. Vom Saal, "Environmental toxins: exposure to bisphenol A advances puberty," *Nature*, vol. 401, no. 6755, pp. 763–764, 1999.

[53] D. Li, Z. Zhou, D. Qing et al., "Occupational exposure to bisphenol-A (BPA) and the risk of self-reported male sexual dysfunction," *Human Reproduction*, vol. 25, no. 2, pp. 519–527, 2010.

[54] D. K. Li, Z. Zhou, M. Miao et al., "Relationship between urine bisphenol-A Level and declining male sexual function," *Journal of Andrology*, vol. 31, no. 5, pp. 500–506, 2010.

[55] R. A. Keri, S. M. Ho, P. A. Hunt, K. E. Knudsen, A. M. Soto, and G. S. Prins, "An evaluation of evidence for the carcinogenic activity of bisphenol A," *Reproductive Toxicology*, vol. 24, no. 2, pp. 240–252, 2007.

[56] C. Leranth, T. Hajszan, K. Szigeti-Buck, J. Bober, and N. J. MacLusky, "Bisphenol A prevents the synaptogenic response to estradiol in hippocampus and prefrontal cortex of ovariectomized nonhuman primates," *Proceedings of the National Academy of Sciences of the United States of America*, vol. 105, no. 37, pp. 14187–14191, 2008.

[57] N. J. MacLusky, T. Hajszan, and C. Leranth, "The environmental estrogen bisphenol A inhibits estradiol-induced hippocampal synaptogenesis," *Environmental Health Perspectives*, vol. 113, no. 6, pp. 675–679, 2005.

[58] J. H. Morrison, "Environmental estrogens impact primate brain," *Proceedings of the National Academy of Sciences of the United States of America*, vol. 105, no. 37, pp. 13705–13706, 2008.

[59] M. Yokosuka, R. Ohtani-Kaneko, K. Yamashita, D. Muraoka, Y. Kuroda, and C. Watanabe, "Estrogen and environmental estrogenic chemicals exert developmental effects on rat hypothalamic neurons and glias," *Toxicology in Vitro*, vol. 22, no. 1, pp. 1–9, 2008.

[60] R. Zhou, Z. Zhang, Y. Zhu, L. Chen, M. Sokabe, and L. Chen, "Deficits in development of synaptic plasticity in rat dorsal striatum following prenatal and neonatal exposure to low-dose bisphenol A," *Neuroscience*, vol. 159, no. 1, pp. 161–171, 2009.

[61] C. Leranth, K. Szigeti-Buck, N. J. MacLusky, and T. Hajszan, "Bisphenol A prevents the synaptogenic response to testosterone in the brain of adult male rats," *Endocrinology*, vol. 149, no. 3, pp. 988–994, 2008.

[62] Y. I. Weng, P. Y. Hsu, S. Liyanarachchi et al., "Epigenetic influences of low-dose bisphenol A in primary human breast epithelial cells," *Toxicology and Applied Pharmacology*, vol. 248, no. 2, pp. 111–121, 2010.

[63] S. Jenkins, N. Raghuraman, I. Eltoum, M. Carpenter, J. Russo, and C. A. Lamartiniere, "Oral exposure to Bisphenol A increases dimethylbenzanthraceneo-induced mammary cancer in rats," *Environmental Health Perspectives*, vol. 117, no. 6, pp. 910–915, 2009.

[64] G. S. Prins, W. Y. Tang, J. Belmonte, and S. M. Ho, "Developmental exposure to bisphenol A increases prostate cancer susceptibility in adult rats: epigenetic mode of action is implicated," *Fertility and Sterility*, vol. 89, no. 2, article e41, 2008.

[65] G. S. Prins, W. Y. Tang, J. Belmonte, and S. M. Ho, "Perinatal exposure to oestradiol and bisphenol A alters the prostate epigenome and increases susceptibility to carcinogenesis," *Basic and Clinical Pharmacology and Toxicology*, vol. 102, no. 2, pp. 134–138, 2008.

[66] G. S. Prins, "Endocrine disruptors and prostate cancer risk," *Endocrine-Related Cancer*, vol. 15, no. 3, pp. 649–656, 2008.

[67] M. D. Anway and M. K. Skinner, "Epigenetic programming of the germ line: effects of endocrine disruptors on the development of transgenerational disease," *Reproductive BioMedicine Online*, vol. 16, no. 1, pp. 23–25, 2008.

[68] S. M. Ho, W. Y. Tang, J. Belmonte De Frausto, and G. S. Prins, "Developmental exposure to estradiol and bisphenol A increases susceptibility to prostate carcinogenesis and epigenetically regulates phosphodiesterase type 4 variant 4," *Cancer Research*, vol. 66, no. 11, pp. 5624–5632, 2006.

[69] T. J. Murray, M. V. Maffini, A. A. Ucci, C. Sonnenschein, and A. M. Soto, "Induction of mammary gland ductal hyperplasias and carcinoma in situ following fetal bisphenol A exposure," *Reproductive Toxicology*, vol. 23, no. 3, pp. 383–390, 2007.

[70] E. Somm, V. M. Schwitzgebel, A. Toulotte et al., "Perinatal exposure to bisphenol A alters early adipogenesis in the rat," *Environmental Health Perspectives*, vol. 117, no. 10, pp. 1549–1555, 2009.

[71] N. Ben-Jonathan, E. R. Hugo, and T. D. Brandebourg, "Effects of bisphenol A on adipokine release from human adipose tissue: implications for the metabolic syndrome," *Molecular and Cellular Endocrinology*, vol. 304, no. 1-2, pp. 49–54, 2009.

[72] F. Grün and B. Blumberg, "Environmental obesogens: organotins and endocrine disruption via nuclear receptor signaling," *Endocrinology*, vol. 147, no. 6, pp. S50–S55, 2006.

[73] F. Grun, "Obesogens," *Current Opinion in Endocrinology, Diabetes and Obesity*, vol. 17, no. 5, pp. 453–459, 2010.

[74] R. R. Newbold, E. Padilla-Banks, W. N. Jefferson, and J. J. Heindel, "Effects of endocrine disruptors on obesity," *International Journal of Andrology*, vol. 31, no. 2, pp. 201–207, 2008.

[75] K. Wada, H. Sakamoto, K. Nishikawa et al., "Life style-related diseases of the digestive system: endocrine disruptors stimulate lipid accumulation in target cells related to metabolic syndrome," *Journal of Pharmacological Sciences*, vol. 105, no. 2, pp. 133–137, 2007.

[76] R. R. Newbold, E. Padilla-Banks, R. J. Snyder, and W. N. Jefferson, "Perinatal exposure to environmental estrogens and the development of obesity," *Molecular Nutrition and Food Research*, vol. 51, no. 7, pp. 912–917, 2007.

[77] J. Miyawaki, K. Sakayama, H. Kato, H. Yamamoto, and H. Masuno, "Perinatal and postnatal exposure to bisphenol A increase adipose tissue mass and serum cholesterol level in mice," *Journal of Atherosclerosis and Thrombosis*, vol. 14, no. 5, pp. 245–252, 2007.

[78] F. S. Vom Saal and J. P. Myers, "Bisphenol A and risk of metabolic disorders," *JAMA—Journal of the American Medical Association*, vol. 300, no. 11, pp. 1353–1355, 2008.

[79] R. M. Sharpe and A. J. Drake, "Bisphenol A and metabolic syndrome," *Endocrinology*, vol. 151, no. 6, pp. 2404–2407, 2010.

[80] P. Alonso-Magdalena, S. Morimoto, C. Ripoll, E. Fuentes, and A. Nadal, "The estrogenic effect of bisphenol a disrupts pancreatic β-cell function in vivo and induces insulin resistance," *Environmental Health Perspectives*, vol. 114, no. 1, pp. 106–112, 2006.

[81] R. R. Newbold, E. Padilla-Banks, and W. N. Jefferson, "Environmental estrogens and obesity," *Molecular and Cellular Endocrinology*, vol. 304, no. 1-2, pp. 84–89, 2009.

[82] D. Sharp, "Environmental toxins, a potential risk factor for diabetes among Canadian Aboriginals," *International Journal of Circumpolar Health*, vol. 68, no. 4, pp. 316–326, 2009.

[83] X. Tian, M. Takamoto, and K. Sugane, "Bisphenol A promotes IL-4 production by Th2 cells," *International Archives of Allergy and Immunology*, vol. 132, no. 3, pp. 240–247, 2003.

[84] H. Yan, M. Takamoto, and K. Sugane, "Exposure to bisphenol A prenatally or in adulthood promotes T_H2 cytokine production associated with reduction of $CD4^+CD25^+$ regulatory T cells," *Environmental Health Perspectives*, vol. 116, no. 4, pp. 514–519, 2008.

[85] Y. Masuo, M. Ishido, M. Morita, and S. Oka, "Effects of neonatal treatment with 6-hydroxydopamine and endocrine disruptors on motor activity and gene expression in rats," *Neural Plasticity*, vol. 11, no. 1-2, pp. 59–76, 2004.

[86] Y. Masuo, M. Morita, S. Oka, and M. Ishido, "Motor hyperactivity caused by a deficit in dopaminergic neurons and the effects of endocrine disruptors: a study inspired by the physiological roles of PACAP in the brain," *Regulatory Peptides*, vol. 123, no. 1–3, pp. 225–234, 2004.
[87] J. Kimura-Kuroda, I. Nagata, and Y. Kuroda, "Disrupting effects of hydroxy-polychlorinated biphenyl (PCB) congeners on neuronal development of cerebellar Purkinje cells: a possible causal factor for developmental brain disorders?" *Chemosphere*, vol. 67, no. 9, pp. S412–S420, 2007.
[88] T. Fujimoto, K. Kubo, and S. Aou, "Prenatal exposure to bisphenol a impairs sexual differentiation of exploratory behavior and increases depression-like behavior in rats," *Brain Research*, vol. 1068, no. 1, pp. 49–55, 2006.
[89] H. B. Patisaul and H. L. Bateman, "Neonatal exposure to endocrine active compounds or an ERβ agonist increases adult anxiety and aggression in gonadally intact male rats," *Hormones and Behavior*, vol. 53, no. 4, pp. 580–588, 2008.
[90] B. C. Ryan and J. G. Vandenbergh, "Developmental exposure to environmental estrogens alters anxiety and spatial memory in female mice," *Hormones and Behavior*, vol. 50, no. 1, pp. 85–93, 2006.
[91] Y. H. Tian, J. H. Baek, S. Y. Lee, and C. G. Jang, "Prenatal and postnatal exposure to bisphenol A induces anxiolytic behaviors and cognitive deficits in mice," *Synapse*, vol. 64, no. 6, pp. 432–439, 2010.
[92] K. H. Cox, J. D. Gatewood, C. Howeth, and E. F. Rissman, "Gestational exposure to bisphenol A and cross-fostering affect behaviors in juvenile mice," *Hormones and Behavior*, vol. 58, no. 5, pp. 754–761, 2010.
[93] S. J. Genuis, "Sensitivity-related illness: the escalating pandemic of allergy, food intolerance and chemical sensitivity," *Science of the Total Environment*, vol. 408, no. 24, pp. 6047–6061, 2010.
[94] S. Dearing, "Canada sets the bar high by declaring Bisphenol A toxic," October 2010, http://www.digitaljournal.com/article/298935#ixzz1R5Q3MJqzhttp://www.digitaljournal.com/article/298935#ixzz12YD1MxcT.
[95] R. W. Snyder, S. C. Maness, K. W. Gaido, F. Welsch, S. C. J. Sumner, and T. R. Fennell, "Metabolism and disposition of bisphenol A in female rats," *Toxicology and Applied Pharmacology*, vol. 168, no. 3, pp. 225–234, 2000.
[96] J. B. Matthews, K. Twomey, and T. R. Zacharewski, "In vitro and in vivo interactions of bisphenol A and its metabolite, bisphenol A glucuronide, with estrogen receptors α and β," *Chemical Research in Toxicology*, vol. 14, no. 2, pp. 149–157, 2001.
[97] L. H. Pottenger, J. Y. Domoradzki, D. A. Markham, S. C. Hansen, S. Z. Cagen, and J. M. Waechter, "The relative bioavailability and metabolism of bisphenol A in rats is dependent upon the route of administration," *Toxicological Sciences*, vol. 54, no. 1, pp. 3–18, 2000.
[98] S. J. Genuis, "Elimination of persistent toxicants from the human body," *Human and Experimental Toxicology*, vol. 30, no. 1, pp. 3–18, 2011.
[99] S. J. Genuis, D. Birkholz, I. Rodushkin, and S. Beesoon, "Blood, Urine, and Sweat (BUS) study: monitoring and elimination of bioaccumulated toxic elements," *Archives of Environmental Contamination and Toxicology*, vol. 61, no. 2, pp. 344–357, 2010.
[100] R. J. Jandacek, N. Anderson, M. Liu, S. Zheng, Q. Yang, and P. Tso, "Effects of yo-yo diet, caloric restriction, and olestra on tissue distribution of hexachlorobenzene," *American Journal of Physiology—Gastrointestinal and Liver Physiology*, vol. 288, no. 2, pp. G292–G299, 2005.
[101] G. W. Yu, J. Laseter, and C. Mylander, "Persistent organic pollutants in serum and several different fat compartments in humans," *Journal of Environmental and Public Health*, vol. 2011, Article ID 417980, 2011.
[102] X. Ye, Z. Kuklenyik, L. L. Needham, and A. M. Calafat, "Quantification of urinary conjugates of bisphenol A, 2,5-dichlorophenol, and 2-hydroxy-4-methoxybenzophenone in humans by online solid phase extraction-high performance liquid chromatography-tandem mass spectrometry," *Analytical and Bioanalytical Chemistry*, vol. 383, no. 4, pp. 638–644, 2005.
[103] E. Kandaraki, A. Chatzigeorgiou, S. Livadas et al., "Endocrine disruptors and Polycystic Ovary Syndrome (PCOS): elevated serum levels of bisphenol A in women with PCOS," *Journal of Clinical Endocrinology and Metabolism*, vol. 96, no. 3, pp. E480–E484, 2011.
[104] L. Cobellis, N. Colacurci, E. Trabucco, C. Carpentiero, and L. Grumetto, "Measurement of bisphenol A and bisphenol B levels in human blood sera from healthy and endometriotic women," *Biomedical Chromatography*, vol. 23, no. 11, pp. 1186–1190, 2009.
[105] V. Padmanabhan, K. Siefert, S. Ransom et al., "Maternal bisphenol-A levels at delivery: a looming problem?" *Journal of Perinatology*, vol. 28, no. 4, pp. 258–263, 2008.
[106] L. N. Vandenberg, I. Chahoud, J. J. Heindel, V. Padmanabhan, F. J. R. Paumgartten, and G. Schoenfelder, "Urinary, circulating, and tissue biomonitoring studies indicate widespread exposure to bisphenol A," *Environmental Health Perspectives*, vol. 118, no. 8, pp. 1055–1070, 2010.
[107] J. Mendiola, N. Jørgensen, A. M. Andersson et al., "Are environmental levels of bisphenol A associated with reproductive function in fertile men?" *Environmental Health Perspectives*, vol. 118, no. 9, pp. 1286–1291, 2010.
[108] S. Moors, M. Blaszkewicz, H. M. Bolt, and G. H. Degen, "Simultaneous determination of daidzein, equol, genistein and bisphenol A in human urine by a fast and simple method using SPE and GC-MS," *Molecular Nutrition and Food Research*, vol. 51, no. 7, pp. 787–798, 2007.

17

Television Watching, Diet Quality, and Physical Activity and Diabetes among Three Ethnicities in the United States

Fatma G. Huffman, Joan A. Vaccaro, Joel C. Exebio, Gustavo G. Zarini, Timothy Katz, and Zisca Dixon

Department of Dietetics and Nutrition, Robert Stempel College of Public Health and Social Work, Florida International University, AHC1-435, Miami, FL 33199, USA

Correspondence should be addressed to Fatma G. Huffman, huffmanf@fiu.edu

Academic Editor: V. Mohan

Diabetes is a world-wide epidemic associated with multiple environmental factors. Prolonged television viewing (TV) time has been related to increased risk of obesity and type 2 diabetes in several studies. TV viewing has been positively associated with cardiovascular disease risk factors, lower energy expenditure, over-eating high-calorie and high-fat foods. The objective of this study was to assess the associations of hours of TV viewing with dietary quality, obesity and physical activity for three ethnic minorities with and without type 2 diabetes. Diet quality and physical activity were inversely related to prolonged TV viewing. African Americans and participants with type 2 diabetes were more likely to watch more than 4 hours of TV per day as compared to their counterparts. Diet quality was inversely associated with physical activity level. Future studies are needed to establish the risk factors of prolonged TV watching in adult populations for the development of diabetes or diabetes-related complications. Although strategies to reduce TV watching have been proven effective among children, few trials have been conducted in adults. Intervention trials aimed at reducing TV viewing targeting people with type 2 diabetes may be beneficial to improve dietary quality and physical activity, which may reduce diabetes complications.

1. Introduction

Diabetes has become a worldwide epidemic. Quality of diet and physical inactivity have been attributed to the rise in prevalence of obesity leading to type 2 diabetes (the most common form) among developed and developing countries. Prolonged television (TV) viewing time has been associated with increased risk of obesity and type 2 diabetes in men from the Health Professionals Follow-Up Study (HPFS) [1] and women from the Nurses' Health Study [2]. Average hours of TV viewing, independent of physical activity, was positively associated with low-density lipoprotein cholesterol and inversely associated with high-density lipoprotein cholesterol and apolipoprotein A1 in an eight-year prospective study of 486 men randomly sampled from the HPFS [3]. Several other studies reported TV watching as positively associated with cardiovascular risk factors such as blood pressure, low-density lipoprotein, triglycerides, and insulin resistance [4–6] and overeating [7]. The average hours of TV viewing was estimated at 2.73 hours per day for all U.S. civilians and 3.44 hours for those who reported watching TV according to the Bureau of Labor Statistics [8]. Estimates for adults are close to 5 hours per day [9].

The association of TV with poor health outcomes may be partially attributed to the role of television. Although sedentary behaviors such as computer use, reading, board and video game-playing, and driving a car require little physical exertion, TV viewing results in a lower metabolic rate than other sedentary activities [10]. Unique to TV, as compared to other sedentary activities, is food commercials. Lower intakes of fruits, vegetables, and whole grains and higher intake of fried foods, processed meat and sugar-sweetened beverages have been associated with TV viewing in adults [11]; and references therein. Exposure to food advertisements has been associated with overeating and choosing foods of poor dietary quality (higher salt, saturated fat, and lower dietary fiber) [1, 2].

Analysis of diet by a dietary index provides a more comprehensive approach to food consumption and health than measurement of single nutrients or diet quantity [12, 13]. Dietary indexes have been developed to measure the degree of adherence to a standard deemed as "healthy eating." A dietary index includes the most important dietary components of a particular diet and then scores adherence to those components. The dietary index chosen for this study, the Healthy Eating Index, 2005 (HEI-05) (discussed in detail in Section 3.2), parallels the dietary recommendations for persons at risk for or with diabetes.

Common types of physical activities consist of leisure-time (including sports and social activities), occupational, transport, and at-home or domestic physical work. While physical inactivity is an established risk factor for obesity and diabetes, TV viewing hours has not been established as a risk factor for obesity and diabetes in adult populations. Despite the evidence by prospective studies that high levels of TV viewing was a risk factor for improper dietary intake, poor lipid profile, and type 2 diabetes in both men and women, public health goals target increasing physical activity, but has not set thresholds for sedentary activities [14]. Little or no correlation has been found for average hours of TV viewing and hours of physical activity for large epidemiological studies in men [3] and women [2]; yet, obesity indicators were positively associated with TV hours in these studies. Evidence suggests that TV watching may be an independent risk factor for obesity and type 2 diabetes.

2. Purpose

The objective of this study was to assess the associations of hours of TV viewing with dietary quality, obesity and physical activity for three ethnic minorities with and without type 2 diabetes. Since median TV viewing was 3 hours and the 75th percentile was 4 hours for the combined sample, high TV viewing was set at more than 4 hours. Sedentary behavior is a risk factor for diabetes. Those persons with diabetes should be more likely to engage in sedentary behavior such as TV viewing. Therefore, the following hypotheses were tested. (1) Persons with type 2 diabetes will be more likely to watch more than 4 hours of TV per day as compared to persons without diabetes, independent of ethnicity; (2a) individuals with type 2 diabetes in the lowest quartile of HEI-05 (poorest diet) will be more likely to watch over 4 hours of TV as compared to those in the highest quartile, independent of ethnicity; and (2b) participants with the highest quartile of physical activity measured as metabolic equivalents (MET) per hour per week ($1\,\text{kcal}\cdot\text{kg}^{-1}\cdot\text{h}^{-1}$) will be less likely to watch more than 4 hours of TV as compared to those in the lowest quartile, independent of diabetes status and ethnicity. Physical activity was estimated by self-reported responses from the Modifiable Activities Questionnaire [15] (further details are provided in Section 3.2). Hypothesis 2 was tested with physical activity and diet as covariates so each variable would adjust for the other. A secondary purpose was to assess differences in dietary components of the HEI across ethnicities, physical activity level, BMI, and TV viewing by ANOVA models.

3. Materials and Methods

3.1. Study Participants. This was a cross-sectional study of $N = 868$ participants: Cuban American (CA) ($N = 361$), Haitian American (HA) ($N = 258$), and African American (AA) ($N = 249$) with ($N = 455$) and without ($N = 410$) type 2 diabetes collected from 2008–2010. By study design, approximately half of each racial/ethnic minority in this study had type 2 diabetes and the rest were free of diabetes. Sample size was determined by a pilot study of cardiovascular risk factors for CA and was based on 80% power to attain a difference with 95% confidence among 7 subgroups [three ethnicities, two genders and diabetes status (with and without diabetes)], for variations in serum glucose, hemoglobin A1C, and blood lipids. Recruitment of CA was conducted based on a target of $N = 350$. Sufficient power was achieved at $N = 250$. The remaining racial/ethnic minority target goal was lowered to $N = 250$. When the target was achieved recruitment efforts were ended. Recruitment was conducted by alternating between selecting potential participants with and then without type 2 diabetes. Participants were initially recruited by randomly generated mailing lists. The lists of addresses were purchased from Knowledge Base Marketing, Inc., Richardson, TX, USA This company provided four mailing lists generated from multiple databases of CA and AA, identified as having or not having type 2 diabetes from Miami-Dade and Broward Counties, Florida, USA During a one year period, approximately 10,000 letters, in English and Spanish, explaining the study and containing contact information with an invitation flyer, were mailed to CA individuals with and without type 2 diabetes. Three percent ($n = 300$) of the letters were returned due to unknown addresses. From the remaining delivered letters, 4% ($n = 388$) responded. About 7,550 letters were mailed to AA participants with and without type 2 diabetes. Approximately, 6.3% ($n = 477$) of the letters were returned due to unknown addresses. From the remaining delivered letters, 4% ($n = 256$) responded. We were not able to recruit HA in the same manner because Knowledge Base Marketing, Inc. did not have a database for the HA community. Therefore, recruitment of HA participants ($n = 258$) were from community-based sources. (a) Local diabetes educators and community health practitioners in Miami-Dade and Broward Counties were contacted: several local diabetes educators who were either former students or in close contact with the Department of Dietetics and Nutrition at Florida International University (FIU). Official letters of invitation outlining the study were mailed to the diabetes educators and health professionals in Miami-Dade and Broward counties requesting their cooperation in recruiting individuals. (b) Invitational flyers were distributed to all university faculty, staff and students using the university-wide e-mail system explaining the research protocol and requesting their assistance in the study. (c) Several residential rental facilities also agreed to help in the recruitment process. (d) Print advertisements were placed in local Haitian newspapers and principal gathering places of these groups such as churches, supermarkets, and restaurants. Radio advertisements on local Creole stations were also aired. When the target recruitment goal was reached for all ethnic groups, efforts to recruit participants were stopped. Interested participants were initially interviewed by telephone, where the study purpose was explained to them. Age, gender, ethnicity, diabetes status and study qualification were determined. To ascertain type 2 diabetes status, each participant who self reported having diabetes was asked for the age of diagnosis, and initial treatment modalities. Participants who did not qualify for the study ($n = 28$) consisted of those being younger than 35 years old ($n = 12$), other ethnicity ($n = 5$), or having other chronic diseases or illnesses ($n = 11$). If a subject was determined to be eligible, then his or her participation was requested at the Human Nutrition Laboratory at Florida International University (FIU). Participants were instructed to refrain from smoking, consuming any food or beverages except water, and engaging in any unusual exercise for at least eight hours prior to their blood collection. This study was approved by the Institutional Review Board at FIU. The purpose and protocol of the study were explained to the participants, and their written consent either in English, Spanish, or Creole was obtained prior to the commencement of the study. Laboratory results showed that nineteen participants (CA = 7; HA = 8; AA = 4) who reported not having diabetes were reclassified as having type 2 diabetes according to American Diabetes Association standards. These participants were given their laboratory results and referred to their physicians. This study adhered to the institutional review board requirements on the use of human subjects. Trained interviewers who were bilingual in English/Creole and English/Spanish administered questionnaires.

3.2. Measures. Sociodemographic data was collected by self-report with a questionnaire constructed by the principal investigator. This questionnaire included questions about age, gender, tobacco use, education, income, language preference, years lived in the United States, and health insurance.

Physical activity and TV viewing were estimated from the Modifiable Activity Questionnaire (MAQ) [15]. The use of this questionnaire to estimate metabolic cost and perform a MET calculation is explained in detail in the compendium of physical activity [16]. The MAQ assesses leisure activities from a popular list, (such as dancing swimming, bicycling, walking/jogging (outdoor, treadmill), strength/weight training, aerobics (water, dance, step), gardening or yard work) over the past year that were performed more than 10 times. TV viewing was reported to the nearest 1/4 hour. The participants, with the help of a trained interviewer, estimate the number of months and frequency per month and duration of each activity. For occupational activity, participants reported all jobs held over the past year. The number of hours sitting at work and usual mode of transportation to work was recorded for each job. Total physical activity was calculated, summing all leisure and occupational activity hours per week. These values were then multiplied by their estimated metabolic cost. Activity was expressed as metabolic equivalents (MET) per hour per week ($1\ \text{kcal}\cdot\text{kg}^{-1}\cdot\text{h}^{-1}$). One MET is the equivalent of sitting quietly.

Anthropometric measures taken included waist circumference, weight, and height. Waist circumference to the nearest 0.1 cm was measured horizontally with a nonstretchable measuring tape. The tape was placed midway between the 12th rib and iliac crest at minimal respiration to determine central obesity. Body mass index(es) (BMI) was calculated by weight divided by height (kg/m^2).

Glycosylated hemoglobin (A1C) was measured from a 20 ml sample of venous blood collected from each participant after an overnight fast (8–10 h) by a certified phlebotomist using standard laboratory techniques. Whole-blood samples for A1C were collected in a tube containing EDTA and A1C percentages were measured using Roche Tina Quant method by the Laboratory Corporation of America (LabCorp, Miami, FL, USA).

Dietary intake was measured using the semiquantitative food-frequency questionnaire, version 97GP 2006, developed by Walter C. Willett (copyrighted at Harvard University, Boston, MA, USA). The FFQ has been extensively validated and standardized in multiethnic population-based prospective and cross-sectional studies [17–19]. Participants self-reported average consumption of specific amounts of various foods over the past year, choosing from a frequency range from "never" to "six or more servings" per day, based on standardized portion sizes. The participants were shown food models and asked to estimate the number of servings that they consumed for each portion. In addition, this FFQ includes questions about type and frequency of vitamin and mineral supplementation, alcohol consumption and details about sugar, salt, and fat used in cooking and as condiments. Open-ended section for ethnically specific foods was included in this version of the FFQ. The questionnaire was reviewed by the interviewer with the participant for omissions at the close of the interview. The Harvard University Food Composition Database was used as the reference for macro- and micro-nutrient calculations. Daily servings of food groups were calculated by summing frequency factors (which corresponded to the reported consumption frequencies) for all food items.

Dietary quality was assessed by the HEI-05, which measures adherence of the individual's overall diet to the Federal Dietary Guidelines of the United States Department of Agriculture (USDA). The HEI-05 was formulated based on the USDA food guide pyramid using the proportions of grains, fruits and vegetables, dairy, meat, and discretionary sweets, fats, and oils. Diet quality from the HEI-05 was calculated from each completed FFQ. The HEI-05 consists of 12 components—total fruit, whole fruit, total vegetables, dark green and orange vegetables and legumes, total grains, whole grains, milk, meat and beans, oils, saturated fat, sodium, and energy from solid fats, alcohol, and added sugars (SoFAAS). Twelve individual components of the HEI-05 represent all of the major food groups found in MyPyramid (an online, interactive counterpart based on the DGA's available to the public). The intakes of foods and nutrients are represented on a density basis, as amounts per 1,000 calories [13]. A minimum score of zero for no intake and a maximum score of either 5 for fruits, vegetables, and grains, 10 for milk and meat/bean products, and 10 for oils was assigned for healthy components. For sugars, saturated fat, and sodium, higher scores were assigned for lower intakes. For SoFAAS the highest score was 20 (representing $\leq 20\%$ of energy) and the maximum for saturated fat and sodium was 10 points each. Saturated fat and sodium received a score of 8 for the intake levels that reflect the 2005 and 2010 DGA's less than 10% of energy from saturated fat, and 1.1 grams of sodium/1,000 kcal, respectively. Total HEI-05 ranges from 0 to 100 points and the higher the score, the more the diet complies with the 2005 DGA's, presuming a better diet quality [13]. For this analysis, missing values ($n = 32$) were assigned to participants with total daily energy (reported dietary intake) of either < 500 or > 5000 Kcal/day. There were missing values for physical activity and TV ($n = 9$) leaving $N = 827$ (224 AA, 246 HA, and 357 CA). There were $n = 439$ with and $n = 388$ without type 2 diabetes.

3.3. Statistical Analysis. Prior to analysis, all continuous variables were tested by the Kolmogorov-Smirnov test and transformed to achieve normality and linearity if needed. The general characteristics of the study population were compared by diabetes status and ethnicity using the Chi-squared test for categorical variables and the Student's t-test for continuous variables. To test the hypotheses, a binary variable for high versus normal hours per day of watching television was determined, using the 75th percentile for the combined group and allowing sufficient marginal means to compare by diabetes status. Ethnicity, diabetes status, dietary quality (HEI), and physical activity were the major independent variables for this study. Full logistic regression models included 2-way interactions for ethnicity, diabetes status, HEI and physical activity. Age, gender, obesity indicators (either waist circumference or BMI due to their collinearity), and smoking were included in the final model due to their clinical significance. A binary variable to indicate risk for diabetes was constructed with A1C = 6% as the cut-off. Potential confounders such as education and marital status were tested. Education was collapsed from 5 to 3 categories to include sufficient numbers in each category. The most parsimonious model was chosen by Hosmer and Lemeshow's recommendation for the elimination of adjustment variables (in this case education and marital status) with P values greater than 0.25 [20]. To assess differences in the dietary components of HEI across ethnicity, physical activity level, BMI, and TV viewing, ANOVA models with post hoc analyses were conducted. All analyses were performed by the *Statistical Package for the Social Sciences* (SPSS) version 19, (Chicago, IL, USA), and a P-value < 0.05 was considered significant.

4. Results

4.1. General Characteristics of the Study Population by Diabetes Status. Descriptive statistics of the study population are presented in Table 1. AA and HA with type 2 diabetes were significantly older than their counterparts without diabetes, whereas for CA there were no differences in age across diabetes status. As a whole, CA were the oldest, followed by HA, and AA. CA had more female participants; however, there were approximately equal numbers of males with and without diabetes within each ethnicity. Participants currently smoking did not differ by diabetes status; conversely, there were significant differences between ethnicities (analysis not shown). There were significant differences in education by ethnicity/race ($P < 0.001$) for the combined sample (with and without diabetes); AA had the highest percent with at least some college (55.1), followed by CA (36.8) and HA (32.9). CA had the highest percent with less than a high school diploma (49.6), followed by HA (46.3) and AA (16.0) (data not shown). Comparisons of each ethnicity by diabetes status are presented in Table 1. HA with diabetes had a lower education level than those without diabetes; however, AA and HA had no differences in education by diabetes status (AA and CA with type 2 diabetes had significantly higher BMI than those without diabetes. AA with type 2 diabetes) had significantly more participants who watched more than 4 hours of TV as compared to those without diabetes. CA with type 2 diabetes had higher HEI scores than those without diabetes. HA without diabetes were more physically active than those with type 2 diabetes. HA without diabetes had a significantly higher percent of persons at risk for diabetes (56.1) as compared to CA (41.2) and AA (37.5) as indicated by A1C ≥ 6.0 ($P_{\text{ethnicity}} = 0.011$) (analysis not shown).

4.2. Television Watching. The likelihood of viewing more than 4 hours of TV/day ("high TV") is shown in Table 2. AA were more likely to watch more than 4 hrs of TV as compared to CA [OR = 5.30 (3.30, 8.49), $P < 0.001$] and HA [OR = 8.55 (4.88, 14.8), $P < 0.001$] (comparison of AA and HA was performed post-hoc by recoding ethnicity). Participants with diabetes were 1.62 (1.12, 2.34) times more likely (odds ratio) to watch more than 4 hours of TV as compared to those without diabetes ($P = 0.010$). A second model was conducted with A1C to account for differences in this risk factor for persons with and without diabetes. The results were consistent between the models for ethnicity. AA were still more likely to watch more than 4 hours of TV as compared to CA [OR = 5.13 (3.18, 8.25), $P < 0.001$]; however, adding A1C to the model negated differences by diabetes status [OR = 1.36 (0.85, 2.17), $P = 0.199$].

The outcome "high TV" was also explored to test the risk of high A1C by ethnicity stratified by diabetes status. Models, adjusted for age, gender, and BMI quartile, were significant [χ^2 (10) ($N = 433$) = 68.4, $P < 0.001$, *with diabetes* and χ^2 (10) ($N = 386$) = 33.9, $P < 0.001$, *without diabetes*]. AA were still more likely to watch more than 4 hours of TV as compared to CA [OR = 4.98 (2.70, 9.18), $P < 0.001$, *with diabetes* and OR = 3.56 (1.27, 9.94), $P = 0.015$, *without diabetes*]. Neither high A1C nor the interaction of high A1C with ethnicity was significant for those with or without diabetes [high A1C: $P = 0.878$, *with diabetes* and $P = 0.503$, *without diabetes*; high A1C by ethnicity: $P = 0.644$, *with diabetes* and $P = 0.914$, *without diabetes*] (data not shown).

Table 1: General characteristics of the study population.

Variable	Ethnicity	Without T2D	With T2D	P-value
Age (years) Mean ± SD	AA	51.1 ± 8.7	54.5 ± 10.2	0.007
	HA	53.5 ± 10.7	57.8 ± 10.1	0.001
	CA	63.0 ± 10.9	65.2 ± 11.8	0.069
Gender N (%)	AA-F	54 (51.9)	64 (53.3)	0.893
	AA-M	50 (48.0)	56 (46.7)	
	HA-F	57 (50.0)	72 (54.5)	0.523
	HA-M	57 (50.0)	60 (45.4)	
	CA-F	113 (66.5)	116 (62.0)	0.439
	CA-M	57 (33.5)	71 (38.0)	
Currently smoking (yes) (N%)	AA	48 (40.0)	47 (36.4)	0.327
	HA	7 (5.8)	9 (6.5)	0.514
	CA	28 (16.2)	30 (16.0)	0.533
Education < HS degree/GED	AA	14 (13.5)	22 (18.2)	0.526
	HA	43 (37.7)	71 (53.8)	0.020
	CA	79 (46.2)	99 (52.7)	0.320
BMI 4th Quartile N (%) (> 34 kg/m^2)	AA	29 (27.9)	61 (51.3)	<0.001
	HA	17 (15.0)	18 (13.6)	0.520
	CA	27 (15.9)	55 (29.4)	0.017
TV hours 4th quartile (> 4.0 hours) N (%)	AA	34 (32.7)	66 (55.0)	0.001
	HA	8 (7.0)	19 (14.4)	0.065
	CA	28 (16.5)	36 (19.3)	0.494
HEI 4th quartile (healthiest diet score) (> 59.3) N (%)	AA	20 (19.2)	14 (11.7)	0.129
	HA	38 (33.3)	37 (28.0)	0.782
	CA	34 (20.0)	63 (33.9)	0.004
PA (MET hr/wk) 4th quartile (highest activity) N (%)	AA	35 (33.7)	29 (24.2)	0.404
	HA	40 (35.1)	23 (17.4)	0.009
	CA	44 (25.9)	31 (16.6)	0.191

Abbreviations. AA: African American; HA: Haitian American; CA: Cuban American; T2D: type 2 diabetes; F: female; M: male; BMI: body mass index; HS: high school; GED: general equivalency diploma; TV: television; HEI: Healthy Eating Index; PA: physical activity; MET: metabolic equivalents.
Notes. Age was compared using the Student t-test and reported in mean ± SD. The Chi-squared test was used to for categorical data and reported as N (%) where % are within diabetes status. A P value of 0.05 was considered significant. Physical activity (PA) was measured in metabolic equivalents (MET) per week. MET = 1 kcal·kg^{-1}·h^{-1}. One MET is the equivalent of sitting quietly.

4.3. Television Watching, HEI, and Physical Activity. The likelihood of diet score quartile and physical activity level with "high" TV viewing is presented in Table 3. Diet quality and physical activity were inversely related to "high TV viewing." AA were 5.27 (3.09, 8.97) times more likely compared to CA and 8.06 (4.48, 14.5) times more likely (odds ratio) to watch more than 4 hours of TV as compared to HA ($P < 0.001$). The comparison of AA with HA was by post-hoc analysis, recoding ethnicity.

4.4. Additional Analysis: Physical Activity and HEI. Diet quality was inversely associated with physical activity level as measured by the Chi-squared test and the z-test. The association of dietary quality with physical activity level was

Table 2: Likelihood of TV viewing more than 4 hour/day comparing ethnicities and diabetes status.

Independents	*B*	SE	df	*P*	OR	95% C.I. OR Lower	95% C.I. OR Upper
				Model 1			
Ethnicity	—	—	2	<0.001	—	—	—
AA	1.67	0.24	1	<0.001	5.29	3.30	8.49
HA	−0.37	0.26	1	0.160	0.69	−0.41	1.16
CA (reference group)	—	—	—	—	—	—	—
With diabetes	0.48	0.19	1	0.010	1.62	1.12	2.34
				Model 2			
Ethnicity	—	—	2	<0.001	—	—	—
AA	1.63	0.24	1	<0.001	5.13	3.18	8.25
HA	−0.40	0.26	1	0.132	0.67	0.40	1.13
CA (reference group)	—	—	—	—	—	—	—
With diabetes	0.31	0.24	1	0.199	1.36	0.85	2.17

Abbreviations. AA: African Americans; *B*: coefficient; SE: standard error; df: degrees of freedom; Q: quartile; CA: Cuban American; HA: Haitian American.
Notes. Television watching was reported to the nearest 0.25 hours. The dependent variable is $\geq$ 4.25 hours of TV versus $\leq$ 4.00 hours of TV. The 4th quartile of BMI is the reference.
Model 1 was adjusted for age ($P = 0.036$), gender ($P = 0.28$), BMI quartiles ($P = 0.331$), currently smoking ($P = 0.111$), and education ($P = 0.019$). Participants who were older and had less education were more likely to watch more than 4 hours of TV per day as compared to their counterparts.
Model 1 parameters. χ^2 (11) = 112.8 ($N = 825$), $P < 0.001$. Nagelkerke R-squared = 0.193 with 78.1% of the cases classified correctly.
Model 2 included age ($P = 0.051$), gender ($P = 0.228$), BMI quartiles ($P = 0.419$), currently smoking ($P = 0.082$), education ($P = 0.023$), and an adjustment for high glycosylated hemoglobin: high A1C $\geq$ 6% ($P = 0.321$), diabetes status by high A1C ($P = 0.134$).
Model 2 parameters. χ^2 (13) = 112.8 ($N = 819$), $P < 0.001$. Nagelkerke R-squared = 0.197 with 78.6% of the cases classified correctly.

Table 3: Effect of diet and physical activity on likelihood of viewing more than 4 hours/day of TV.

Independents	*B*	S.E	df	*P*	OR	95% C.I. OR Lower	95% C.I. OR Upper
Quartiles HEI	—	—	3	0.014	—	—	—
Q1	0.80	0.29	1	0.006	2.22	1.25	3.92
Q2	0.25	0.29	1	0.337	1.29	0.74	2.25
Q3	0.69	0.28	1	0.015	1.98	1.14	3.45
Quartiles physical activity (MET/wk)	—	—	3	<0.001	—	—	—
Q1	1.18	0.28	1	<0.001	3.25	1.86	5.68
Q2	0.80	0.29	1	0.005	2.23	1.27	3.91
Q3	0.39	0.30	1	0.195	1.47	0.82	2.64
Ethnicity	—	—	2	<0.001	—	—	—
AA	1.66	0.27	1	<0.001	5.27	3.09	8.97
HA	−0.42	0.27	1	0.125	0.66	0.38	1.12
Diabetes (yes)	0.45	0.19	1	0.020	1.56	1.08	2.27

Abbreviations. BMI: body mass index; *B*: coefficient; SE: standard error; Q: quartile; HEI: Healthy Eating Index; AA: African American; HA: Haitian American.
Notes. Cuban Americans were the reference. The 4th quartile was the reference for HEI, physical activity, and BMI. Physical activity was measured in metabolic equivalents (MET) per week. MET = 1 $\text{kcal}\cdot\text{kg}^{-1}\cdot\text{h}^{-1}$. One MET is the equivalent of sitting quietly. Television watching was reported to the nearest 0.25 hours. The dependent variable is $\geq$ 4.25 hours of TV versus $\leq$ 4.00 hours of TV. Education and currently married were tested. Education remained in the final model. The model was adjusted for age ($P = 0.058$), gender ($P = 0.705$), BMI quartile ($P = 0.207$), currently smoking ($P = 0.221$), and education ($P = 0.019$). Compared to persons with at least college, those with less than a high school education were 1.54 times more likely to watch more than 4 hours of TV/day.
Model parameters. χ^2 (17) = 147 ($N = 827$), $P < 0.001$. Nagelkerke R-squared = 0.247 with 79.6% of the cases classified correctly.

examined by the Chi-squared test [χ^2 (9) ($N = 826$) = 28.1, $P = 0.001$] and proportions were estimated by the z-test. The z-test results are shown in Table 4.

4.5. Additional Analysis. Of interest were the differences in consumption of each food group of the HEI across ethnicities, physical activity, TV viewing, and obesity. First, the results of ANOVA and post-hoc analyses were performed for ethnicities. There were differences across ethnicities in dietary components of the HEI for all categories ($P < 0.001$). For most categories, post-hoc analysis showed differences between all three ethnicities from each other. The results are presented in Table 5. Healthier scores in SoFAAS and saturated fat were found for HA as compared to CA and AA. Of concern is the high sodium intake for CA. Proportionally, average servings from the fruit and vegetable groups were

Table 4: Cross tabulations of percentiles of HEI by percentiles of PA.

Quartiles of physical activity (MET/wk)		Quartiles of Healthy Eating Index, 2005				Total
		19.3–41.85	41.86–50.20	50.21–58.06	58.07–84.1	
	N	67[a]	56[a,b]	50[a,b]	36[b]	209
1	% within PA	32.1	26.8	23.9	17.2	100.0
	% within HEI	32.5	27.1	24.2	17.5	25.3%
	N	46[a]	51[a]	46[a]	64[a]	207
2	% within PA	22.2	24.6	22.2	30.9	100.0
	% within HEI	22.3	24.6	22.2	31.1	25.1
	N	43[a]	43[a]	53[a,b]	69[b]	208
3	% within PA	20.7	20.7	25.5	33.2	100.0
	% within HEI	20.9	20.8	25.6	33.5	25.2
	N	50[a]	57[a]	58[a]	37[a]	202
4	% within PA	24.8	28.2	28.7	18.3	100.0
	% within HEI	24.3	27.5	28.0	18.0	24.5
	N	206	207	207	206	826
Total	% within PA	24.9	25.1	25.1	24.9	100.0
	% within HEI	100.0	100.0	100.0	100.0	100.0

Notes. Each superscript letter denotes a subset of quartiles of Healthy Eating Index (HEI) categories whose column proportions do not differ significantly from each other at the alpha = 0.05 level. This option computes pairwise comparisons of column proportions and indicates which pairs of columns (for a given row) are significantly different, applying the Bonferroni correction. Different superscripts represent quartiles that differ at the alpha = 0.05 level. Quartiles of HEI score presented are rounded versions for informational purpose. Actual quartiles were calculated to the 0.001 place. Missing values (n = 32) were participants with total energies of either <500 or >5000 Kcal. The range of HEI-05 was 19.3–84.1 (based on a possible range of 0–100).
Model parameters. χ^2 (9) (N = 826) = 28.1, P = 0.001.

lower than those from the meat and bean group across ethnicities; however, HA had the highest total vegetable intake and the lowest meat and bean consumption as compared to CA and AA.

Next, food groups were compared by ethnicity across PA quartiles by ANOVA. Significant differences were found in all fruit and vegetable groups (total fruit, $P < 0.001$; whole fruit, $P < 0.001$; total vegetables, $P = 0.009$; whole grains, $P = 0.008$; and, saturated fat, $P = 0.030$). Healthier eating patterns with increased PA were found only with the fruits and vegetables, and saturated fat categories, but not for whole grains. As PA increased, fruit and vegetable intake increased. For whole grains and saturated fat, healthier patterns were not observed with increased PA. The highest level of PA (Q4) as compared to the second level (Q2) had a lower consumption of whole grains (0.49, $P = 0.008$). The second level of PA (Q2) had a higher score (lower consumption) for saturated fat as compared to the first level (Q1) (0.75, $P = 0.036$).

The third ANOVA and post-hoc analyses evaluated the HEI food groups across quartiles of TV viewing. There were differences in all food categories: total fruit, $P < 0.001$; total vegetables, $P < 0.001$; green vegetables, $P < 0.001$, grains $P < 0.001$, milk, $P < 0.001$, oils, $P = 0.022$; sodium, $P = 0.005$; and SoFAAS, $P = 0.022$, except the meat and bean group ($P = 0.337$) and the whole fruit group ($P = 0.060$). Those that watched TV, 3-4 hr/day (Q3) consumed less total fruits than those that watched the least TV (0–1.75 hr/day) (-0.46, $P = 0.023$). Total vegetable intake was lower for Q3 as compared to Q1 (-1.20, $P < 0.001$); Q4 as compared to Q3 (0.059; $P = 0.003$); and, Q4 as compared to Q1 (0.61, $P = 0.003$). Total grain intake was less in Q2 as compared to Q1 (-0.51, $P < 0.001$) and less for Q3 as compared to Q1 (-0.59, $P < 0.001$). Less whole grain consumption was associated with Q3 as compared to Q1 (-0.51, $P = 0.003$) and Q4 as compared to Q1 (-0.61, $P = 0.001$). More servings from the milk group were found for Q2 (0.92, $P = 0.009$) and Q3 (1.04, $P = 0.001$) as compared to Q1. Lower intake of oils was associated with Q3 as compared to Q1 (-1.09, $P = 0.016$). A lower score for saturated fat (higher saturated fat consumption) was associated with Q3 and Q4 as compared to Q1 (-1.01, $P = 0.001$) and (-1.26, $P < 0.001$), respectively. For sodium, the highest quartile of TV viewing (Q4) had a lower score (higher than recommended intake) as compared Q1 (-0.79, $P = 0.50$), Q2 (-1.00, $P = 0.007$) and Q3 (-0.85, $P = 0.021$); although Q4–Q1 is marginally significant. The third quintile of TV viewing was associated with less adequate scores as compared to the lowest quintile (-1.63, $P = 0.03$) for SoFAAS.

The food groups were also compared across quartiles of BMI. There were no significant differences in any food groups except for the meat and bean group ($P < 0.001$). The trend was as expected, the two highest quartiles of BMI consumed higher mean portions of meat and beans as compared to the two lower quartiles.

5. Discussion

Participants with and without diabetes who watched more than 4 hours of TV per day were more likely to have poorer quality diets and engage in less physical activity than those who viewed less hours of TV. Poorer quality diets, including

TABLE 5: Healthy Eating Index (HEI) food group scores by ethnicity.

Food group	Ethnicity	Mean (SD)	CA-HA	CA-AA	AA-HA
Total fruit	CA	2.68 (1.70)			
	HA	4.34 (1.25)	−1.57*	−1.23*	−0.34*
	AA	3.91 (1.46)			
Whole fruit	CA	2.71 (1.94)			
	HA	4.20 (1.35)	−1.49*	−0.93*	−0.56*
	AA	3.64 (1.63)			
Total vegetable	CA	1.59 (1.40)			
	HA	4.56 (0.89)	−2.97*	−2.21*	−0.76*
	AA	3.64 (1.81)			
Green vegetables	CA	3.44 (1.54)			
	HA	3.54(1.60)	−0.94	1.25*	−1.34*
	AA	2.20 (1.50)			
Total grains	CA	2.58 (1.04)			
	HA	3.94 (1.18)	−1.35*	−0.91*	−0.44*
	AA	3.49 (1.07)			
Whole grains	CA	1.23 (1.50)			
	HA	2.46 (1.59)	−1.23*	−0.44*	−0.79*
	AA	1.66 (1.21)			
Milk	CA	5.51 (2.69)			
	HA	4.14 (3.03)	1.36*	1.13*	0.45
	AA	4.19 (2.72)			
Meat/beans	CA	5.17 (1.67)			
	HA	5.64 (1.39)	−0.47*	−0.59*	0.12
	AA	5.76 (1.29)			
Oils	CA	4.80 (1.48)			
	HA	5.64 (1.39)	−1.46	−1.90*	0.44
	AA	5.76 (1.29)			
Saturated fat	CA	5.54 (2.80)			
	HA	8.26 (2.06)	−2.72*	−0.83*	−1.89*
	AA	6.37 (2.51)			
Sodium	CA	7.85 (1.57)			
	HA	5.74 (3.11)	2.11*	3.85*	−1.73*
	AA	4.00 (3.06)			
SoFAAS	CA	10.3 (4.69)			
	HA	13.4 (6.78)	−3.06*	−0.20	−2.86*
	AA	10.6 (6.85)			

Abbreviations. CA: Cuban American; HA: Haitian American; CA: Cuban American; SoFAAS: energy from solid fats, alcohol, and added sugars.
Note. An asterisk* denotes a significant difference at $P < 0.05$.

higher amounts of processed foods (high calorie, high salt, low nutrition foods such as cold-cuts/lunch meat, sausages, fast food nuggets and burgers) and fried foods, refined grains, sugar, and lower fruit and vegetable intake, were associated with TV watching in adults [1, 2, 11]. The findings of a 6-year follow-up study suggest that participants free of diabetes who engage in prolonged TV viewing may be at risk for developing diabetes [2]. Our results were in agreement with several studies that found persons with type 2 diabetes have been shown not to follow recommended exercise and dietary practices independent of ethnicity. There were no significant differences in physical activity levels and dietary practices between a lower-income sample of approximately equal numbers of White non-Hispanics and AA with type 2 diabetes ($N = 196$) and 75% of both groups did not meet the government recommendations for physical activity and about 50% of both groups reported following recommended dietary practices (at that time was 30 minutes of exercise at least 3 times per week) [21]. These results were corroborated in a larger, multiethnic survey ($n = 1560$ Whites, $n = 279$ Blacks, and $n = 125$ Hispanics) of persons with diabetes enrolled in managed care where there were no differences across groups and approximately 55% reported exercising at least 3 times per week [22].

In our study AA with and without diabetes with poorest diet quality (lowest quartile of HEI-05) were most likely to watch more than 4 hours of TV as compared to those with better diet quality. Daily TV viewing has been estimated 7 hours for AA as compared to 5 hours for the total population [9]. Similar to the national trend, AA had a higher percent of participants classified in the obese categories. Obesity could be a limiting factor to performing physical activity due to physical and psycho-social factors. TV programs and commercials may influence eating behavior partly through a stimulus for food and overeating [23]. Certain populations may be more susceptible to the adverse effects of TV advertising [23]. More commercials for unhealthy foods were shown on TV programs aimed at AA audiences as compared to TV programs for the general population [24].

Our finding that physical activity was inversely associated with TV watching was in agreement with a large male population with type 2 diabetes ($N = 37,918$; aged 40–75 years) which indicated that men who spent more time watching TV were less likely to exercise [1]. Conversely our results were in discord with a population of approximately half Caucasian and half African American women ($N = 189$) [25] as well as a large study of French adults ($n = 5028$ men aged 45–60 and $n = 7713$ women aged 35–60) [26] and a large primarily Caucasian study of women ($N = 50,277$) [2].

Our results for no differences in physical activity comparing ethnicities may be inconclusive, since there has been a great variation in self-reported measures of physical activity and indices of cardiorespiratory fitness [27]; and references therein. The authors suggest that these variations may be greater for AA males as compared to other groups; however, they used a modified version of *CHAMPS Physical Activity Questionnaire among African-Americans* which assessed moderate and vigorous leisure activities, only [27]. In a US representative population of Hispanics, non-Hispanic Whites, and AA with diabetes, more AA males were exercising regularly as compared to other race and gender groups [28]. Yet, AA men had the lowest MET-minutes/week based on the *International Physical Activity Questionnaire* (IPAQ) suggesting discordance with perceptions and performance of exercise [28]. The IPAQ is a less-detailed physical activity questionnaire designed for developing countries and may not accurately capture physical activity for AA.

Our measure of physical activity included the total of all activities in the past year and the average per week was used for comparison. Accuracy of self-reported measurement of light activities, which occur during leisuretime and employment, may be a confounder in studies of physical activity level and TV viewing. Recreational activities and more intense sports are more accurately recalled than daily or lighter-intensity activities [27]. To its merit, the Modifiable Activity Questionnaire used in this study was designed to assess extreme levels of activity and validated to assess physical activity in populations with diabetes and at high risk for diabetes [6]. Since the majority of our participants engaged in light activity and did not meet the current recommendations for physical activity [29], a major strength of this questionnaire was the consideration of all types of physical activity performed by the individual including domestic choirs, transportation, employment, and leisure pursuits.

5.1. Limitations. It is important to note the limitations of this research. The study was cross-sectional and TV viewing cannot be said to cause dietary and physical activity choices. Another possible limitation was nonresponse bias; participants who responded and agreed to be in this study may have different characteristics from those who were not reached or declined. Diet, physical activity and TV viewing were by self-report and the accuracy depends on the participant's ability to recall their behaviors. Consequently, there may have been over- or under-reporting biases.

5.2. Recommendations for Interventions. Future studies are needed to establish prolonged TV watching in adult populations as a detrimental behavior and risk factor for the development of diabetes or diabetes-related complications. Although strategies to reduce TV watching have been proven effective among children, few trials have been conducted in adults [23]. A two-phase (3-week observation and 3-week intervention) randomized trial of 36 obese adults who normally watched a minimum of 3 hours of TV agreed to a 50% reduction in TV viewing per week using a lockout monitor showed promising results [30]. The intervention group showed an increase in energy expenditure without energy intake difference and decrease in BMI [30]. The findings from their study can be used to design future interventions. The investigators chose an intervention period of a short duration (3 weeks); albeit, increase in energy expenditure over time may prove to augment weight reduction. The influence of high-calorie, high-fat food advertisements may also be minimized by reducing TV viewing. Persons at risk for or having type 2 diabetes should be targeted for altering TV viewing habits in an effort to increase energy expenditure and reduce the influence of over-eating high-calorie, high-sodium, and high-fat-foods. In addition, strategies to substitute cheaper high calorie dense (low-nutrient) foods with cost-effective healthy foods are needed to reach communities in lower socio-economic neighborhoods.

Acknowledgment

This study was funded by a Grant to the first author from the National Institutes of Health: NIH/NIDDK no. ISC1DK083060-03.

References

[1] F. B. Hu, M. F. Leitzmann, M. J. Stampfer, G. A. Colditz, W. C. Willett, and E. B. Rimm, "Physical activity and television watching in relation to risk for type 2 diabetes mellitus in men," *Archives of Internal Medicine*, vol. 161, no. 12, pp. 1542–1548, 2001.

[2] F. B. Hu, T. Y. Li, G. A. Colditz, W. C. Willett, and J. E. Manson, "Television watching and other sedentary behaviors in relation to risk of obesity and type 2 diabetes mellitus in women," *Journal of the American Medical Association*, vol. 289, no. 14, pp. 1785–1791, 2003.

[3] T. T. Fung, F. B. Hu, J. Yu et al., "Leisure-time physical activity, television watching, and plasma biomarkers of obesity and cardiovascular disease risk," *American Journal of Epidemiology*, vol. 152, no. 12, pp. 1171–1178, 2000.

[4] M. Aadahl, M. Kjær, and T. Jørgensen, "Influence of time spent on TV viewing and vigorous intensity physical activity on cardiovascular biomarkers. The Inter 99 study," *European Journal of Cardiovascular Prevention and Rehabilitation*, vol. 14, no. 5, pp. 660–665, 2007.

[5] D. W. Dunstan, J. Salmon, N. Owen et al., "Associations of TV viewing and physical activity with the metabolic syndrome in Australian adults," *Diabetologia*, vol. 48, no. 11, pp. 2254–2261, 2005.

[6] R. W. Jakes, N. E. Day, K. T. Khaw et al., "Television viewing and low participation in vigorous recreation are independently associated with obesity and markers of cardiovascular disease risk: EPIC-Norfolk population-based study," *European Journal of Clinical Nutrition*, vol. 57, no. 9, pp. 1089–1096, 2003.

[7] M. L. Granner and A. Mburia-Mwalili, "Correlates of television viewing among African American and Caucasian women," *Women and Health*, vol. 50, no. 8, pp. 783–794, 2010.

[8] United States Bureau of Labor Statistics (BLS), "American time use survey–2010 results," 2010, Table 1. "Time spent in primary activities 1 and percent of the civilian population engaging in each activity, averages per day by sex, 2010 annual averages," News Release, June 22, 2011. U.S. Department of Labor, USDL-11-0919, http://www.bls.gov/news.release/pdf/atus.pdf.

[9] The Nielson Company, "State of the media: trends in TVviewing—2011 TV upfronts," http://blog.nielsen.com/nielsenwire/.

[10] B. E. Ainsworth, W. L. Haskell, A. S. Leon et al., "Compendium of physical activities: classification of energy costs of human physical activities," *Medicine and Science in Sports and Exercise*, vol. 25, no. 1, pp. 71–80, 1993.

[11] A. Grøntved and F. B. Hu, "Television viewing and risk of type 2 diabetes, cardiovascular disease, and all-cause mortality: a meta-analysis," *Journal of the American Medical Association*, vol. 305, no. 23, pp. 2448–2455, 2011.

[12] A. K. Kant and B. I. Graubard, "A comparison of three dietary pattern indexes for predicting biomarkers of diet and disease," *Journal of the American College of Nutrition*, vol. 24, no. 4, pp. 294–303, 2005.

[13] J. Reedy, S. M. Krebs-Smith, and C. Bosire, "Evaluating the Food Environment. Application of the healthy eating index-2005," *American Journal of Preventive Medicine*, vol. 38, no. 5, pp. 465–471, 2010.

[14] United States Department of Health and Human Services, Healthy People, 2020, "Leading health indicators: Nutrition and physical activity," 2010, Washington DC, USA, http://healthypeople.gov/2020/LHI/nutrition.aspx.

[15] A. M. Kriska, W. C. Knowler, R. E. LaPorte et al., "Development of questionnaire to examine relationship of physical activity and diabetes in Pima Indians," *Diabetes Care*, vol. 13, no. 4, pp. 401–411, 1990.

[16] B. E. Ainsworth, W. L. Haskell, S. D. Herrmann et al., "2011 compendium of physical activities: a second update of codes and MET values," *Medicine and Science in Sports and Exercise*, vol. 43, no. 8, pp. 1575–1581, 2011.

[17] B. J. Caan, "Comparison of the block and the Willett self-administered semiquantitative food frequency questionnaires with an interviewer—administered dietary history," *American Journal of Epidemiology*, vol. 148, no. 12, pp. 1137–1147, 1998.

[18] S. D. Nath and F. G. Huffman, "Validation of a semiquantitative food frequency questionnaire to assess energy and macronutrient intakes of Cuban Americans," *International Journal of Food Sciences and Nutrition*, vol. 56, no. 5, pp. 309–314, 2005.

[19] W. C. Willett, L. Sampson, and M. J. Stampfer, "Reproducibility and validity of a semiquantitative food frequency questionnaire," *American Journal of Epidemiology*, vol. 122, no. 1, pp. 51–65, 1985.

[20] D. W. Hosmer and S. Lemeshow, *Applied Logistic Regression*, John Wiley & Sons, New York, NY, USA, 2nd edition, 2000.

[21] R. H. Cox, J. P. Carpenter, F. A. Bruce, K. P. Poole, and C. K. Gaylord, "Characteristics of low-income African-American and Caucasian adults that are important in self-management of type 2 diabetes," *Journal of Community Health*, vol. 29, no. 2, pp. 155–170, 2004.

[22] V. L. Welch, N. V. Oster, J. A. Gazmararian et al., "Impact of a diabetes disease management program by race and ethnicity," *Disease Management and Health Outcomes*, vol. 14, no. 4, pp. 245–252, 2006.

[23] J. A. Foster, S. A. Gore, and D. S. West, "Altering TV viewing habits: an unexplored strategy for adult obesity intervention?" *American Journal of Health Behavior*, vol. 30, no. 1, pp. 3–14, 2006.

[24] M. A. Tirodkar and A. Jain, "Food messages on African American television shows," *American Journal of Public Health*, vol. 93, no. 3, pp. 439–441, 2003.

[25] M. L. Granner and A. Mburia-Mwalili, "Correlates of television viewing among African American and Caucasian women," *Women and Health*, vol. 50, no. 8, pp. 783–794, 2010.

[26] H. Charreire, E. Kesse-Guyot, S. Bertrais et al., "Associations between dietary patterns, physical activity (leisure-time and occupational) and television viewing in middle-aged French adults," *The British journal of nutrition*, vol. 105, no. 6, pp. 902–910, 2011.

[27] K. Resnicow, F. McCarty, D. Blissett, T. Wang, C. Heitzler, and R. E. Lee, "Validity of a modified CHAMPS physical activity questionnaire among African-Americans," *Medicine and Science in Sports and Exercise*, vol. 35, no. 9, pp. 1537–1545, 2003.

[28] J. R. Gavin, K. M. Fox, and S. Grandy, "Race/Ethnicity and gender differences in health intentions and behaviors regarding exercise and diet for adults with type 2 diabetes: a cross-sectional analysis," *BMC Public Health*, vol. 11, article no. 533, 2011.

[29] United States Department of Health and Human Services, "Physical Activity Guidelines for Americans," 2008, Washington, DC, http://www.health.gov/PAGuidelines/.

[30] J. J. Otten, K. E. Jones, B. Littenberg, and J. Harvey-Berino, "Effects of television viewing reduction on energy intake and expenditure in overweight and obese adults: a randomized controlled trial," *Archives of Internal Medicine*, vol. 169, no. 22, pp. 2109–2115, 2009.

Built Environment and Its Influences on Walking among Older Women: Use of Standardized Geographic Units to Define Urban Forms

Vivian W. Siu,[1] William E. Lambert,[2] Rongwei Fu,[2] Teresa A. Hillier,[3] Mark Bosworth,[4] and Yvonne L. Michael[5]

[1] *Population Research Center and Institute of Metropolitan Studies, Portland State University, P.O. Box 751, Portland, OR 97207, USA*
[2] *Department of Public Health and Preventive Medicine, Oregon Health & Science University, 3181 SW Sam Jackson Park Road, Mail Code CB 669, Portland, OR 97239, USA*
[3] *Kaiser Permanente Center for Health Research, Northwest/Hawaii, 3800 N. Interstate Avenue, Portland, OR 97227, USA*
[4] *Metro Data Resource Center, 600 NE Grand Avenue, Portland, OR 97232, USA*
[5] *Department of Epidemiology and Biostatistics, Drexel University School of Public Health, 1505 Race Street, MS 1033, Philadelphia, PA 19102, USA*

Correspondence should be addressed to Vivian W. Siu, vsiu@pdx.edu

Academic Editor: David Strogatz

Consensus is lacking on specific and policy-relevant measures of neighborhood attributes that may affect health outcomes. To address this limitation, we created small standardized geographic units measuring the transit, commercial, and park area access, intersection, and population density for the Portland, Oregon metropolitan area. Cluster analysis was used to identify six unique urban forms: central city, city periphery, suburb, urban fringe with poor commercial access, urban fringe with pool park access, and satellite city. The urban form information was linkable to the detailed physical activity, health, and socio-demographic data of 2,005 older women without the use of administrative boundaries. Evaluation of the relationship between urban forms and walking behavior indicates that older women residing in city center were more likely to walk than those living in city periphery, suburb communities, and urban fringe with poor commercial access; however, these women were not significantly more likely to walk compared to those residing in urban fringe with poor park access or satellite city. Utility of small standardized geographic units and clusters to measure and define built environment support research investigating the impact of built environment and health. The findings may inform environmental/policy interventions that shape communities and promote active living.

1. Introduction

Urban forms, or areas with different combinations of built environment characteristics, are believed to influence people's daily physical activities. Urban sprawl correlates with increasing automobile dependency and sedentary lifestyle over the past half century [1]. In response, planning efforts to promote New Urbanism and Smart Growth have grown in recent years [2]. At the same time, the number and proportion of older adults in the United States are also increasing [3]. Older adults represent a population that could benefit from these planning efforts; in general, older adults engage in relatively low levels of physical activity [4, 5] and in low intensity activities such as walking and gardening for exercise [6], compared to younger adults. Older women are of particular concern, since women tend to have lower levels of physical activity than men in any age group [4, 7]. Women also tend to live longer than men, so they constitute a large share of the vulnerable population. Positive associations were found between accessibility of facilities, housing density, population density, and the level of walking in several studies that focused on older populations [8–12], and particularly among older women [13, 14] in different neighborhoods and cities across the United States.

Challenges with quantifying built environment measurements, including inconsistent attribute definitions, different scales of data, and varying data quality by jurisdictions, make it difficult to compare between studies designed to quantify the benefits of certain urban form in relation to physical activity. Studies with built environments measured at the individual level typically gathered information by surveying individuals' perceptions of the environment [11, 12, 15, 16], by aggregating neighborhood measures from secondary data such as Census [10, 13, 15–21], or by measuring these characteristics within a certain distance of the subjects' residences [11, 13, 16, 22–25]. Few previous studies have quantified the built environment attributes objectively at high resolution or used cluster analysis to identify different urban forms [17, 26–28].

These research gaps provided an opportunity for the current study to expand on the existing literature investigating the association between built environments and walking among older women by developing refined built environment measures in order to identify distinct urban forms. A better understanding of the relationship between built environments and walking behaviors could lead to urban design and planning policies that promote walking, thereby generating public health benefits.

We hypothesized that a compact urban form promotes walking among older women. Compact neighborhoods with high population density, high street connectivity, and close proximity to transit services, commercial areas, and parks were posited to be favorable to pedestrian activity. High connectivity and convenient access to amenities were hypothesized to shape transportation choices and encourage utilitarian and leisure walking, and high population density was anticipated to support investment of infrastructure and amenities. Older women residing in these compact areas are expected to walk more than those residing in remote areas with low population density, poor street connectivity, and poor accessibility to transit services, commercial areas, and park areas.

2. Materials and Methods

Our analysis used data from participants in the Portland, Oregon, site of the Study of Osteoporotic Fractures (SOF), a national multicenter observational study of healthy, community-dwelling women age 65 years and older recruited in 1986 from four metropolitan areas in the United States. Women were recruited irrespective of bone mineral density and fracture history; those unable to walk without assistance and those with bilateral hip replacements were excluded. All women provided written consent, and the SOF study was approved by each site's institutional review board. Although only baseline data were examined for the current study, prospective data collection included clinical exams and questionnaires to assess longitudinal change in anthropometric and demographic factors, medical history, and information on functioning, quality of life, and lifestyle [29]. Measurement and quality control procedures for the SOF cohort are detailed elsewhere [30].

The subset of SOF participants from Portland, Oregon, totaled 2,419 subjects. In the current analysis, we excluded 347 women (14.3%) who resided outside of the urban growth boundary (UGB) and 67 women (2.8%) whose residence could not be geocoded (e.g., P.O. Box given for address). Thus, the analytic sample was restricted to 2,005 subjects who resided within the Portland UGB, representing 82.9% of the total Portland, Oregon, SOF cohort.

2.1. Built Environment Measures. Six neighborhood measures were created using the existing Portland Metro's Regional Land Information System (RLIS) administrative data and ArcGIS 9.3 (ESRI, Redlands, CA, USA). Among this set of six measures, two measures of accessibility to transit services were included: distance to bus stop and distance to light rail station. Two measures of residential/commercial/recreational land use mix were included: distance to commercial area and distance to park area. One measure of street connectivity was created: street intersection density. One measure of residential distribution was created: population density. Spatial information was unavailable for 1986; therefore data from the earliest available year were used. The 1988 archival transit data from TriMet, the local transit agency, was digitized to develop the distance to bus stop and light rail station variables. Metro-maintained zoning and park data from 1990 were used to create the distance to commercial area and park area variables. A 1988 streets file was established for measuring the intersection density variable, and 1990 Census block population data was adopted for developing the population density variable.

The six built environment variables were developed in a raster environment for the entire Portland metro area. Each grid cell was set at 264 feet^2 (or 80 meters^2), the length for each side of the grid would take roughly one minute of brisk walking to complete. Usage of high-resolution grid cells to quantify built environment attributes minimized the geographic unit of measure. The refined geographic units for establishing built environment measures lessened the potential bias associated with the use of coarsely grouped measures, in which neighborhood characteristics might be wrongly assumed as the experience for the individuals (i.e., the ecological fallacy). The high-resolution cell size also facilitated linkage of localized resident neighborhood measures to the subjects based on their mapped residential address location.

The neighborhood measures were standardized to ensure comparability among measures with different scales. The four distance variables (accessibility to the closest bus stop, light rail station, commercial area, and park area) were measured in Euclidean distance; shorter distance indicated better accessibility. The two density variables, intersection density and population density, were created using the kernel density function, accounting for the number of street intersections within a quarter mile buffer from each grid cell and the number of persons in a one mile buffer; higher number indicated greater density.

The reliability and validity of the built environment measures were evaluated using a combination of GIS analysis processes and statistical tests. Vector/direct distance and density measurements for the six attributes were established for the study sample and compared to the raster approach. Various tests and graphs used for assessing the level of agreement between built environment measures developed through the raster method, and the vector method indicated reasonable agreement [31], meaning that the distance and density measurements created using the raster and the more standard and commonly adopted vector approaches were similar.

2.2. Walking. SOF participants reported the total number of blocks walked daily (12 blocks = 1 mile) for utilitarian and for leisure purposes; we added these measures to create the overall number of blocks walked daily. Since a fair share of the participants (11%) reported no walking at all, this variable was dichotomized into walking less than five blocks a day, and walking five or more blocks a day. Five blocks is equivalent to about 400 meters or a quarter of a mile. This amount of walking has been found to provide health benefit to sedentary older adults [32]. As a result of this classification, 65% of our subjects ($n = 1,572$) walked five or more blocks a day.

2.3. Statistical Analysis. We used k-median statistical clustering to group grid cells with similar values of accessibility to transit, land use mix, street connectivity, and residential density into clusters representing types of urban-form. The Calinski-Harabasz stopping rule was used to determine the optimal number of clusters that would maximize the between group differences while minimizing the within group differences of the built environment measures considered [33]. Grid cells with similar composition of neighborhood attributes were aggregated into the same group, converting the six continuous built environment measures into six categories of exposure corresponding to distinct urban forms.

Subject characteristics were summarized using descriptive statistics. Multivariable logistic regression models were used to assess the association between urban-form and walking while controlling for confounding variables. Potential confounding variables included individual characteristics of the women: age, years of education, marital status, overall exercise (Kcal/week), BMI (kg/m^2), smoking (pack years), self-reported health, history of stroke, and history of arthritis/rheumatism. Additional potential confounding variables included block group level neighborhood characteristics from the Census: demographic composition, education, occupation, poverty, income, and household type. All potential confounders with a univariate P value less than 0.25 were considered in the preliminary model. Variables were removed from the model one by one beginning with the variable with the highest P value until all variables in the model were significant at $\alpha = 0.05$. The pairwise comparisons of the impact on walking by different urban forms were also explored to identify urban forms that might have impacted walking differently. All statistical analyses were conducted using Stata 11 (StataCorp, College Station, TX, USA).

3. Results

The k-median cluster analysis resulted in six distinct urban-form clusters across the metro region. The medians and interquartile ranges of built environment measures for each cluster are summarized in Table 1. Clusters 1, 2, and 3 showed a gradual decrease in accessibility and density for all built environment attributes: with Cluster 1 being the "best" urban-form with close proximity to transit, commercial areas, and park areas. Intersection and population density in Cluster 1 were also the highest of the six clusters. The accessibility and density decreased from the central core to Cluster 2 and dropped even further for Cluster 3. Although Clusters 4, 5, and 6 generally had poorer accessibility to amenities and lower density than Cluster 3, there were certain attributes in each of these clusters that were similar to another cluster and that provide some insight as to how specific attributes influence walking habits. For instance, Clusters 4 and 5 shared low intersection and population density, and they had similar measures for access to bus or light rail services; they differed in that Cluster 4 had the greatest distance to commercial areas while Cluster 5 had the greatest distance to park areas. Cluster 6 was similar to Cluster 3 in terms of access to commercial areas and density, but it had the greatest distance to transit services among the six clusters.

The resulting clusters were mapped into ArcGIS to evaluate face validity (Figure 1). The map demonstrates reasonable clustering with grid cells assigned to the same group being spatially continuous; the distribution of the six clusters was also sensible and consistent with our knowledge of the environmental characteristics of the metro region.

The walking behavior of older women varied by purpose of walking and type of cluster (Table 2). Generally, older women who walked for leisure purposes tend to walk more than those who walked only for utilitarian purpose in each of the six clusters. The relative variation in walking by urban-form typology demonstrated a similar pattern for those who walked for utilitarian purposes, for leisure purposes, as well as for both purposes combined. Specifically, the central city consistently ranked one of the highest while the urban fringe with poor commercial area access ranked the lowest among the six clusters in median number of daily blocks walked, regardless of walking purposes.

Table 3 provides results from the multivariable logistic regression estimating the association between urban-form and walking. Compared to women who lived in the central city, those who lived in the urban fringe with poor commercial area access, city periphery, and suburbs were significantly less likely to walk each day (adjusted odds ratios (ORs) ranged from 0.40 for urban fringe to 0.69 for city periphery and suburbs). Women who lived in the satellite city were also less likely to walk (OR: 0.53) compared to those who live in the central city, but the difference was not statistically significant. There was also no difference in walking among

TABLE 1: Summary of built environment attributes by cluster, Portland metro area.

Urban-form cluster	Median (interquartile range) distance in meters to the nearest:				Median (interquartile range) density per km²	
	Bus stop	Light rail station	Commercial area	Park	Intersections	Population
Cluster 1: central city	161 (80–241)	2968 (1451–5465)	228 (80–341)	402 (241–569)	111 (92–138)	2591 (2062–3027)
Cluster 2: city periphery	241 (114–402)	3817 (2037–7701)	332 (161–580)	433 (241–688)	53 (38–69)	1473 (1125–1793)
Cluster 3: suburb	433 (228–809)	12876 (9927–15253)	628 (322–995)	410 (180–688)	24 (10–42)	777 (407–1199)
Cluster 4: urban fringe with poor commercial area access	1778 (1048–2680)	11273 (7816–15331)	2255 (1835–2747)	724 (402–1074)	5 (0–13)	62 (0–334)
Cluster 5: urban fringe with poor park area access	1821 (1018–3030)	8459 (5413–12436)	1049 (613–1527)	1884 (1479–2421)	7 (2–17)	166 (10–367)
Cluster 6: satellite city	6112 (4474–8697)	23356 (21622–26551)	515 (241–900)	764 (433–1249)	26 (8–50)	641 (280–1093)

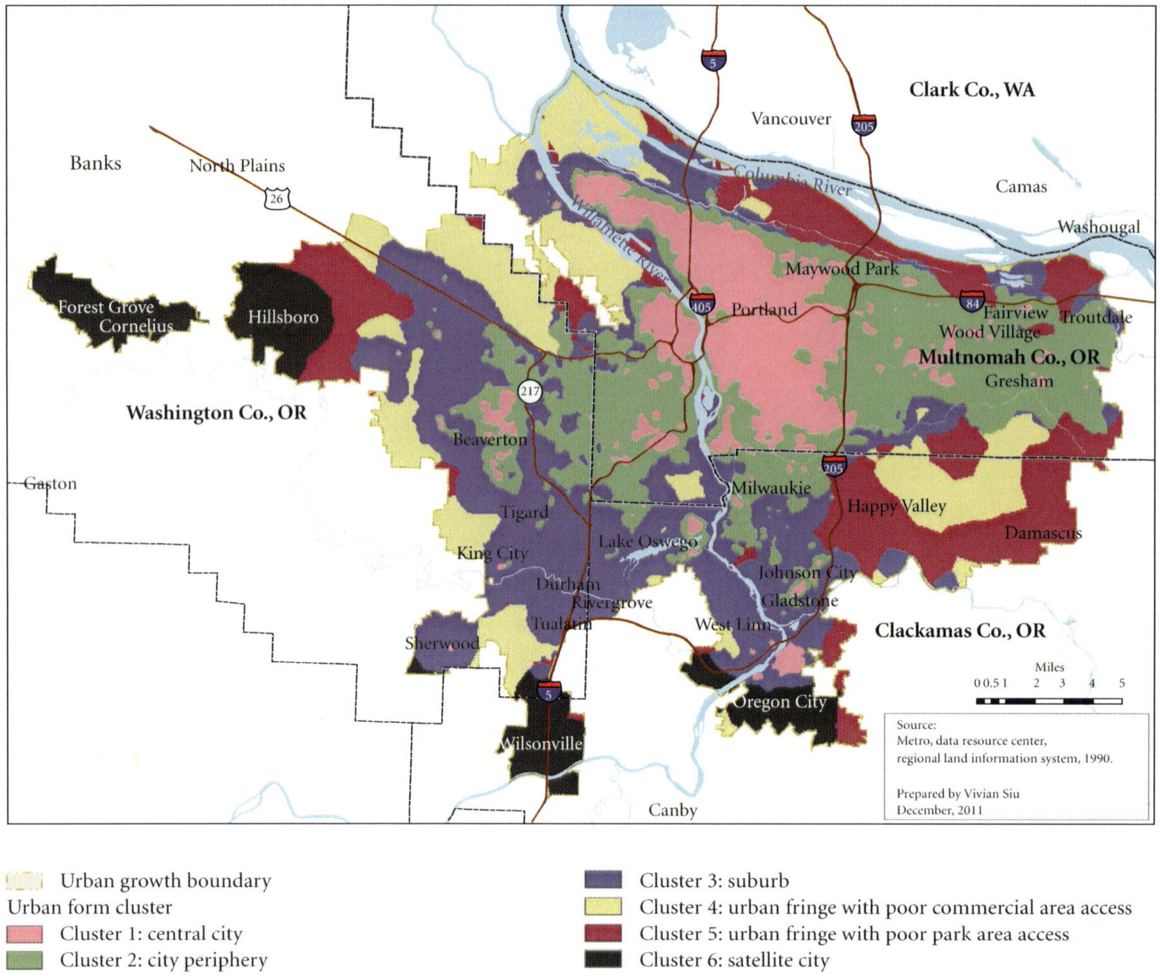

Figure 1: Spatial representation of urban-form clusters, Portland metro area.

older women residing in the urban fringe with poor park areas access compared to those in the central city (OR: 0.98). Pairwise comparison between other clusters did not identify other significant differences.

In addition, the likelihood of women walking decreased with increasing age or increasing neighborhood block group share of live-alone population in poverty. Likelihood of walking increased for older women with more than 12 years of education compared to those with 12 years or less education (OR: 1.32) or who burned more than 2500 kcal per week through exercise compared to those who exercise less (OR: 2.49). On the other hand, the likelihood of walking as compared to the reference group decreased for women who rate their health fair, poor, or very poor (OR: 0.52); smoked 1–40 pack-years (OR: 0.88) or over 40 pack-years (OR: 0.66); were overweight (OR: 0.83), or obese (OR: 0.59); had a history of stroke (OR: 0.57).

4. Discussion

Few studies have either quantified built environment characteristics using high-resolution geographic unit or have used clusters to classify attributes of the built environment as urban forms. Our analysis pulls together various objective, high-resolution, and standardized measures to identify neighborhood clusters that portray the walking potential for individuals. Cluster analysis identified six homogeneous zones optimizing the joint distribution of built environment characteristics: accessibility to transit, land use mix, street connectivity, and residential density. The analytic process classified the Portland metro area into six unique urban-forms clusters: central city, city periphery, suburb, urban fringe with poor commercial area access, urban fringe with poor park area access, and satellite city. These urban-form clusters accounted for multiple built environment measures jointly without tying to an arbitrary administrative or neighborhood boundary which arguably fails to accurately represent the complex mix of urban forms.

Our analytic approach builds upon theory related to the urban built environment and physical activity; empirical use of built environment measures in combination to create a summary characterization of neighborhood type provided greater contextual meaning about the composition of different built environments without committing to a predefined neighborhood boundary. Our successful application of these

TABLE 2: Summary of self-reported daily walking by older women living in Portland metropolitan area according to urban-form cluster.

Urban-form cluster	Number of blocks walked per day					
	Mean	Standard deviation	Median	Minimum	Maximum	*N*
Walking for utilitarian purposes						
Cluster 1: central city	6.39	5.68	5	1	48	694
Cluster 2: city periphery	5.76	5.65	4	1	60	573
Cluster 3: suburb	6.67	7.13	4.5	1	48	170
Cluster 4: urban fringe with poor commercial area access	5.65	5.35	4	1	24	20
Cluster 5: urban fringe with poor park area access	6.95	7.60	4	1	36	41
Cluster 6: satellite city	5.33	4.30	5	1	15	9
Walking for leisure purposes						
Cluster 1: central city	14.69	10.85	12	1	82	492
Cluster 2: city periphery	13.88	10.30	12	1	72	457
Cluster 3: suburb	14.28	10.52	12	1	48	151
Cluster 4: urban fringe with poor commercial area access	9.79	8.40	8	1	24	14
Cluster 5: urban fringe with poor park area access	11.66	8.55	10	1	36	29
Cluster 6: satellite city	15.00	10.20	13.5	5	28	6
Walking for leisure and utilitarian purposes combined, excluding those who do not walk regularly						
Cluster 1: central city	14.60	13.36	11	1	102	799
Cluster 2: city periphery	13.98	12.88	10	1	96	690
Cluster 3: suburb	15.59	13.45	12	1	66	211
Cluster 4: urban fringe with poor commercial area access	10.00	9.65	5	1	30	25
Cluster 5: urban fringe with poor park area access	13.84	11.12	12	1	44	45
Cluster 6: satellite city	13.80	11.83	9.5	2	36	10
Walking for leisure and utilitarian purposes combined, including those who do not walk regularly						
Cluster 1: central city	13.24	13.41	9	0	102	881
Cluster 2: city periphery	12.26	12.91	8	0	96	787
Cluster 3: suburb	13.43	13.60	9	0	66	245
Cluster 4: urban fringe with poor commercial area access	8.93	9.63	4.5	0	30	28
Cluster 5: urban fringe with poor park area access	12.22	11.37	10	0	44	51
Cluster 6: satellite city	10.62	11.90	6	0	36	13

methods to evaluate likelihood of walking in older women suggests potential utility for future studies. Although a variety of methods have been used to define and quantify characteristics of the built environment, challenges remain with the dissemination of spatial information at refined geographic units. We created objective and localized built environment measures using standardized geographic units that were not bigger than a city block. This measurement scale allowed for geographically relevant built environment measures that were linkable to individual-level data.

In previously published research, Riva and colleagues [10] used cluster analysis to identify exposure to built environment characteristics that promote physical activity such as access, land use, and density. Similar to our analysis, Riva et al. observed that the number of 10-minute episodes of walking was significantly higher in the central urban zone compared to the low density suburban zone. While the specific methods to quantify built environment variables varied slightly from our approach, they obtained similar findings suggesting that the methodology of cluster analysis is robust and useful. Differences in data availability and the specific ways in which variables can be operationalized will exist, but cluster analysis as a method appears to be able to identify meaningful areas with distinct characteristics.

In our analysis, older women living in neighborhoods characterized by high population density, high street connectivity, convenient access to amenities, especially transit and commercial areas were most likely to walk for exercise and transport. Our findings are consistent with previous studies that indicate that good infrastructure and design, such as availability of transit services and high street connectivity, encourage people to navigate around the area [20, 28, 34]. The existence of commercial businesses and parks appears to provide destinations that attract people to visit [2, 11, 26], and in turn, the high population density provides the capacity to support businesses and transportation services [2, 11, 20, 26]. It is reasonable to hypothesize that these components act similarly to support a greater likelihood of walking among older women. Comparison between the clusters suggested that access to destinations, such as park or commercial areas, increases the likelihood of walking. Residents in the urban fringe with poor access to commercial areas were more likely to walk compared to residents in the urban fringe with poor park access, suggesting that proximity

TABLE 3: Estimated odds ratios and 95% confidence intervals for the association of variables with walking.

Variable	Adjusted OR	95% CI	*P*-value
Built environment			<0.01
Cluster 1: central city	Reference		
Cluster 2: city periphery	0.69	(0.55, 0.85)	
Cluster 3: suburb	0.69	(0.50, 0.95)	
Cluster 4: urban fringe w/poor commercial area access	0.40	(0.18, 0.88)	
Cluster 5: urban fringe w/poor park area access	0.98	(0.52, 1.84)	
Cluster 6: satellite city	0.53	(0.16, 1.71)	
Percent live alone population in poverty, 1989	0.28	(0.11, 0.70)	<0.01
Age	0.95	(0.93, 0.96)	<0.01
Education level			<0.01
12 years or less	Reference		
More than 12 years	1.32	(1.08, 1.62)	
Self-rated health			<0.01
Excellent/good	Reference		
Fair/poor/very poor	0.52	(0.41, 0.67)	
Smoking			0.04
0 pack-years	Reference		
1–40 pack-years	0.88	(0.70, 1.11)	
More than 40 pack-years	0.66	(0.48, 0.92)	
Exercise (kcal per week)			<0.01
2500 kcal or less	Reference		
More than 2500 kcal	2.49	(1.84, 3.37)	
BMI			<0.01
Underweight/normal (less than 25.0)	Reference		
Overweight (25.0–29.9)	0.83	(0.66, 1.03)	
Obese (30.0 or above)	0.59	(0.46, 0.77)	
Stroke			0.01
No history of stroke	Reference		
With history of stroke	0.57	(0.37, 0.88)	

to a commercial area might play a stronger role in promoting walking than proximity to a park in this age group.

Several limitations in the current study must be recognized. Given the cross-sectional nature of our study, it is not possible to determine whether association reflects a preference among active older women to live in the central city areas for reasons such as greater transportation options or better access to amenities. However, neighborhood selection is only one of the many factors affecting mobility of the older population. Generally, factors determining the mobility of the elderly population include life cycle events, environmental factors, and economic status [35]. Moreover, diversity in the older population, including age, gender, and resources, also accounts for varying housing preferences and mobility levels [3, 35–37]. Some literature suggests that an individual's preference may not be consistent with the actual living environment or affect walking habits [38, 39]. In other studies, intraurban migration pattern among elderly suggests that older adults who are wealthy and socially active tend to move away from central city, while more diverse individuals of lower income relocate within similar neighborhoods [40]. Also, neighborhood preferences may not play a strong role in the relocation decision among those who moved [3]. While self-selection cannot be ruled out, it may have limited impact on the observed association in our analysis.

The age of our data may limit its generalizability to the present day. The geographic and health data used for this study were collected or recorded 26 years ago. The urban process and development experienced in Portland might have since altered the clusters and the composition of neighborhood factors. Some of the findings from the current study may not be directly applicable in contemporary sense due to changes in urban forms occurred since 1986; however, the findings and relative associations may be useful to areas that remained unchanged or have transformed to different urban forms identified. Additionally, the process is still relevant and useful for analysis of the association between built environment and walking using current data or data from other places and regions. This information provides general guidance and direction to changes in built environment that can encourage walking among older women.

5. Conclusions

In conclusion, we found that urban areas with the best access to transit services, close proximity to amenities such as businesses and parks, high street connectivity, and high population density were most likely to promote walking in older women. The use of cluster analysis synthesized the information to account for the complex interactions between multiple built environment attributes. The built environment characteristics of the central city were associated with increased utilitarian and leisure walking among older women relative to the city periphery, the suburb, or the urban fringe with poor commercial area access. The long-term benefits of shifting urban form to be more pedestrian-friendly are critically important with the aging population; changes in built environment would promote higher levels of physical activity among older adults and likely among people of other age groups. This change, in turn, may lower the risk of diseases related to the lack of physical activity in the population. Our analysis approach contributes to the theory related to urban-form typology and promotion of physical activity via the use of methods that quantify built environment characteristics without committing to a predefined neighborhood boundary.

Acknowledgments

The authors are grateful for the financial support from the National Institutes of Health/National Institute on Aging (AG028254-04). They thank Corey Nagel for the extraction of the Study of Osteoporotic Fracture data and the staff at the Metro Data Resource Center (DRC) for the maintenance of the Regional Land Information System, which provides spatial data necessary for this project. The authors acknowledge the contribution of the study participants and the support of the SOF staff and investigators. The Study of Osteoporotic Fractures (SOF) is supported by the National Institutes of Health funding. The National Institute on Aging (NIA) provides support under the following grant numbers: R01 AG005407, R01 AR35582, R01 AR35583, R01 AR35584, R01 AG005394, R01 AG027574, and R01 AG027576.

References

[1] R. C. Brownson, T. K. Boehmer, and D. A. Luke, "Declining rates of physical activity in the United States: what are the contributors?" *Annual Review of Public Health*, vol. 26, pp. 421–443, 2005.

[2] S. L. Handy, M. G. Boarnet, R. Ewing, and R. E. Killingsworth, "How the built environment affects physical activity: views from urban planning," *American Journal of Preventive Medicine*, vol. 23, no. 2, pp. 64–73, 2002.

[3] M. B. Neal, N. Chapman, J. Dill et al., *Age-Related Shifts in Housing and Transportation Demand*, College of Urban and Public Affairs, Portland State University, 2006.

[4] R. C. Brownson, P. L. Remington, and J. R. Davis, *Chronic Disease Epidemiology and Control*, American Public Health Association, Washington, DC, USA, 2nd edition, 1998.

[5] C. Mathers, G. Stevens, and M. Mascarenhas, "Global health risks: mortality and burden of disease attributable to selected major risks," Department of Health Statistics and Informatics, World Health Organization, 2009, http://www.who.int/healthinfo/global_burden_disease/GlobalHealthRisks_report_full.pdf.

[6] T. Prohaska, E. Belansky, B. Belza et al., "Physical activity, public health, and aging: critical issues and research priorities," *Journals of Gerontology B*, vol. 61, no. 5, pp. S267–S273, 2006.

[7] T. J. Bungum and M. Thompson-Robinson, "Modes and locales of physical activity: older adults," *Californian Journal of Health Promotion*, vol. 1, pp. 40–48, 2008.

[8] A. Forsyth, J. Michael Oakes, B. Lee, and K. H. Schmitz, "The built environment, walking, and physical activity: is the environment more important to some people than others?" *Transportation Research D*, vol. 14, no. 1, pp. 42–49, 2009.

[9] C. L. Nagel, N. E. Carlson, M. Bosworth, and Y. L. Michael, "The relation between neighborhood built environment and walking activity among older adults," *American Journal of Epidemiology*, vol. 168, no. 4, pp. 461–468, 2008.

[10] M. Riva, L. Gauvin, P. Apparicio, and J. M. Brodeur, "Disentangling the relative influence of built and socioeconomic environments on walking: the contribution of areas homogenous along exposures of interest," *Social Science and Medicine*, vol. 69, no. 9, pp. 1296–1305, 2009.

[11] D. A. Rodríguez, K. R. Evenson, A. V. Diez Roux, and S. J. Brines, "Land use, residential density, and walking. The multi-ethnic study of atherosclerosis," *American Journal of Preventive Medicine*, vol. 37, no. 5, pp. 397–404, 2009.

[12] R. Shigematsu, J. F. Sallis, T. L. Conway et al., "Age differences in the relation of perceived neighborhood environment to walking," *Medicine and Science in Sports and Exercise*, vol. 41, no. 2, pp. 314–321, 2009.

[13] W. C. King, S. H. Belle, J. S. Brach, L. R. Simkin-Silverman, T. Soska, and A. M. Kriska, "Objective measures of neighborhood environment and physical activity in older women," *American Journal of Preventive Medicine*, vol. 28, no. 5, pp. 461–469, 2005.

[14] M. S. Mujahid, A. V. D. Roux, M. Shen et al., "Relation between neighborhood environments and obesity in the multi-ethnic study of atherosclerosis," *American Journal of Epidemiology*, vol. 167, no. 11, pp. 1349–1357, 2008.

[15] H. M. Badland, G. M. Schofield, K. Witten et al., "Understanding the relationship between activity and neighbourhoods (URBAN) Study: research design and methodology," *BioMed Central Public Health*, vol. 9, pp. 224–234, 2009.

[16] E. Cerin, E. Leslie, L. D. Toit, N. Owen, and L. D. Frank, "Destinations that matter: associations with walking for transport," *Health and Place*, vol. 13, no. 3, pp. 713–724, 2007.

[17] J. Lin and L. Long, "What neighborhood are you in? Empirical findings of relationships between household travel and neighborhood characteristics," *Transportation*, vol. 35, no. 6, pp. 739–758, 2008.

[18] M. G. Boarnet, M. Greenwald, and T. E. McMillan, "Walking, urban design, and health: toward a cost-benefit analysis framework," *Journal of Planning Education and Research*, vol. 27, no. 3, pp. 341–358, 2008.

[19] R. Boer, Y. Zheng, A. Overton, G. K. Ridgeway, and D. A. Cohen, "Neighborhood design and walking Trips in Ten U.S. Metropolitan areas," *American Journal of Preventive Medicine*, vol. 32, no. 4, pp. 298–304, 2007.

[20] P. F. Coogan, L. F. White, T. J. Adler, K. M. Hathaway, J. R. Palmer, and L. Rosenberg, "Prospective study of urban form and physical activity in the black women's health study," *American Journal of Epidemiology*, vol. 170, no. 9, pp. 1105–1117, 2009.

[21] L. Gauvin, M. Riva, T. Barnett et al., "Association between neighborhood active living potential and walking," *American Journal of Epidemiology*, vol. 167, no. 8, pp. 944–953, 2008.

[22] D. T. Duncan, J. Aldstadt, J. Whalen, S. J. Melly, and S. L. Gortmaker, "Validation of WalkScore for estimating neighborhood walkability: an analysis of four US metropolitan areas," *International Journal of Environmental Research and Public Health*, vol. 8, no. 11, pp. 4160–4179, 2011.

[23] L. D. Frank, J. F. Sallis, T. L. Conway, J. E. Chapman, B. E. Saelens, and W. Bachman, "Many pathways from land use to health: associations between neighborhood walkability and active transportation, body mass index, and air quality," *Journal of the American Planning Association*, vol. 72, no. 1, pp. 75–87, 2006.

[24] F. Li, K. J. Fisher, R. C. Brownson, and M. Bosworth, "Multilevel modelling of built environment characteristics related to neighbourhood walking activity in older adults," *Journal of Epidemiology and Community Health*, vol. 59, no. 7, pp. 558–564, 2005.

[25] G. R. McCormack, B. Giles-Corti, and M. Bulsara, "The relationship between destination proximity, destination mix and physical activity behaviors," *Preventive Medicine*, vol. 46, no. 1, pp. 33–40, 2008.

[26] B. E. Saelens and S. L. Handy, "Built environment correlates of walking: a review," *Medicine and Science in Sports and Exercise*, vol. 40, no. 7, supplement, pp. S550–566, 2008.

[27] L. Huang, D. G. Stinchcomb, L. W. Pickle, J. Dill, and D. Berrigan, "Identifying clusters of active transportation using spatial scan statistics," *American Journal of Preventive Medicine*, vol. 37, no. 2, pp. 157–166, 2009.

[28] R. Ewing and R. Cervero, "Travel and the built environment," *Journal of the American Planning Association*, vol. 76, no. 3, pp. 265–294, 2010.

[29] S. R. Cummings, D. M. Black, M. C. Nevitt et al., "Appendicular bone density and age predict hip fracture in women," *Journal of the American Medical Association*, vol. 263, no. 5, pp. 665–668, 1990.

[30] S. R. Cummings, M. C. Nevitt, W. S. Browner et al., "Risk factors for hip fracture in white women," *The New England Journal of Medicine*, vol. 332, no. 12, pp. 767–773, 1995.

[31] V. Siu, "Reliability and validity of spatially derived neighborhood design measures for the Portland metro area, 1988–2006," Internship Report for Oregon Health & Science University Master of Public Health Degree, 2009.

[32] P. Diehr and C. Hirsch, "Health benefits of increased walking for sedentary, generally healthy older adults: using longitudinal data to approximate an intervention trial," *Journals of Gerontology A*, vol. 65, no. 9, pp. 982–989, 2010.

[33] T. Calinski and J. Harabasz, "A dendrite method for cluster analysis," *Communications in Statistics-Theory and Methods*, vol. 3, no. 1, pp. 1–27, 1974.

[34] M. Schlossberg, A. W. Agrawal, K. Irvin, and V. L. Bekkouche, "How far, by which route, and why? A spatial analysis of pedestrian preference," Report 06-06, Mineta Transportation Institute, San Jose State University, 2007.

[35] R. F. Wiseman and C. C. Roseman, "A typology of elderly migration based on the decision making process.," *Economic Geography*, vol. 55, no. 4, pp. 324–337, 1979.

[36] J. F. Sergeant, D. J. Ekerdt, and R. Chapin, "Measurement of late-life residential relocation: why are rates for such a manifest event so varied?" *Journals of Gerontology B*, vol. 63, no. 2, pp. S92–S98, 2008.

[37] G. Lin, "Elderly migration: household versus individual approaches," *Papers in Regional Science*, vol. 76, no. 3, pp. 285–300, 1997.

[38] L. D. Frank, B. E. Saelens, K. E. Powell, and J. E. Chapman, "Stepping towards causation: do built environments or neighborhood and travel preferences explain physical activity, driving, and obesity?" *Social Science and Medicine*, vol. 65, no. 9, pp. 1898–1914, 2007.

[39] S. Handy, X. Cao, and P. L. Mokhtarian, "Self-selection in the relationship between the built environment and walking: empirical evidence from Northern California," *Journal of the American Planning Association*, vol. 72, no. 1, pp. 55–74, 2006.

[40] R. F. Wiseman and M. Virden, "Spatial and social dimensions of intraurban elderly migration," *Economic Geography*, vol. 53, no. 1, pp. 1–13, 1977.

Changes in Peak Flow Value during Immunotherapy Administration

Diego Saporta

Associates in ENT & Allergy, PA 470 North Aveue, Elizabeth, NJ 07208, USA

Correspondence should be addressed to Diego Saporta, saporta.allergy@gmail.com

Academic Editor: Janette Hope

Nasal allergies are prevalent affecting a large percentage of the population. Not only the upper respiratory tract but the whole body is involved. Allergies produce morbidity (and even occasional mortality) as they can lead to asthma development, and increased number of accidents. Immunotherapy results can be evaluated by following symptom scores, medication use, and objective measurements. Using a Peak Flow Meter (PFM) to evaluate immunotherapy results, it became evident that patients with and without asthma exhibited an improvement in the Peak Flow (PF) value, suggesting that lower airway involvement in allergic patients could be more prevalent than assumed. A consecutive chart review was performed including patients of any age with nasal allergies (with or without asthma) treated with immunotherapy for at least 6 months that had at least 2 complete evaluations. When immunotherapy was successful, most patients exhibited an increase in the PF value regardless of asthma status. A very significant finding was that most allergy sufferers may have lower airway inflammation. The use of the PF value to assess immunotherapy results and the potential failure to diagnose asthma in allergy sufferers are discussed. A better diagnosis of lower airway inflammation could be substantial in the management of these patients.

1. Introduction

Nasal allergies are common and their prevalence in industrialized societies appears to be increasing. While nasal allergies were rarely diagnosed in the 19th century, their occurrence markedly increased during the 20th century. For example, studies show the incidence of nasal allergies in parts of the United States at 10% in 1974, 20% in 1986, and 42% in 1994 [1]. Similar figures of up to 40% have been reported in other parts of the world too [2]. In addition, similar increases have occurred in conditions not usually associated with allergies but with clear allergic etiology, such as eczema and asthma. These figures indicate an explosive increase. It is possible that an increasingly polluted environment is a causative factor [1].

Asthma is a common chronic disorder of the airways characterized by an underlying inflammation that leads to bronchial hyperresponsiveness and recurring airflow obstruction. In some cases patients develop persistent changes in airway structure, including fibrosis, smooth muscle hypertrophy, and angiogenesis. In the United States asthma affects more than 22 million people. It is one of the most common chronic diseases of childhood, affecting more than six million children in the USA [3].

The occurrence of asthma also has increased. Hospitalization rates are higher among young children. Collectively, individuals with asthma account for more than 497,000 hospitalizations annually. The onset of asthma for most patients begins early in life with the pattern of disease persistence. Recognizable risk factors include atopic disease. Current asthma treatment with anti-inflammatory therapy does not appear to prevent progression of the underlying disease severity [3].

The allergic disease affects the whole body. Fatigue is one of the most common complaints of the allergy sufferer, [4] and nasal congestion is recorded as the most bothersome symptom of allergic rhinitis [5]. Nasal obstruction is often the most severe symptom in patients with nasal allergies and it can lead to the onset or worsening of obstructive sleep apnea (OSA) [6].

Sleep-related symptoms are extremely common in patients with allergic rhinitis. Sleep impairment associated with allergic rhinitis is likely a major contributor to the overall disease morbidity, health care costs, and loss of work productivity [7].

Individuals with OSA are at an increased risk for motor vehicle accidents [8] and lack of sleep has been implicated in job related accidents as well. [9] In addition, there are patients where the influence of nasal obstruction in sleep disordered breathing is critical [10]. Nasal obstruction also is a contributing factor to development of dentofacial abnormalities in the developing child [11].

So it is clear that having allergies means dealing with more than just nasal congestion, rhinorrhea, and itchy eyes. Not only can quality of life be significantly impaired for those with allergies, but also this condition can be potentially life threatening given that a patient with allergies is susceptible to fatigue, sleep deprivation, a higher incidence of accidents, and lower airway inflammation with bronchoconstriction.

While medical management of nasal allergies will control symptoms in the best of circumstances, immunotherapy is the only treatment modality available that can potentially cure the allergic condition [12, 13]. Immunotherapy works by modifying the immunological response of the allergic individual through stimulating the production of IgG (usually known as a "blocking antibody") and eliciting more complex changes in the activity of the T-cells [14], where T-cell tolerance is attained mainly by generation of allergen-specific Treg cells leading to suppressed T-cell proliferation and Th1 and Th2 cytokine responses against the allergen. This is accompanied by a significant increase in allergen-specific IgG_4, IgG_1, and IgA and a decrease in IgE in the late stage of the disease [13].

In the clinical setting immunotherapy treatment is usually evaluated by following changes in symptoms scores. Specifically, the patient rates his/her symptoms usually using a numerical scale, and the change of this value over time is followed to assess improvement or lack thereof. Even though this is a subjective tool, different symptoms scores have been scientifically validated as useful [15–17]. Some of the objective measurements of symptomatic improvement include use of acoustic rhinomanometry [18].

In our office we use a symptom questionnaire (see Figure 1) based on the scoring method followed by Fell [17]. We added objective measurements including nasal resistance determined by acoustic rhinomanometry and determination of PF value. While acoustic rhinomanometry requires significant training of the technician, it is time consuming, and yields results that are difficult to interpret, using a PFM device requires minimal training and yields easy-to-interpret results in seconds. It became clear that determining the PF value was a simpler procedure that could be easily incorporated in a private practice clinical setting. Soon after the use of the PFM was incorporated in our practice, it was observed that patients with allergies exhibited an improvement in PF value if immunotherapy was successful (as measured by a decrease in symptom scores and medication use) and that such improvement occurred not only in the patients with asthma but also in the allergy sufferer without any asthma symptoms.

Table 1: Symptoms considered for scoring.

Sneezing
Runny nose
Nasal obstruction
Post nasal drip
Watery eyes
Itchy eyes
Itchy ears
Itchy nose
Itchy throat
Itchy skin
Clogged ears
Facial pain/pressure
Headaches
Cough
Sensation of tight chest
Wheezing
Shortness of breath
Exercise-induced SOB
Exercise-induced cough
Exercise-induced wheezing
Waking up with symptoms

To verify this hypothesis, we collected the data presented herein, with the understanding that this is only an observational study that lacks the rigor of a prospective randomized study with a control group.

2. Methods

A consecutive chart review was performed. Inclusion criteria for the study were patients of any age with nasal allergies (with or without asthma) treated with immunotherapy for at least six months that had at least two complete evaluations. A complete evaluation included symptom scoring, evaluation of medication use, and determination of PF value.

Ethical Considerations. Subjects' privacy was assured by the way data was collected and recorded so that subjects could not be directly or indirectly identified. In other words, a patient's privacy was protected by entering data for statistical analysis in a simple spreadsheet with nonspecific identifiers, such as patient number 1 and patient number 2, with subsequent refiling of the patient's chart according to usual procedure.

In our practice we follow Fell's method [17] for symptom scoring, which classifies each symptom with a numerical analog from 0 through 3 as follows:

0: symptom is not present,

1: symptom is mild,

2: symptom is moderate,

3: symptom is severe.

There were 21 symptoms considered for this evaluation (see Table 1). The symptom score was obtained by adding the

Diego saporta MD. Allergy symptom assessment Starting date:

Name: DOB AGE SEX

Symptoms	PRE-RX								
Date SLIT/SCIT									
Sneezing									
Runny nose									
Nasal obstruction									
Post nasal drip									
Watery eyes									
Itchy eyes									
Itchy ears									
Itchy nose									
Itchy throat									
Itchy skin									
Hives-rash									
Sorethroat									
Clogged ears									
Facial pain/pressure									
Headaches intensity									
*Headaches frequency									
Dizziness									
Tinnitus (noise in ears)									
Diag ASTHMA Y N									
Cough									
Sensation of tight chest									
Wheezing									
SOB									
Exercise-cough									
Exercise-SOB									
Exercise-wheezing									
*Wake at night w/symptom									
*Bronchodilators(Pro/Max Albut/Xopen/Prove/Vent/Alup)									
Last time used									
*ICS (advair//pulmic/asmanex)									
*Allergy pills									
*Intranasal sprays									
Fatigue									
Poor sleep									
Snoring									
Difficulty concentrating									
Problems/complications									
FEV 1									
PFM									
SNR									

Symptoms:
0: Never,
1: Mild,
2: Moderate,
3: Severe;

Frequency (*):
0: Never,
1: 1 time/wk (or less),
2: 2-3 times per week,
3: 4 or more per week.

FIGURE 1

values of each symptom (0–3) in each patient; the maximum total symptom score was 63. The total number of symptoms also was considered for monitoring clinical response.

When considering clinical response to immunotherapy, the use of medications is monitored as well. Patients that do not exhibit a decrease in medication use with the administration of immunotherapy are reassessed. For this evaluation we considered use of allergy pills (antihistamines or leukotriene receptor antagonists), intranasal topical steroids, and short acting bronchoagonists. No patient in this study was on oral or systemic steroids or decongestants.

For evaluation of medication use we use a similar numerical scale as follows:

0: medication is not being used,

1: medication is being used once a week or less,

2: medication is being used 2 to 3 times per week,

3: medication is being used 4 or more times per week.

The maximum total medication score was 9 and the maximum total number of medications was 3. When immunotherapy is successful, medication use will decrease regardless of the type of medication. In the asthmatic patient, asthma inhalers will be used less frequently or even discontinued entirely in the more successful outcomes.

The value of the PFM determination is used as the parameter to be recorded during each patient's visit.

The sample included adults and children with or without asthma treated with subcutaneous injection immunotherapy (SCIT) or sublingual immunotherapy (SLIT). Antigens were mixed according to results of an intradermal dilutional test. The data presented here was not analyzed according to test results. Patients on SCIT were treated according to American Academy of Otolaryngic Allergy (AAOA) guidelines [19]. Patients on SLIT were treated according to a previously published protocol [20]. The formulation of both injectable and oral allergy-vaccines was the same; based on allergy test results, all positive allergens were included in the treatment mixture.

Asthma symptoms considered included cough, sensation of tight chest, wheezing, shortness of breath (SOB), exercise-induced symptoms (cough, SOB, wheezing), or waking up at night with any of those symptoms. Presence of asthma symptoms in patients who considered themselves "nonasthmatic" was also analyzed.

Sixty charts that met inclusion conditions were identified. They were analyzed using the same criteria regardless if patients were treated with SCIT or SLIT. For each patient we evaluated total symptoms score, total number of symptoms, medication score, total number of medications used, and the PF value, which was obtained before treatment initiation and at least once more at the time of data collection.

The changes of the above parameters during the administration of immunotherapy were evaluated. In determining the results between two or more groups of patients, an ANOVA (Analysis of Variance) was performed using the PF performance as the dependent variable. When determining significance between continuous variables, a bivariate correlation analysis was performed.

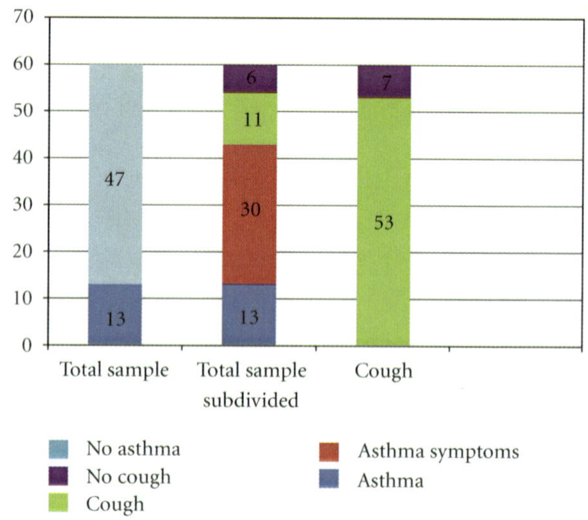

FIGURE 2: Total sample and subgroups. *Total sample*: 60 subjects, 13 report asthma, 47 do not. *Total sample subdivided*: 13 report asthma, Remainder 47: 30 have cough and other asthma symptoms, 11 have cough only, and 6 have no cough or other asthma symptoms. *Cough*: 53/60 subjects had cough.

3. Results

3.1. Demographics. The total sample included 60 subjects, ages 4 through 75 (mean 41.1 ± 17.5). Mean length of treatment was 22.9 ± 13.1 months. In 42 of 60 patients (70%), treatment extended for more than 12 months.

3.2. Asthma. A diagnosis of asthma was self-reported by 13 subjects (21% of the total sample), and only 1 of these subjects did not report cough as one of the symptoms. The remaining 47 subjects denied having asthma, although 30 reported asthma symptoms (30/47 = 63.8%) (see Figure 2).

The group of 47 patients that did not report asthma were divided into three subgroups (see Figure 2):

(a) patients with cough and other asthma symptoms: 30,

(b) patients with cough but no other asthma symptoms: 11,

(c) patients without cough (and no other asthma symptoms): 6.

3.3. Cough. Cough was reported by 53 out of 60 patients in this sample (88%). Eleven out of these 53 (subgroup b) had no other symptoms suggestive of lower airway inflammation. While it can be assumed that a patient with cough and other symptoms of lower airway inflammation has asthma, a patient with cough and no other symptoms is a different situation. Even though it is proven that cough can be the only symptom a patient with asthma may present, no further conclusions can be made without information on spirometric results or response to bronchodilator and/or anti-inflammatory therapy (see Figure 2).

Because all the information in this report comes from the symptom scoring sheet and not from office notes, we

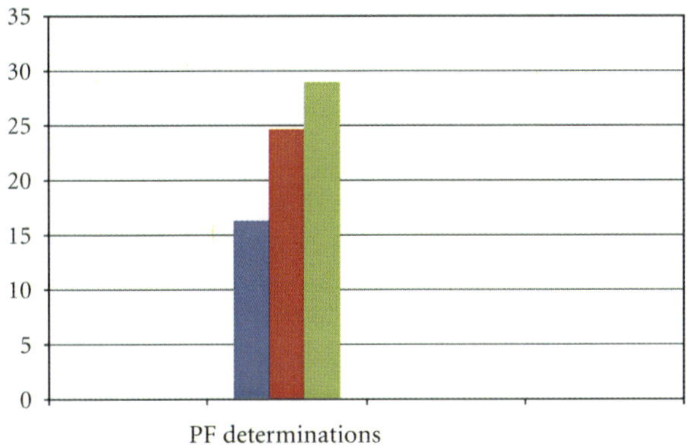

Figure 3: Percentage of PF value change in relation to the number of PF determinations. 2PF: two PF determinations. 3PF: three PF determinations. 4+PF: four or more PF determinations. The number of PF measurements is positively associated with the percentage of PF change ($r = 0.357$, $P < 0.01$).

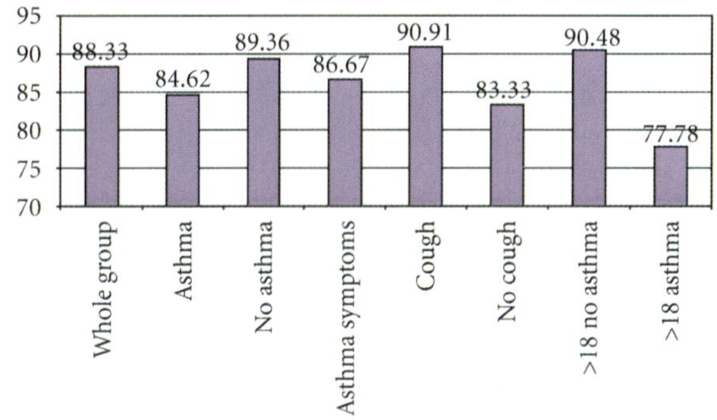

Figure 4: Number of subjects that had improved PF values in different groups. Whole group: 53/60; Asthma: Self-reported asthma patients: 11/13; No asthma: Patients that denied asthma: 42/47; Asthma Symptoms: Patients that denied asthma but had asthma symptoms: 26/30; Cough: Patients that denied asthma and had cough but no other asthma symptoms: 10/11; No cough: Patients that denied asthma and had NO cough and NO other asthma symptoms: 5/6. ANOVA showed no significant difference in average percentage of PF change of the aforementioned groups ($F = 0.975$, $P =$ N/S). >18 No Asthma: Patients older than 18 years of age that did not report asthma: 38/42. >18 Asthma: Patients older than 18 years of age that reported asthma: 7/9.

decided to consider the group "cough but no other asthma symptoms" as a separate group (see Discussion).

Adding the number of patients with asthma to the number of patients with cough and other asthma symptoms (13 + 30 = 43) suggests that 72% (43/60 = 71.6%) of the patients in a group of nonselected allergy patients are indeed asthmatic, and this is, at best, a conservative number as some of patients with "cough only" could also be asthmatic.

3.4. PF Changes. Average PF change for all 60 patients during immunotherapy increased from 376.23 (±115.01) at the beginning of treatment to 472.65 (±127.47) at the time of data collection for an overall improvement of 25.63%. From the total sample, 53 out of the 60 subjects (88.33%) showed an improvement in PF value, 4 had a worsening of PF value, and 3 had no change. Of the 53 subjects that showed an improvement in PF value, 48 had a decrease in symptoms score and number of symptoms. Therefore a PF increase has a predictor value of 90.57% for clinical improvement of the patient.

While an increase in the PF value is strongly associated with a symptomatic improvement (48/53), a decrease in the PF value is not necessarily associated with clinical worsening: of the 4 subjects with a worse PF value, all still had a decreased symptom score and 3 had a decrease in the number of symptoms. Of the 3 subjects with no change in the PF value, 2 got better (decrease in symptoms scores and number of symptoms) and 1 got worse.

3.5. PF Changes in Relation to the Number of Measurements. In 11 patients there were 2 PF value measurements, one at the beginning of the treatment and the second one at the time of data collection (see Figure 3). Average PF change during immunotherapy for these patients ranged from 390.00 (±115.84) to 453.55 (±161.36), for an overall improvement of 16.29%.

In 13 patients there were 3 PF value measurements. Average PF change during immunotherapy for these patients ranged from 368.46 (±109.76) to 459.23 (±103.23), for an overall improvement of 24.63%.

In 36 patients there were 4 or more PF value measurements. Average PF change during immunotherapy for these patients spanned from 374.83 (±119.37) to 483.33 (±126.49), for an overall improvement of 28.95%.

A bivariate correlation analysis showed that the number of PF measurements is positively associated with the percentage of PF change ($r = 0.357$, $P < 0.01$). Therefore when more PF measurements are obtained, it is more likely to obtain a greater improvement in the PF value.

3.6. PF Value in Relation to Length of Treatment. There is a positive correlation between the change in the PF value and the number of months that the patient was treated ($r = 0.253$, $P < 0.05$). In other words, the longer a patient receives immunotherapy the more likely the PF value will increase.

3.7. PF Changes in Different Groups. PF changes were evaluated in patients that reported asthma and in the subgroups of the patients that did not report asthma (see Figure 4).

Patients That Reported Asthma. In the 13 patients who self-reported having asthma, the average PF value increased from 315.69 (±124.85) to 385.38 (±85.40), for an overall improvement of 18.08%. Eleven out of the 13 patients had an improvement in the PF value (84.62%). Two got worse (15.38%).

Patients That Did Not Report Asthma. In the group of 47 patients that did not report asthma, 42 (89.36%) had an improvement in the PF value, 3 did not improve (6.38%), and 2 decreased (4.26%). This group of 47 patients can be divided in 3 subgroups.

(a) For the thirty patients that did not report asthma but had asthma symptoms, the average PF value increased from 398.33 (±114.11) to 492.30 (±139.40), for an overall improvement of 23.59%. Twenty-six out of the 30 patients had an improvement in the PF value (86.67%). Three patients did not show any improvement (10.00%), and 1 got worse (3.33%).

(b) For the eleven patients that had cough but no other symptoms suggestive of lower airway inflammation, the average PF value increased from 376.36 (±109.39) to 510.91 (±105.49), for an overall improvement of 35.75%. Ten out of the 11 patients had an improvement in the PF value (90.91%). In 1 patient the PF value decreased (9.09%).

(c) For the six patients that had no cough or any other symptom suggestive of lower airway inflammation, the average PF value increased from 396.67 (±79.16) to 493.33 (±115.87) for an overall improvement of 24.37%. Five out of 6 patients had an improvement in the PF value (83.33%). In 1 patient the PF value decreased (16.67%).

An ANOVA showed that there is no significant difference among the average percentage of PF change of the aforementioned groups ($F = 0.975$, $P =$ N/S).

3.8. Age. Because children can grow during a multiyear treatment (e.g., children between 3 and 13 years of age grow approximately 2 inches per year, and 2 inches can determine an increase of 15 to 25 points in PF value depending on the patient's sex), the same calculations were done excluding patients younger than 18 years of age. There were 51 patients older than 18 years of age.

The average PF value in these 51 patients (see Figure 4) changed from 395.76 (±110.01) to 495.49 (±120.97), for an overall improvement of 25.20%. In this group there were 9 patients (17.65%) that reported asthma and 42 patients (82.35%) that did not report asthma.

In the 42 patients that did not report asthma the PF value improved from 404.29 (±106.84) to 515.48 (±118.02), for an overall improvement of 27.50%. Thirty-eight out of the 42 showed an improvement in PF value (90.48%). The PF value did not change in 2 patients (4.76%) and decreased in 2 others (4.76%).

In the 9 patients that reported asthma, the PF value improved from 356.00 (±122.38) to 402.22 (±90.52), for an overall improvement of 12.98%. In 7 out of the 9 patients the PF value showed an improvement (77.78%). The PF value decreased in 2 (22.22%).

3.9. Pattern of PF Change. It was observed that patients could be divided into 2 groups according to the way the PF value changed during the administration of immunotherapy: in the first group the PF determination increased each time it was obtained, and in the second group the PF value fluctuated during the course of immunotherapy even though the value at the time of data collection was generally higher than the initial value.

Thirty-six patients (36/60: 60%) belonged to the first group (sustained improvement), and twenty-one patients (21/60: 35%) belonged to the second group (PF value cycled up and down). Three patients did not have any changes in the PF value (3/60: 5%).

In the first group 35 out of 36 patients (97%) had a decrease in the symptoms score, and 34 out of 36 patients (94%) had a decrease in the number of symptoms (coincident with an increase in the PF value).

For patients that consistently improved (35 of 60), the difference in symptom scores for those that had 5 or more PF value measurements was statistically higher than that for those that had fewer than 5 determinations ($F = 5.02$, $P < 0.05$). Number of symptoms also exhibited a similar pattern when comparing the same 2 groups ($F = 6.42$, $P < 0.05$).

4. Discussion

Patients with symptoms suggestive of lower airway inflammation may not consider themselves as asthmatic, but it is likely they are. A patient that only exhibits cough could be asthmatic, but unless an improvement in spirometric values after administration of bronchodilators is demonstrated or symptom improvement occurs after administration of asthma drugs, it is not possible to establish that patient as asthmatic.

Our sample consisted of 60 patients with allergies that were not screened for the presence of asthma. Of those patients, 13 self-reported having asthma and 30 reported experiencing asthma symptoms but did not report asthma, meaning that an impressive 71.67% of our sample potentially could be asthmatic. If the patients with cough but no other asthma symptoms were also considered, then this percentage could be even higher. If this finding is extrapolated to all allergy sufferers, it can then be assumed that the majority of allergy sufferers consulting an allergy practice might be asthmatic. It is clear that asking a patient if he/she is asthmatic is not sufficient; rather the presence of each symptom of asthma needs to be addressed. Patients with asthma are often at higher risk for severe reactions not only during the administration of immunotherapy [21, 22] but also during testing, and these patients should be considered more sensitive [23]. Fatalities from immunotherapy, although rare, are more common in asthmatics [24, 25]. Given all this, it is important to establish if an allergy patient is asthmatic or not, as a diagnosis of asthma affects quality of life as well as morbidity, and it can also potentially impact the life expectancy of that patient.

There is a tendency to consider asthma and allergic rhinitis (AR) as two separate entities, but there is strong evidence that this is not so. The term rhinobronchitis has been proposed to help recognize the concept of chronic inflammation throughout the entire airway in the patient with concurrent allergic rhinitis and asthma [26]. Up to 19% of hay fever sufferers develop asthma later in life [27]. Nasal challenge with environmental stimuli (such as cold air) leads to bronchoconstriction [26, 28]. Some AR patients with no perceived asthma develop bronchial hyperreactivity during AR exacerbation [26]. All this data supports the concept that the upper and lower airways are a unique entity impacted by a common, evolving inflammatory process. Therefore from an immunotherapeutic point of view, AR and asthma should be considered a single entity [29], and the results reported here support the concept of the Unified Airway [30]. If the allergic reaction influences the whole body, it is only logical that the bronchi will be involved in the widespread inflammation that affects the allergy sufferer.

There were 6 patients in the sample of 60 that were definitely not asthmatic. In these patients the average PF value improved 24.37%, and the PF value increased in 5 of 6 cases (83.33%). Both of these figures are in range with the other groups, which supports the idea that even nonasthmatic patients with nasal allergies still have lower airway inflammation. This explains why, even when a patient reports no asthma symptoms, the pulmonary function as assessed by the PF value improves with treatment. With this in mind, nasal allergies and asthma should be considered a continuum of the same disease that expresses itself differently in each patient; for certain individuals this means that the nose and the eyes will be more affected, and for others it means that the lower respiratory system will be more substantially impacted. However, it is a disease that at all times, even if to a minimal degree, probably involves all the organ systems.

This concept is difficult for patients to accept, and we find that when patients with hyperreactive airway are told they have asthma, the usual response is to deny the possibility. Still this is an important concept when treating patients with immunotherapy, since, as mentioned earlier, asthmatic patients are more likely to experience reactions [21, 22].

These results should contribute to raising awareness that potentially any patient presenting with allergy symptoms could also have lower airway hyperreactivity. As previously stated, the figure of 72% is possibly a conservative estimate; and if patients that had cough but no other asthma symptoms were considered as patients with airway hyperreactivity, the number could be even higher. In other words, in a sample of 60 nonselected allergy patients, it is possible that up to 90% ([13 + 30 + 11]/60) were asthmatic.

Having any symptoms suggestive of lower airway inflammation (and cough is one that is very frequently found) should lead to a work up to rule out the presence of a hyperreactive lower airway. We feel that if this was the case, the frequency of asthma-related diagnoses would markedly increase.

The fact that when more PF measurements are obtained the PF value will be higher could be related to the finding that the longer the number of months the patient is treated with immunotherapy the higher the PF value will be. This suggests that the longer the treatment, the better the results, regardless of the presence of asthma symptoms and age of the patient. In other words it appears that immunotherapy, when successful, leads to improvement of pulmonary function in all patients with allergies.

Immunotherapy is a treatment that can modify the immunological mechanisms that cause allergy symptoms [12]. It is an old treatment modality [31] that is proven to be effective [32–34]. With immunotherapy, it is expected that medication use will decrease, regardless of when the medication was started and which medication was used. When the treatment is fully successful, medications can be stopped. We only analyzed medication use, as the purpose of this study was not to address potential differences in effects of various medications, but to demonstrate that with immunotherapy medication use diminishes.

This is a retrospective study and, as such, it lacks the value of a prospective, randomized study with controls, which is very difficult to perform in private practice settings. The information reported in this study suggests that a PFM device could be useful in monitoring a patient's progress during immunotherapy, as changes in PF value can predict how a patient is doing from a clinical standpoint. The information it provides is available immediately, offering a quick assessment of patient's progress.

When PF value consistently improves, the predictor value of the PF change is very high. However, in a few cases these findings are relative: in some cases we observed that with an unchanged or decreased PF value, a patient can still experience some improvement (decreased symptom/medication score). We also found that with a better PF value, the patient can have clinical worsening (increased symptom/medication score). Overall, it appears that following a patient's PF value during immunotherapy is a good indicator of how he/she is responding to the treatment: a decrease in PF value can be used to predict that a patient is not doing well, and an increase in PF value can be used to predict that a patient is doing well, particularly if the increase in PF value is sustained over time.

We hope that this information will serve as a stimulus for authors in research facilities to plan a randomized prospective study with a control group where the usefulness of a PFM can be more properly evaluated.

5. Conclusion

Patients with nasal allergies that deny having asthma often have asthma symptoms. In our study, this occurred in at least 72% of the patients that denied having asthma. Therefore when taking a patient's history, it is critical to ask about the presence of each symptom of asthma, regardless of the patient's perception of asthmatic status.

If it is accepted that the allergic condition affects the whole organism, then it is only logical that the lower airway of an allergy sufferer will be involved. While the degree of involvement varies according to the individual, it appears from this data that the proportion of individuals with affectation of the lower airway is staggering. Perhaps then it is time to reassess the definition of asthma. A "looser" term such as lower airway inflammation or airway hyperreactivity would be more inclusive of all patients with asthma symptoms. Even the term rhinobronchitis [26] should be considered, as patients often reject the label of asthmatic. Regardless, it appears that lower airway inflammation is common and treatment of this inflammation either by anti-inflammatory inhaled corticosteroids, immunotherapy, or detoxifying interventions [35] could not only treat the present condition but perhaps, more importantly, prevent the development of irreversible lower airway remodeling.

Change in PF value can give a rapid assessment of how a patient is responding to treatment. When PF value increases, it is likely that a patient will improve in the majority of cases. In cases where the PF value is better in each determination, the PF has a 94% to 97% predictor value that the patient is doing well.

When PF value improves during the administration of immunotherapy, these changes are independent of asthmatic condition, the presence of any or no asthma symptoms, or the patient's age. Only length of treatment and number of PF measurements are related to an improved PF value.

Acknowledgment

The statistical analyses were performed by Y. M. Samra, Ph.D. Dr. Samra is a member of the faculty at Manhattan College where he teaches operations management and strategic management.

References

[1] J. H. Krouse, "Seasonal and perennial rhinitis," in *Allergy and Immunology. An Otolaryngic Approach*, Williams & Wilkins, Philadelphia, Pa, USA, 2002.

[2] C. E. Baena-Cagnani and P. Patel, "Efficacy and long-term safety of mometasone furoate nasal spray in children with perennial allergic rhinitis," *Current Medical Research and Opinion*, vol. 26, no. 9, pp. 2047–2055, 2010.

[3] "Expert Panel Report 3: Guidelines for the Diagnosis and Management of Asthma," http://www.nhlbi.nih.gov/guidelines/asthma/asthgdln.pdf, Full Report 2007.

[4] E. Boyd, "Patient history," in *Allergy and Immunology. An Otolaryngic Approach*, Williams & Wilkins, Philadelphia, Pa, USA, 2002.

[5] D. E. Stull, E. O. Meltzer, J. H. Krouse et al., "The congestion quantifier five-item test for nasal congestion: refinement of the congestion quantifier seven-item test," *American Journal of Rhinology and Allergy*, vol. 24, no. 1, pp. 34–38, 2010.

[6] J. P. Corey, S. M. Houser, and B. A. Ng, "Nasal congestion: a review of its etiology, evaluation, and treatment," *Ear, Nose and Throat Journal*, vol. 79, no. 9, pp. 690–693, 2000.

[7] R. J. Soose, "Role of allergy in sleep-disordered breathing," *Otolaryngologic Clinics of North America*, vol. 44, no. 3, pp. 625–635, 2011.

[8] S. Tregear, J. Reston, K. Schoelles, and B. Phillips, "Obstructive sleep apnea and risk of motor vehicle crash: systematic review and meta-analysis," *Journal of Clinical Sleep Medicine*, vol. 5, no. 6, pp. 573–581, 2009.

[9] G. C. Gauchard, J. M. Mur, C. Touron et al., "Determinants of accident proneness: a case-control study in railway workers," *Occupational Medicine*, vol. 56, no. 3, pp. 187–190, 2006.

[10] T. Verse and W. Pirsig, "Impact of impaired nasal breathing on sleep-disordered breathing," *Sleep and Breathing*, vol. 7, no. 2, pp. 63–76, 2003.

[11] J. C. Posnick and N. Agnihotri, "Consequences and management of nasal airway obstruction in the dentofacial deformity patient," *Current Opinion in Otolaryngology and Head and Neck Surgery*, vol. 18, no. 4, pp. 323–331, 2010.

[12] H. S. Nelson, "Allergen immunotherapy: where is it now?" *Journal of Allergy and Clinical Immunology*, vol. 119, no. 4, pp. 769–777, 2007.

[13] M. Akdis and C. A. Akdis, "Mechanisms of allergen-specific immunotherapy," *Journal of Allergy and Clinical Immunology*, vol. 119, no. 4, pp. 780–789, 2007.

[14] R. C. Haydon and B. R. Gordon, "Aeroallergen immunotherapy," in *Allergy and Immunology. An Otolaryngic Approach*, Williams & Wilkins, Philadelphia, Pa, USA, 2002.

[15] E. F. Juniper, G. H. Guyatt, R. S. Epstein, P. J. Ferrie, R. Jaeschke, and T. K. Hiller, "Evaluation of impairment of health related quality of life in asthma: development of a questionnaire for use in clinical trials," *Thorax*, vol. 47, no. 2, pp. 76–83, 1992.

[16] M. A. Pynnonen, H. M. Kim, and J. E. Terrell, "Validation of the sino-nasal outcome test 20 (SNOT-20) domains in nonsurgical patients," *American Journal of Rhinology and Allergy*, vol. 23, no. 1, pp. 40–45, 2009.

[17] W. R. Fell, R. L. Mabry, and C. S. Mabry, "Quality of life analysis of patients undergoing immunotherapy for allergic rhinitis," *Ear, Nose and Throat Journal*, vol. 76, no. 8, pp. 528–536, 1997.

[18] G. Ciprandi, C. Klersy, I. Cirillo, and G. L. Marseglia, "Quality of life in allergic rhinitis: relationship with clinical, immunological, and functional aspects," *Clinical and Experimental Allergy*, vol. 37, no. 10, pp. 1528–1535, 2007.

[19] R. C. Haydon and B. R. Gordon, "Aeroallergen immunotherapy," in *Allergy and Immunology, an Otolaryngic Approach*, J. H. Krouse, S. J. Chadwick, B. R. Gordon, and M. J. Derebery, Eds., pp. 151–182, Williams & Wilkins, Philadelphia, Pa, USA, 2002.

[20] D. Saporta and A. B. McDaniel, "Efficacy comparison of multiple-antigen subcutaneous injection immunotherapy and multiple-antigen sublingual immunotherapy," *Ear, Nose and Throat Journal*, vol. 86, no. 8, pp. 493–497, 2007.

[21] W. E. Davis, P. R. Cook, M. S. McKinsey, and J. R. Templer, "Anaphylaxis in immunotherapy," *Otolaryngology: Head and Neck Surgery*, vol. 107, no. 1, pp. 78–83, 1992.

[22] A. T. Borchers, C. L. Keen, and M. E. Gershwin, "Fatalities following allergen immunotherapy," *Clinical Reviews in Allergy and Immunology*, vol. 27, no. 2, pp. 147–158, 2004.

[23] B. R. Gordon, "Prevention and management of office allergy emergencies," *Otolaryngologic Clinics of North America*, vol. 25, no. 1, pp. 119–134, 1992.

[24] R. F. Lockey, L. M. Benedict, P. C. Turkeltaub, and S. C. Bukantz, "Fatalities from immunotherapy (IT) and skin testing (ST)," *Journal of Allergy and Clinical Immunology*, vol. 79, no. 4, pp. 660–677, 1987.

[25] D. I. Bernstein, M. Wanner, L. Borish, G. M. Liss, and Immunotherapy Committee, American Academy of Allergy, Asthma and Immunology, "Twelve-year survey of fatal reactions to allergen injections and skin testing: 1990–2001," *Journal of Allergy and Clinical Immunology*, vol. 113, no. 6, pp. 1129–1136, 2004.

[26] F. E. R. Simons, "Allergic rhinobronchitis: the asthma-allergic rhinitis link," *Journal of Allergy and Clinical Immunology*, vol. 104, no. 3 II, pp. 534–540, 1999.

[27] O. Linna, J. Kokkonen, and M. Lukin, "A 10-year prognosis for childhood allergic rhinitis," *Acta Paediatrica*, vol. 81, no. 2, pp. 100–102, 1992.

[28] S. S. Braman, A. A. Barrows, and B. A. DeCotiis, "Airway hyperresponsiveness in allergic rhinitis. A risk factor for asthma," *Chest*, vol. 91, no. 5, pp. 671–674, 1987.

[29] J. Bousquet, P. Demoly, and F. B. Michel, "Specific immunotherapy in rhinitis and asthma," *Annals of Allergy, Asthma and Immunology*, vol. 87, no. 1, pp. 38–42, 2001.

[30] J. H. Krouse, R. W. Brown, S. M. Fineman et al., "Asthma and the unified airway," *Otolaryngology: Head and Neck Surgery*, vol. 136, no. 5, pp. S75–S106, 2007.

[31] C. S. Smith, "Allergen immunotherapy practice parameter update," *The Journal of the Kentucky Medical Association*, vol. 102, no. 2, pp. 53–56, 2004.

[32] L. Cox, "Allergen immunotherapy and asthma: efficacy, safety, and other considerations," *Allergy and Asthma Proceedings*, vol. 29, no. 6, pp. 580–589, 2008.

[33] Joint Task Force on Practice Parameters; American Academy of Allergy, Asthma and Immunology; American College of Allergy, Asthma and Immunology; Joint Council of Allergy, Asthma and Immunology, "Allergen immunotherapy: a practice parameter second update," *Journal of Allergy and Clinical Immunology*, vol. 120, supplement 3, pp. S25–S85, 2007.

[34] J. L. Broek, J. Bousquet, C. E. Baena-Cagnani et al., "Allergic Rhinitis and its Impact on Asthma (ARIA) guidelines: 2010 revision," *Journal of Allergy and Clinical Immunology*, vol. 126, no. 3, pp. 466–476, 2010.

[35] S. J. Genuis, "Sensitivity-related illness: the escalating pandemic of allergy, food intolerance and chemical sensitivity," *Science of the Total Environment*, vol. 408, no. 24, pp. 6047–6061, 2010.

The Prevalence of Very Frequent Physical Fighting among Boys and Girls in 27 Countries and Cities: Regional and Gender Differences

Monica H. Swahn, Lindsay Gressard, Jane B. Palmier, Huang Yao, and Melissa Haberlen

Institute of Public Health, Georgia State University, P.O. Box 3995, Atlanta, GA 30302-3995, USA

Correspondence should be addressed to Monica H. Swahn; mswahn@gsu.edu

Academic Editor: Pam R. Factor-Litvak

Objective. Using nationally representative data, this study examined the prevalence of very frequent physical fighting (≥12 times per year) among youth in 27 countries and cities. Frequent physical fighting has rarely been reported in the previous literature despite the implications for research and practice. *Methods.* Analyses were based on the Global School-based Student Health Survey (2003–2008) and the 2009 US Youth Risk Behavior Survey. Multinomial regression analyses were conducted to determine gender differences in frequent fighting. Countries were categorized into five regions (Sub-Saharan Africa, Central and South America, Asia, Eastern Mediterranean, and the United States), and one-way ANOVA tests were used to determine regional differences. *Results.* The prevalence of frequent fighting was highest in Zambia (7.7%) and lowest in Myanmar (0.5%). Gender differences were found in 20 countries, with boys being more likely to report frequent fighting than girls. The prevalence of frequent fighting varied by region ($F(3, 22) = 4.78$, $P = .01$), with the Eastern Mediterranean having a significantly higher prevalence of frequent fighting than Asia ($P < .01$). *Conclusion.* The prevalence of frequent fighting varies by gender in many countries and varies across world regions. More cross-national research is needed to better understand the sociocultural context of frequent fighting and to inform youth violence prevention efforts.

1. Introduction

Youth violence is a major international public health concern [1, 2]. In nearly every region of the world, adolescents and young adults comprise the majority of violent death victims [3], resulting in significant losses in the world's most productive citizens. Indeed, global surveillance efforts estimate that an average of 565 youth between the ages of 10 and 29 years old are victims of homicide each day, with an additional 20–40 youth violence-related injuries occurring for each homicide [1]. Apart from the potential for death or serious injury, youth experiencing violence, namely, physical fighting, are more likely than their nonviolent counterparts to engage in further risk and violence-related behaviors and to suffer from a myriad of negative physical and emotional health outcomes [1, 4–6]. Considering the magnitude and severity of these consequences, a growing body of the literature has sought to better understand the prevalence and risk factors for youth involvement in physical fighting both in the USA and internationally [1, 2, 7–12]. Most recently, the trends and social correlates of physical fighting among youth in 30 countries were presented [13].

One facet of physical fighting among youth that remains underexamined, however, is the phenomenon of very frequent physical fighting. Although a recent US study indicates that frequent physical fighting (at least 12 times per year) is a relatively rare behavior among high school students, the well-being of those youth engaged in frequent fighting is of concern; adolescents reporting frequent physical fighting are at a heightened risk for suicide and other psychosocial problems when compared to students who engage in less frequent fighting or who do not fight [14]. Furthermore, adolescents who are frequent fighters may be more likely to become chronic offenders, a group that accounts for more than half of all the serious crimes committed by juveniles in the USA [15]. Stark gender differences in the prevalence of frequent fighting are also of note. Among US youth, 4% of boys versus 1% of girls report frequent physical fighting [14].

Internationally, comparative studies examining the occurrence of physical fighting among youth are nearly absent from the current literature, and even fewer studies have examined frequent fighting, most of which limit analyses to youth in Europe and North America [10, 12, 13]. A lack of nationally representative samples of youth has been particularly problematic in producing cross-national comparisons [10, 13]. Moreover, although some studies have been able to examine cross-national patterns of adolescent physical fighting, especially using the Health Behaviour in School-aged Children Survey (HBSC), the measure of frequent fighting has been restricted by survey designs with a maximum value of "3 or more" [13] or "4 or more" fights per year [10, 12]. Nevertheless, findings from these studies indicate that more frequent fighting is linked to an increased risk for both injury and additional risk behaviors across different countries and regions of the world [10, 12]. Prevention and intervention efforts targeted to this specific population may therefore have the potential to maximize limited resources, particularly in low income countries.

In order to better inform global youth violence prevention efforts, additional research examining the prevalence of frequent fighting is clearly needed, in particular in low and middle income countries. Both nationally representative data and surveys that enable participants to report a greater range of fighting frequency will allow for a more detailed examination of youth violence patterns across countries and world regions. Furthermore, considering the significant gender differences found in the prevalence of frequent fighting among US adolescents [14], the assessment of gender patterns in countries with differing cultural practices and gender norms may be particularly informative. Accordingly, the current study seeks to determine the prevalence of very frequent physical fighting (at least 12 times per year) among boys and girls in 27 countries and cities using the Global School-based Student Health Survey [16, 17] and the US Youth Risk Behavior Study [18]. The study will also examine the regional differences by categorizing the countries and cities into five world regions: Sub-Saharan Africa, Central and South America, Asia, Eastern Mediterranean, and the United States (data were not available from Europe). A better understanding of frequent fighting from large, representative cross-national comparisons will inform the development of violence prevention strategies and intervention programs.

2. Methods

The current study is based on data from the Global School-based Student Health Survey (GSHS) [16, 17]. The GSHS was developed and supported by the World Health Organization in collaboration with the United Nations Children's Fund, the United Nations Educational, Scientific, and Cultural Organization, the Joint United Nations Programme on HIV/AIDS, and with technical assistance from the Centers for Disease Control and Prevention. The goal of the GSHS is to provide data on health behaviors and relevant risk and protective factors among students across all regions served by the United Nations. Country-specific questionnaires, fact sheets, public-use data files, documentation, and reports are publicly available from the Centers for Disease Control and Prevention and the World Health Organization and have been described in more detail elsewhere [19]. Briefly, the GSHS is comprised of a self-report questionnaire, administered primarily to students aged 13 to 16 years old within the time period of 2003 to 2008. The survey uses a standardized scientific sample selection process, common school-based methodology, and a combination of core questionnaire modules, core-expanded questions, and country-specific questions.

This study conducted secondary analyses of the publicly available data files for 25 countries and 2 cities (see Table 1 for list). The 25 countries were selected because a complete nationally representative data file was publicly available. Two cities (Beijing, China and Dar es Salam, Tanzania) were also included to expand the regional comparisons. All selected countries and cities used a two-stage cluster sample design. The first stage selected schools with probability proportional to enrollment size, and the second stage randomly selected classrooms in participating schools. All students in selected classrooms were eligible to participate in the survey. The number of study participants and response rates for each country and the two cities are provided in Table 1.

As a means of comparison, this study also included information from the biannual, nationally representative Youth Risk Behavior Survey (YRBS) of high school students in the United States [18]. For this study, data from the 2009 YRBS ($N = 16,410$) were analyzed. The US high school students voluntarily completed the anonymous, self-administered questionnaire in school following local parental permission procedures. All 9th through 12th grades students in public, Catholic, or other private schools in the 50 states and District of Columbia were included in the sampling frame [20]. Approval to conduct these analyses was obtained from the Georgia State University Institutional Review Board.

The measure of very frequent fighting was based on one survey question which asked students to report the number of times they had been involved in a physical fight during the past 12 months. Question wording in the GSHS and YRBS was equivalent. Response options reflected 8 levels ranging from 0 times to 12 or more times. To measure the prevalence of "any fighting," the variable was coded dichotomously to indicate either no physical fights or one or more physical fights. To measure "very frequent physical fighting," the variable was coded again to indicate no physical fights, 1–11 physical fights, or 12 or more fights. Multinomial regression analyses were conducted to determine gender differences in the frequency of fighting across the selected countries and cities, with girls used as the reference group.

To facilitate regional comparisons, the 27 countries and cities were divided into five world regions: Sub-Saharan Africa, Central and South America, Asia, Eastern Mediterranean, and the USA. Table 1 outlines the countries and cities that are included within each region and an overview of the sample characteristics. Although Trinidad and Tobago is considered to be within the continent of North America, it was included in the Central and South America region for

TABLE 1: Characteristics of Global School-based Student Health Surveys for selected countries and the US 2009 Youth Risk Behavior Survey.

Country	Year	Total sample	Type of representation	School response Rate	Student response rate	Participation rate	Boys (Wtd.%)	Girls (Wtd.%)
				Sub-Saharan Africa				
Botswana	2005	2,197	National	100%	95%	95%	45.0%	55.0%
Ghana	2007	6,236	National	97%	86%	83%	53.4%	46.6%
Kenya	2003	3,691	National	96%	87%	84%	48.7%	51.3%
Namibia	2004	6,367	National	95%	86%	82%	45.2%	54.8%
Swaziland	2003	7,341	National	97%	99%	96%	36.2%	63.8%
Uganda	2003	3,215	National	90%	76%	69%	51.2%	48.8%
Tanzania	2006	2,176	Dar Es Salaam	100%	87%	87%	47.9%	52.1%
Zambia	2004	2,257	National	94%	75%	70%	48.9%	51.1%
				Central and South America				
Argentina	2007	1,980	National	94%	82%	77%	48.0%	52.0%
Guyana	2004	1,212	National	100%	80%	80%	49.0%	51.0%
Trinidad and Tobago	2007	2,969	National	100%	78%	78%	49.8%	50.2%
Uruguay	2006	3,406	National	95%	75%	71%	45.2%	54.8%
				ASIA				
Indonesia	2007	3,116	National	98%	95%	93%	49.9%	50.1%
Myanmar	2007	2,806	National	100%	95%	95%	50.8%	49.2%
Sri Lanka	2008	2,611	National	100%	89%	89%	50.0%	50.0%
Thailand	2008	2,767	National	100%	93%	93%	48.5%	51.5%
China	2003	2,348	Beijing	100%	99%	99%	50.5%	49.5%
Philippines	2003	7,338	National	99%	85%	84%	43.2%	56.8%
				Eastern Mediterranean				
Egypt	2006	5,349	National	100%	87%	87%	51.9%	48.1%
Djibouti	2007	1,777	National	85%	98%	83%	60.2%	39.8%
Jordan	2004	2,457	National	100%	95%	95%	50.3%	49.7%
Lebanon	2005	5,115	National	92%	96%	88%	47.7%	52.3%
Libyan Arab Jamahiriya	2007	2,242	National	100%	98%	98%	50.1%	49.9%
Morocco	2006	2,670	National	100%	84%	84%	54.7%	45.3%
Oman	2005	2,979	National	100%	97%	97%	52.6%	47.4%
United Arab Emirates	2005	15,790	National	97%	91%	89%	50.0%	50.0%
				United States				
US	2009	16,410	National	81%	88%	71%	47.8%	52.2%

the purposes of this study. One-way ANOVA and Tukey's HSD post hoc testing were then used to determine any significant regional differences in the prevalence of physical fighting and very frequent physical fighting. The USA was omitted from ANOVA and post hoc testing due to the lack of multiple data points in that region.

3. Results

The prevalence of any fighting and very frequent fighting for each country is presented in Table 2. The prevalence of any fighting among students ranged from 15.9% in Myanmar to 57.7% in Djibouti. Similarly, the prevalence of very frequent fighting varied across countries and cities ranging from 0.53% in Myanmar to 7.7% in Zambia. Statistically significant gender differences among students reporting any fighting were observed in 21 countries and 2 cities; no gender differences were found among students in Kenya, Uganda, Zambia, or Philippines (Table 2). Among students, boys were significantly more likely to report very frequent physical fighting than girls in 18 countries and 2 cities. Six countries and one city demonstrated a relatively strong likelihood for very frequent physical fighting among boys versus girls, with odds ratios ranging from 7.56 to 15.60 (Uruguay, Myanmar, Beijing, Jordan, Lebanon, Libya, and Morocco). Three countries (Trinidad and Tobago, United Arab Emirates, and USA) reported moderate odds ratios for boys versus girls, including the USA in which boys were 5.13 times more likely than girls to report engaging in very frequent fighting (95% CI: 3.46–7.60). Several other countries and one city noted significant, but less marked gender differences, with odds ratios ranging from 1.57 to 4.02

TABLE 2: The prevalence of involvement in any and frequent physical fighting overall and by gender across 27 countries and cities.

Country	Prevalence of any fighting %			Prevalence of frequent fighting (>12) %			Multinomial logistic regression analysis of the association between sex and frequent fighting			
							Fought < 12		Fought ≥ 12	
	Overall	Boys	Girls	Overall	Boys	Girls	OR	OR (95% CI)*	OR	OR (95% CI)*
Sub-Saharan Africa										
Botswana	47.17	53.13	41.51	3.74	4.18	3.32	**1.60**	**1.30–1.97**	**1.57**	**1.03–2.39**
Ghana	53.50	52.18	55.01	4.31	4.55	4.04	**0.88**	**0.78–0.99**	1.06	0.78–1.43
Kenya	49.71	52.39	47.15	5.32	6.43	4.25	1.19	0.92–1.53	**1.68**	**1.08–2.61**
Namibia	50.26	55.18	46.19	5.32	6.43	4.40	**1.40**	**1.23–1.59**	**1.75**	**1.32–2.34**
Swaziland	27.99	37.58	22.62	1.65	2.97	0.92	**1.98**	**1.70–2.29**	**4.02**	**2.46–6.55**
Uganda	34.99	37.88	31.94	2.94	3.50	2.36	1.27	0.98–1.65	1.63	0.94–2.81
Tanzania	40.53	45.37	36.65	1.81	2.54	1.21	**1.40**	**1.17–1.68**	**2.43**	**1.09–5.40**
Zambia	51.45	49.28	54.01	7.66	6.29	9.28	0.87	0.64–1.18	0.61	0.37–1.03
Central and South America										
Argentina	31.27	43.83	19.63	2.93	4.36	1.61	**3.13**	**2.36–4.16**	**3.87**	**2.05–7.30**
Guyana	34.14	46.28	22.46	2.58	3.22	1.97	**3.03**	**2.33–3.95**	2.37	0.86–6.50
Trinidad and Tobago	41.84	55.89	27.88	5.81	8.90	2.75	**3.06**	**2.47–3.78**	**5.29**	**3.14–8.92**
Uruguay	31.32	46.09	19.16	2.05	3.70	0.69	**3.44**	**2.76–4.29**	**8.09**	**4.17–15.69**
ASIA										
Indonesia	33.76	46.95	20.63	1.83	2.28	1.39	**3.47**	**2.77–4.34**	**2.46**	**1.19–5.07**
Myanmar	15.86	21.71	9.80	0.53	0.98	0.07	**2.46**	**1.83–3.30**	**15.60**	**1.65–147.93**
Sri Lanka	47.28	60.27	34.34	2.69	3.26	2.12	**2.92**	**2.44–3.50**	**2.54**	**1.52–4.25**
Thailand	33.30	45.61	21.73	2.52	3.36	1.73	**3.04**	**2.41–3.84**	**2.80**	**1.56–5.04**
China	16.59	26.98	5.98	1.93	3.48	0.34	**5.36**	**3.74–7.70**	**13.10**	**4.58–37.47**
Philippines	50.02	51.63	48.80	3.22	3.59	2.94	1.11	0.92–1.34	1.29	0.86–1.95
Eastern Mediterranean										
Egypt	54.78	65.25	43.46	4.58	5.41	3.67	**2.45**	**1.65–3.62**	2.40	0.66–8.72
Djibouti	57.65	63.95	48.08	5.96	7.99	2.87	**1.78**	**1.45–2.19**	**4.01**	**2.56–6.28**
Jordan	45.91	64.09	27.55	5.33	8.39	2.24	**4.44**	**3.32–5.95**	**7.56**	**3.87–14.75**
Lebanon	45.98	64.56	28.99	5.24	8.92	1.87	**4.11**	**3.62–4.67**	**9.54**	**6.79–13.40**
Libyan Arab Jamahiriya	41.54	57.95	25.11	6.11	10.29	1.92	**3.66**	**2.82–4.76**	**9.52**	**5.66–16.03**
Morocco	43.69	62.18	21.31	2.78	4.39	0.82	**5.87**	**4.70–7.34**	**11.12**	**5.31–23.28**
Oman	41.10	45.73	35.97	5.31	5.75	4.83	**1.51**	**1.23–1.87**	1.40	0.91–2.18
United Arab Emirates	43.20	56.93	29.54	5.45	8.25	2.65	**2.96**	**2.64–3.32**	**5.09**	**4.02–6.44**
United States										
USA	31.41	39.26	22.90	2.55	3.99	0.99	**2.04**	**1.84–2.27**	**5.13**	**3.46–7.60**

*The multinomial logistic regression analyses predicted the odds for engaging in frequent and any fighting relative to not fighting, with girls as the reference group.

(Botswana, Kenya, Namibia, Swaziland, Tanzania, Argentina, Indonesia, Sri-Lanka, and Thailand). Seven countries did not demonstrate a significantly higher risk for very frequent fighting among boys versus girls (Ghana, Uganda, Zambia, Guyana, Philippines, Egypt, and Oman).

The distribution of fighting across the regions is presented in Figure 1. These distributions of the prevalence of student involvement in physical fighting by region are based on the number of times students reported fighting in the past year (1, 2-3, 4-5, 6-7, 8-9, 10-11, 12, or more). The mean prevalence of any fighting (one or more times) by region is presented in Figure 2. The Eastern Mediterranean region demonstrated the highest mean prevalence of any fighting (46.7%), while the USA had the lowest prevalence (31.4%). With the USA excluded, one-way ANOVA determined that the prevalence of any fighting varies significantly by region ($F(3, 22) = 3.43$, $P < .05$), however, post hoc testing did not find significant differences between individual regions.

The mean prevalence of very frequent fighting (12 or more times) by region is presented in Figure 3. The Eastern Mediterranean region had the highest mean prevalence of very frequent fighting (5.1%), while the Asian region had

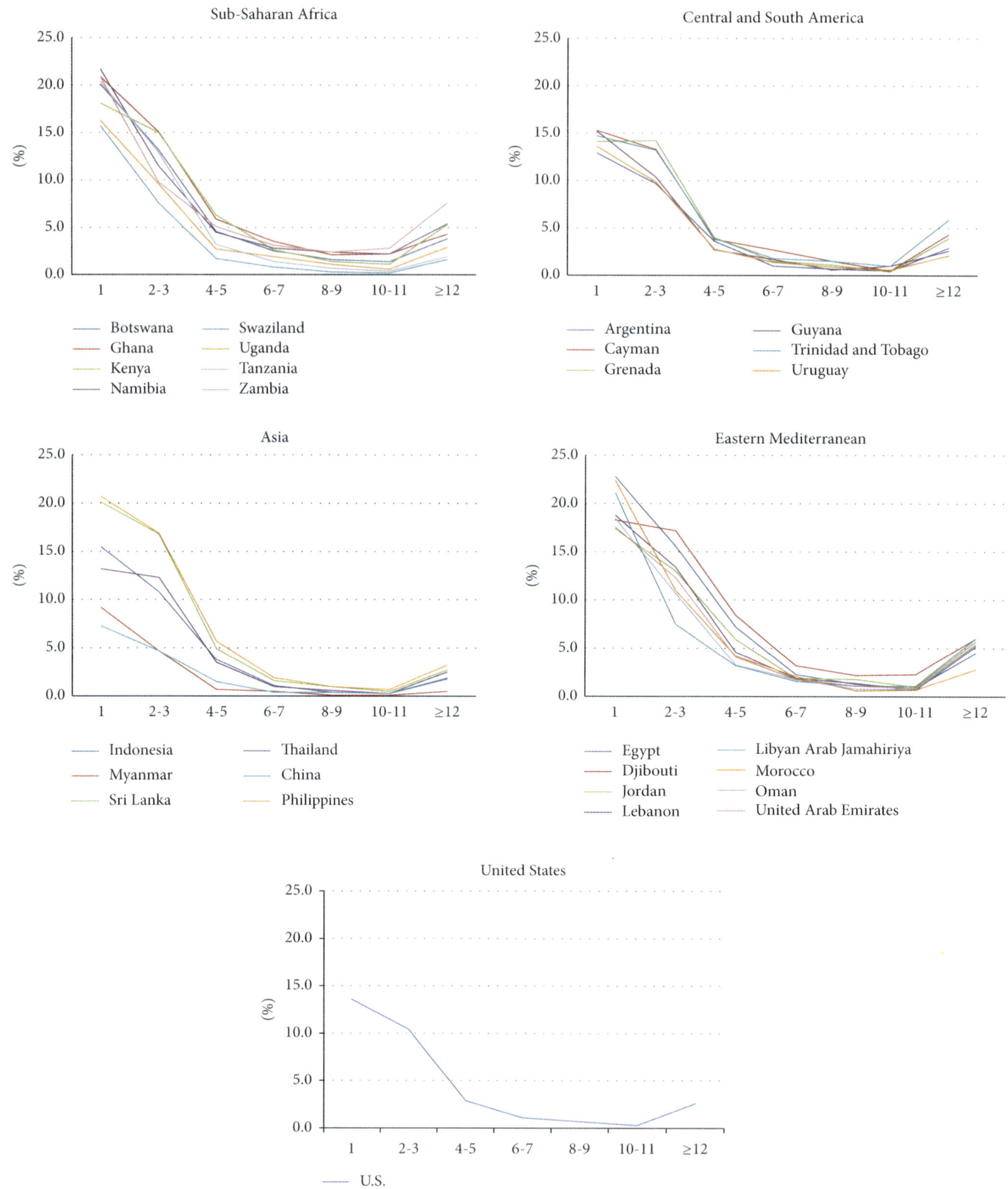

FIGURE 1: Distributions of the prevalence of fighting among students in selected countries, by region.

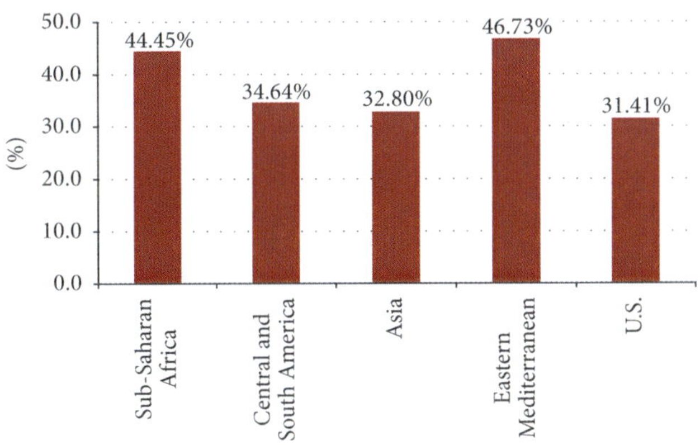

FIGURE 2: The Mean prevalence of any physical fighting (1 or more times) by region, GSHS and YRBS, 2009.

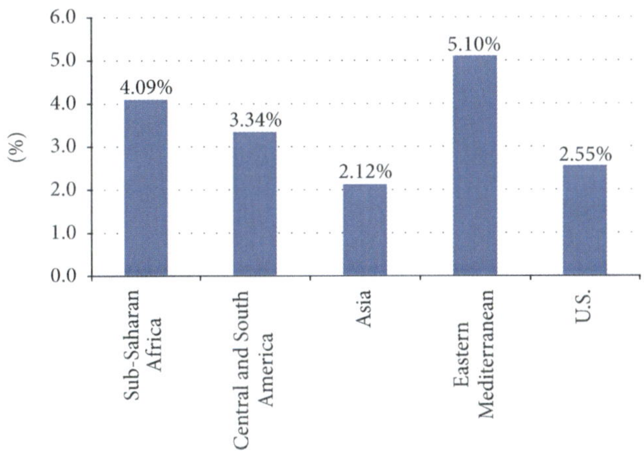

FIGURE 3: The mean prevalence of very frequent physical fighting (12 or more times) by region, GSHS and YRBS, 2009.

the lowest prevalence (2.1%). With the U.S. excluded, one-way ANOVA determined that the prevalence of frequent fighting varies significantly by region ($F(3, 22) = 4.78$, $P = .01$). Tukey's HSD post hoc testing showed that the Eastern Mediterranean region has a significantly higher prevalence of frequent fighting than the Asian region ($P < .01$).

4. Discussion

This study examines cross-national population-based data on the prevalence of very frequent physical fighting across countries and regions of the world. Although involvement in any physical fighting is a common behavior, with over half of students reporting the behavior in some countries, the findings of this study indicate that very frequent physical fighting is a relatively rare behavior. Nevertheless, regional differences in the prevalence of very frequent fighting exist; countries representing the Eastern Mediterranean region exhibit a significantly higher prevalence of very frequent fighting than countries in the Asian region. As Smith-Khuri and Colleagues suggest [12], regional differences in the prevalence of frequent fighting indicate that frequent fighting may not simply be the product of "normal" developmental processes among adolescents. Instead, certain cultural norms and practices may either buffer against or contribute to the occurrence of very frequent fighting. Certain sociopolitical environments, such as political unrest or state of war, may also be a factor [2]. Further research should seek to determine those sociocultural factors that may affect youth reports of very frequent fighting and therefore provide a greater understanding to the associated risk factors. Providing a methodological example, a recent meta-analysis of cross-national research found that several sociocultural factors, such as age structure and income inequality, are significant predictors of criminal behavior, including homicide [21].

Supporting previous research [13, 14], the current study found that, in most countries selected for analyses, very frequent fighting was more likely to be reported by boys than girls. The magnitude of these gender differences, however, differed by country. The potential influence of gender norms on the report of very frequent fighting should thus be explored. Although the relationship context of the fighting reported in this study was not assessed, understanding the contribution of physical dating violence to the prevalence of frequent fighting may offer some important insight into the observed variation in the magnitude of gender differences. Previous cross-national research suggests that girls are particularly likely to fight within the context of intimate relationships, while boys more often fight with strangers [10]. Whether girls living in countries or cultures with stricter dating practices are less involved in frequent fighting may warrant exploration.

An additional aim of future research should be to determine whether higher rates of very frequent fighting among youth are associated with higher injury or death rates among young people in those countries. Previous cross-national research has found that youth reporting fighting four or more times a year are typically two to three times more likely than nonfighters to be hospitalized for an injury [10]. In this same study, the risk for injury among US youth was even greater; frequent fighters were more than 10 times likely than nonfighters to be hospitalized. While differences in health care access may be a factor, these findings suggest that cultural norms and practices may not only influence the frequency of fighting, but perhaps the severity of fighting or use of lethal weapons as well.

Interpretation of the findings in this report is subject to several limitations. First, all participants were school-attending youth, and as such, the findings may not reflect the experiences of youth who have dropped out of school or may not be able to attend school. Findings from a US study indicate that school attendance may be a protective factor for involvement in violence for both male and female students, thereby indicating a potential for underreporting of violent behaviors among school-attending youth [22]. The status of school attendance as a financial privilege in some countries may further affect these findings. Second, involvement in physical fighting may be considered a socially undesirable behavior, for girls in particular, thus potentially affecting the validity of self-report data. Third, the GSHS uses a single survey item to assess the frequency of physical fighting and, as such, does not assess the context of the fighting. The measure may or may not include incidents of fighting with siblings or other close relatives or friends in which there was no intent to harm. Fourth, comparisons across regions may be biased by the countries selected for inclusion, as well as the year for which data were collected. Lastly, the analyses and comparisons do not consider other demographic characteristics or societal level factors that may be relevant to frequent fighting.

Despite these limitations, the findings of this study maintain important implications for expanding and improving future research on frequent fighting among youth. Of utmost importance is the need to establish uniform guidelines for assessing involvement in frequent fighting that would allow comparisons across populations and countries. Researchers currently use a broad range of classifications to assess frequent fighting (e.g., 4 or more times) [10, 12–14]. Validation studies are thus indicated to determine meaningful fighting frequency benchmarks that are associated with an increased risk for injury or other harmful outcome. Standardization of these benchmarks would aid epidemiologic research that may otherwise examine peer violence as a dichotomized construct, dividing youth into those who report no involvement in fighting versus those who report any involvement in fighting, thus ignoring the characteristics, circumstances, and precursors of frequent fighting. It is clear from this study and previous findings that focusing specifically on frequent fighting may elucidate important patterns and differences that may otherwise be missed when describing youth violence more broadly.

5. Conclusion

Given the variability in the prevalence of frequent fighting across countries and regions in this study, future research should examine the risk factors for fighting from an international and comparative perspective in order to inform prevention strategies that may have broader global relevance. Moreover, given recent cross-national comparisons outlining a decline in fighting across primarily European countries [13], research examining fighting trends in other countries and regions is also needed. Considerable gaps in research regarding the correlates and risk factors of frequent fighting specifically also remain. This study, which employed cross-sectional analyses of recent population-based surveillance data to understand the current prevalence and context of frequent fighting, provides insight for addressing these gaps. Furthermore, this study provides a starting point for further research to determine whether youth violence prevention interventions that specifically target frequent fighters present the opportunity for increased impact, particularly in areas with limited resource.

References

[1] United States Department of Health and Human Services, "Youth violence," A Report of the Surgeon General, Centers for Disease Control and Prevention, Substance Abuse and Mental Health Services Administration, National Institute of Mental Health, Rockville, Md, USA, 2001, http://www.surgeongeneral.gov/library/youthviolence/.

[2] World Health Organization, "Youth violence," World Report on Violence and Health, Geneva, Switzerland, 2002, http://www.who.int/violence_injury_prevention/violence/global_campaign/en/chap2.pdf.

[3] A. Reza, J. A. Mercy, and E. Krug, "Epidemiology of violent deaths in the world," *Injury Prevention*, vol. 7, no. 2, pp. 104–111, 2001.

[4] R. Boynton-Jarrett, L. M. Ryan, L. F. Berkman, and R. J. Wright, "Cumulative violence exposure and self-rated health: longitudinal study of adolescents in the United States," *Pediatrics*, vol. 122, no. 5, pp. 961–970, 2008.

[5] D. L. Haynie, R. J. Petts, D. Maimon, and A. R. Piquero, "Exposure to violence in adolescence and precocious role exits," *Journal of Youth and Adolescence*, vol. 38, no. 3, pp. 269–286, 2009.

[6] S. Walsh, M. Molcho, Y. Harel-Fisch et al., "Physical and emotional health problems experienced by youth engaged in violent behaviour," *Injury Prevention*, vol. 16, supplement 1, pp. A64–A64, 2010.

[7] W. Craig, Y. Harel-Fisch, H. Fogel-Grinvald et al., "A cross-national profile of bullying and victimization among adolescents in 40 countries," *International Journal of Public Health*, vol. 54, no. 2, pp. S216–S224, 2009.

[8] Y. Harel-Fisch, S. D. Walsh, H. Fogel-Grinvald et al., "Negative school perceptions and involvement in school bullying: a universal relationship across 40 countries," *Journal of Adolescence*, vol. 34, no. 4, pp. 639–652, 2011.

[9] W. Pickett, H. Schmid, W. F. Boyce et al., "Multiple risk behavior and injury: an international analysis of young people," *Archives of Pediatrics and Adolescent Medicine*, vol. 156, no. 8, pp. 786–793, 2002.

[10] W. Pickett, W. Craig, Y. Harel et al., "Cross-national study of fighting and weapon carrying as determinants of adolescent injury," *Pediatrics*, vol. 116, no. 6, pp. e855–e863, 2005.

[11] W. Pickett, M. Molcho, K. Simpson et al., "Cross national study of injury and social determinants in adolescents," *Injury Prevention*, vol. 11, no. 4, pp. 213–218, 2005.

[12] E. Smith-Khuri, R. Iachan, P. C. Scheidt et al., "A cross-national study of violence-related behaviors in adolescents," *Archives of Pediatrics and Adolescent Medicine*, vol. 158, no. 6, pp. 539–544, 2004.

[13] W. Pickett, M. Molcho, F. J. Elgar et al., "Trends and socioeconomic correlates of adolescent physical fighting in 30 countries," *Pediatrics*, vol. 131, no. 1, pp. e18–e26, 2013.

[14] M. H. Swahn, R. M. Bossarte, J. B. Palmier, H. Yao, and M. H. M. V. Dulmen, "Psychosocial characteristics associated with frequent physical fighting: findings from the 2009 National Youth Risk Behavior Survey," *Injury Prevention*, vol. 19, no. 2, pp. 143–146, 2013.

[15] R. Loeber and D. P. Farrington, Eds., *Serious and Violent Juvenile Offenders: Risk Factors and Successful Interventions*, Sage, Thousand Oaks, Calif, USA, 1999.

[16] Centers for Disease Control and Prevention, "Global School-based Student Health Survey (GSHS)," http://www.cdc.gov/gshs/, 2009.

[17] World Health Organization, "Global School-based Student Health Survey (GSHS)," http://www.who.int/chp/gshs/en/, 2009.

[18] Centers for Disease Control and Prevention, "Youth Risk Behavior Surveillance System (YRBSS): Youth Online," http://apps.nccd.cdc.gov/youthonline/App/Default.aspx, 2009.

[19] World Health Organization, "Global School-based Student Health Survey (GSHS) purpose and methodology," http://www.who.int/chp/gshs/methodology/en/index.html, 2009.

[20] N. D. Brener, L. Kann, S. A. Kinchen et al., "Methodology of the youth risk behavior surveillance system," *Morbidity and Mortality Weekly Report*, vol. 53, no. RR-12, pp. 1–13, 2004.

[21] A. E. Nivette, "Cross-national predictors of crime: a meta-analysis," *Homicide Studies*, vol. 15, no. 2, pp. 103–131, 2011.

[22] J. Blum, M. Ireland, and R. W. Blum, "Gender differences in juvenile violence: a report from Add Health," *Journal of Adolescent Health*, vol. 32, no. 3, pp. 234–240, 2003.

Involuntary and Persistent Environmental Noise Influences Health and Hearing in Beirut, Lebanon

Marjaneh M. Fooladi[1, 2, 3]

[1] *Council for International Exchange of Scholars, A Division of the Institute of International Education, 3007 Tilden Street NW, Suite 5-L, Washington, DC 20008, USA*
[2] *College of Nursing, Florida State University, Vivian M. Duxbury Hall, 98 Varsity Way, P.O. Box 3064310, Tallahassee, FL 32306-4310, USA*
[3] *School of Nursing, American University of Beirut, P.O. Box 11-0236, Riad El Solh, Beirut 1107 2020, Lebanon*

Correspondence should be addressed to Marjaneh M. Fooladi, fooladi@hotmail.com

Academic Editor: Mohammad Mehdi Amin

Objective. This study was conducted to assess the effects of involuntary and persistent noise exposure on health and hearing among Lebanese adults in Beirut, Lebanon, where people are exposed to noise from construction sites, power generators, honking cars, and motorcycles. *Methods.* Using a descriptive and exploratory design with mixed methods, participants were surveyed, interviewed, and tested for hearing while street noise levels were measured near their residents and work places. *Results.* Self-reports of 83 Lebanese adult, who lived and worked in Beirut, helped identify common patterns in experiences such as irritability, anger, headaches, and sleep disturbances due to noise annoyance. Of those tested, 30% suffered from high-frequency hearing impairment. Our results showed that environmental sound dB had increased by 12% and sound intensity by 400% above the maximum standard level when compared to the WHO report of 1999. *Conclusion.* Environmental noise contributes to premature hearing loss and potentiates systemic diseases among Lebanese.

1. Introduction

The unrecognized effects of persistent exposure to environmental noise on health and hearing and the unexplored nonspecific responses to noise pollution in Beirut, Lebanon, were the focus of this study. Literature [1] reports have identified excessive external noise and smoking as a major cause of hearing loss and impairment among children and young adults. The nonmodifiable contributing risk factors are listed as age, genetic trends, male gender, and race. Modifiable factors are voluntary exposure to loud music, smoking, sports, diet, dental hygiene, and systemic diseases [1, 2].

The city of Beirut is a metropolitan and multicultural venue with high-rise buildings erected to replace traditional one-family dwelling and occupy a vast portion of the Mediterranean shores in condensed populated areas. The environmental noise associated with ongoing power generators and construction sites begins at dawn and continues through the night as honking cars and motorcycles zigzag through crowded narrow streets. There is no escape from noise since commercial and residential zones are adjacent in close proximity where people live above the shops and businesses. Incessant honking is an expression of frustration when narrow streets are blocked by parked cars on both sides and fruit venders at each intersection.

In a surveyed community response to noise in Beirut, Lebanon [2], participants identified the main sources as motorcycles (70.4%), traffic (63.1%), and car horns (56.3%). Reported construction and generator annoyance were 42% and 55.1%, respectively. This study aims to identify the current level of persistent environmental noise effect on hearing and overall health among Lebanese living and working on Hamra in Beirut, Lebanon.

In a study of 440 local residents of Beirut, ages 21–50, researchers examined the effects of environmental noise and smoking on hearing loss [2]. They divided the participants into 4 groups of smokers and nonsmokers living in noisy (70–90 dBA) and quiet areas (45–55 dBA) and found hearing loss among the smokers when exposed to 8000 Hz at high frequencies and more hearing impairment among smokers above age 40^+. Younger nonsmokers (21–39) showed significant hearing impairment at low frequencies.

Environmental noise and health were found [3] closely related when researchers assesses 105 adults living near Auckland International Airport in New Zealand for noise sensitivity and annoyance for any adverse health effects. They identified that noise contributed to sleep disturbance and reduced health-related quality of life. Similarly, 2,312 people living near Frankfurt Airport [4] were given environmental (EQoL) and health-related (HQoL) quality of life instruments to assess their experiences with aircraft noise annoyance and disturbances to their life quality. Researchers compared their findings from aircraft noise with exposure to road traffic and railway noise, and results suggested a recursive relationship between noise and health.

Numerous empirical studies have identified long-term exposure to noise as a major health concern. Noise from siren or ambulance can generate an immediate protective reaction known as fight or flight. In a substantial review [5] traffic noise effects were found as a source of environmental annoyance. Referencing the Environmental Expert Council (EEC) of Germany, noise was reported as a major source of severe annoyance and distress. The fastest and most urgent signal to noise is mediated by a subcortical area on amygdala. Even during sleep, the environmental noise from airplanes or heavy equipments can generate dangerous brain signals to release stress hormones. The chronic release of stress hormone from long-term exposure to environmental noise increases the endogenous risk factors such as ischemic heart disease and myocardial infarction [5]. Because each individual study on the adverse health effects of noise in most cases does not reach statistical significance, meta-analysis of multiple studies [5] according to EEC shows a consistent trend towards cardiovascular risk when daytime noise level exceeds 65 dB(A). However, the urgent call for public health safety to reduce extra-aural occupational noise remains misclassified and warnings ignored.

Unprotected and regular exposure to occupational loud noise in the daytime interferes with nocturnal sleep patterns. Researchers [6] divided 3 groups of 8 subjects ($n = 24$) and exposed them to continuous noise at >75 dB for 1–2 years, 5–10 years, and over 15 years and matched them with corresponding healthy control groups who worked in a quiet environment. After using PolySomnoGraphy (PSG) for an all-night sleep study, subjects rated their sleep quality on a Visual Analogue Scale (VAS), and the results showed that workers who were exposed to occupational noise had poor quality sleep and over the years adapted to noise. However, the long-term adverse health effects of noise hidden in an adaptive process or subsequent systemic diseases were not investigated. Assessing the sleep quality of air travelers and their exhaustion level after sleeping on flights may better reveal brain responses to unrecognized and constant noise.

According to the 1998 WHO report [7], Lebanon occupies 10, 452 square kilometers (Km^2) of land strip with a population of 4.5 million residents. Over 80% of Lebanese reside in crowded urban areas in high-rise buildings. Researchers [8] have examined the quality of life in high-rise buildings or controlled built environments (CBE) and found them incompatible with the psychological needs of women and children. The recent social architects place multiple families in one high-rise building, and residents exposed to overcrowding, external loud noise from proximate airports or railroads, air pollution, toxins, and malodorous sewer are those experiencing nonspecific stress manifested as irritability and aggression similar to patients in hospitals and convalescent centers or air travelers kept in CBEs such as airports who experience stress.

Farmers using farming equipment are at risk for noise-induced hearing loss [9]. Ninety three industrial farmers between the ages of 18–75 were surveyed after complete health history and demographic data on noise exposure. Their bilateral hearing sensitivity was assessed, using air conduction audiometric testing at 500–800 Hz frequencies. Farmers completed the self-assessment of communication (SAC) hearing handicap scale, and their hearing threshold was less than 25 dB HL. Subjects had high-frequency hearing loss, and those older than age 50 had a higher perceived hearing handicap and damage from external noise. Among other noise-related health effects researchers [10, 11] have identified impaired cognitive abilities as reflects in Table 1, when at various noise levels there is annoyance, speech and sleep interference, reduced work productivity, hearing impairment, and physiological changes [10–13].

Noise at a certain frequency and decibel is detrimental to hearing and according to the United States Environmental Protection Agency (USEPA) and World Health Organization (WHO) (see Table 2) outdoor exposure to the environmental noise should remain within an acceptable range to avoid hearing loss [10–13]. According to the WHO report published by the Lebanese Ministry of Environment, the noise level in Beirut, Lebanon could have adverse health effects on the local residents (see Table 3). The physiological effects of environmental noise have been associated with the endocrine changes [14, 15].

2. Methodology

The purpose of this study was to examine the local perceptions on environmental noise levels and how exposure to involuntary and persistent noise affected young Lebanese health and hearing. To assess street noise level and its health and hearing effects, a cross-sectional design was adopted using mixed methods and the critical theory of participatory action according to Freire [16]. This exploratory and descriptive investigation was focused on individual experiences with persistent noise.

Assured of anonymity and confidentiality participants willingly engaged in informal dialogues and interviews for 30–60 minutes. Interviews took place at various locations including workplace, shops, dormitories, or outdoors. Interviewers helped participants recall and explain past and present experiences with noise at different peak hours and

Table 1: Physiological and psychological effects of noise pollution.

Effect	Comment
Annoyance	Even relatively low levels of noise can cause annoyance and frustration. A tranquil background can make noise more intrusive. Natural sounds are generally less annoying than unnecessary or controllable sound such as car horns. For instance, intermittent sounds such as a tap dripping on a quiet night can be more disturbing than the sound of falling rain.
Speech interference	Noise can interfere with speech. When the background noise level is 50 dBA, normal conversation can be easily carried with someone up to 1 m away. Any more than that, problems will arise.
Sleep interference	Noise can wake people from sleep and keep them awake. Even if not actually woken, a person's sleep pattern can be disturbed, resulting in a reduced feeling of well-being the next day. External noise measuring up to 30 dBA in a bedroom is appropriate for sleep.
Decreasedwork performance	Noise pollution can make people nervous. Accordingly, it can prevent people from concentrating on their work. As noise levels increase, ability to concentrate and work efficiently and accurately reduces. Louder noise bursts can be more disruptive. Noise is more likely to reduce the accuracy of the work than reduce the total quantity of work done. Complex tasks are more likely to be impaired.
Hearing loss	Prolonged exposure to noise levels above 85 dBA can damage inner ear cells and lead to hearing loss. At first, hearing loss is usually temporary and recovery takes place over a few days. After further exposure, people may not fully recover and develop deafness. The extent of deafness depends on the degree of exposure and individual susceptibility. Even brief exposure to very high levels of 130 dBA or more can cause instant, irreversible hearing damage. Research has shown that noise is one of the leading causes of hearing loss for millions of people with impaired hearing in the United States.
Physiological changes	Noise can change a man's physiological state by speeding up pulse and respiratory rates. There is medical evidence that noise can cause heart attacks in individuals with existing cardiac injury and that continued exposure to loud noises could cause such chronic effects as hypertension or ulcers. According to medical studies, there is an increased risk to the cardiovascular system from a sound pressure level of above 65 dBA.
References	[12–15]

Table 2: Brief USEPA and WHO recommended sound levels for community noise.

Level	Effect	Area
USEPA		
Leq(24) < 70 dB*	Hearing outdoor activity	All outdoor areas including residential zones, farms, and other places where people spend varying amount of time and places in which quiet is the basis for use.
Ldn < 55 dB**	Interference and annoyance	
Leq (24) < 55 dB	Outdoor activity interference and annoyance	Outdoor areas where people spend limited amount of time such as school yards, and playgrounds.**
WHO		
Leq (24) = 55 dB	Serious to moderate annoyance	Outdoor living area
Leq (24) = 70 dB	Hearing impairment	Industrial, commercial shopping, and traffic areas, indoors and outdoors
References		[10–13]

*Level equivalent of sound (Leq) is the energy average noise level (usually A-weighted) integrated over some specified time. Also referred to as Equivalent sound pressure levels.
**Ldn = loudness.

describe how noise influenced their lives and probed for any pattern changes in sleep quality, appetite, and unrecognized stress. This study was initiated in September 2009 and ended in May 2010. Written consent in English and Arabic emphasized no risk for voluntary participation. Basic human rights to freedom were closely observed, and participants were given an opportunity to withdraw from the study at any time.

2.1. Data collection. A multidisciplinary research team of nursing, medicine, and engineering with cultural literacy retrieved ethnographic data according to Spradley [17]. Standard demographic survey questionnaire obtained personal data on education, employment, income, and interviews using open-ended questions focused on past and present health and hearing status and personal approach to stress management. Verbal description and self-report

Table 3: 1999 WHO assessment of community noise problem in greater Beirut area.

Land use	Noise standard dBA	
	Day time*	Evening time**
Commercial, administrative, or downtown	55–65	50–60
Residential/commercial centers on highways	50–60	45–55
City residential areas	45–55	40–50

*7:00 a.m. to 6:00 p.m., **6:00 p.m. to 10:00 p.m.
Lebanese ambient noise limits for intensity in different land use zones [14, 15].

offered valuable personal experiences and concurrently were compared with literature. Recorded and expanded data reached saturation upon two rounds of transcription and were analyzed. Further networking with participants provided sufficient opportunities for clarification. Data were safely stored for future reference.

The initial proposal was aimed to include 100 equally divided men and women, and after randomly approaching residents and shop keepers on Hamra Streets we could only recruit 83 volunteer adult Lebanese (46 men and 37 women). Researcher and two graduate assistants from nursing administered survey questionnaire and interviewed participants for personal experiences with noise. One research assistant from engineering measured street noise levels in areas where participants worked and lived. Research team worked in rotations and frequently compared data to match participants with locations for increased data accuracy. Informal and semistructured interviews using open-ended questions helped retrieve participants' experiences and perceptions with noise to identify their ways of coping or adjusting to environmental noise. Participants were offered a small incentive to compensate for their time and cooperation. Anonymity was assured, and raw data was secured in locked office cabinets.

Demographic data provided age range, the number of years working and/or living on premises, income, and education level. Interviews helped obtain information on health habits such as diet, sleep, and coping techniques. Later, participants were tested for hearing using pure tone screening to determine hearing impairment or loss. The street noise levels were measured at 4 busy intersections near participant's home and workplace using sound level meter (SLM).

Our inclusion criteria consisted of Lebanese men and women between the ages 18–38 who lived and worked on Hamra Street for longer than 6 months. We chose a younger age group to eliminate age-related hearing loss or impairment and health complications associated with advanced age. Because this study was conducted in a metropolitan area and the majority of people in Beirut are trilingual (Arabic, English, and French) we chose to include people with basic language literacy (read and write) and unexposed to voluntary noise such as loud music.

2.2. Findings/Results. Data were analyzed through an immediate debriefing after each interview and compared with field notes and visual clues. Data was reviewed line by line and coded using the four phases of qualitative study by Polit and Hungler [18]. Author's personal experiences with noise annoyance verified published literature to substantiate scientific adequacy and data credibility. Verified data were compiled upon saturation and analysis. The inquiry audit and neutrality were established for dependability and data conformity. Transferability of the framework was unanimous among scholarly colleagues and their personal reflections on noise annoyance.

Researcher and two assistants randomly approached people at various shops, stores, apartment buildings, and dormitories on Hamra Street where residents and shopkeepers often gathered to visit. Consenting participants were later met at a location of their choosing to be surveyed and interviewed. On the same day an appointment was made for each participant to meet individually or as a group for hearing test at the audiology clinic. In three occasions when 4-5 participants were waiting for hearing test, focus group discussion was held ranging from 60–90 minutes to explore more experiences with noise. At other occasions interviews were held at the store, at home, in dormitory, or outdoors.

Standard demographic data revealed an average age of 26.5 for men and 27.3 for women, with mixed educational, income, and employment backgrounds. At interviews participants were asked to elaborate on their daily experiences with environmental noise, and 70% (58) had difficulty sleeping at night, and according to the noise meter results they were exposed to Leq 12 hr >65 dBA. In support of our findings multiple studies [7, 19, 20] have reporting the degree of annoyance, sleep disturbance, and hearing loss related to traffic noise in residential urban communities. Using a questionnaire on the influence of environmental noise on health, researchers [19] sampled 1000 individuals ages 19–80 in a heavy traffic area in Stockholm and found frequent annoyance among 13% of subjects exposed to Leq 24 hr >50 dBA when compared to the 2% who were exposed to <50 dBA. Sleep disturbance were reported by 23% at Leq 24 hr >50 dBA and by 13% exposed to <50 dBA. Habituation to noise has been more related to sleep rather than annoyance. Annoyance and sleep problems were prevalent among those with bedroom windows facing the streets or living in apartments [21].

Most studies on noise report human responses, and few have explored coping with constant noise. Our study focused on finding various forms of coping skills when participants shared experiences with increased craving for sweets 55% (45), caffeine intake 62% (51), and smoking 78% (65). More women 81% (30) in the study reported frustration, anger, and feeling helpless as an aftereffect of persistent noise. Men 93% (43) revealed habituation to noise by unrecognized and later described techniques such as chewing gums or tooth picks, snacking at work, and managing to sleep at night by using other incessant noise such as bathroom fan, radio, and television. Afternoon headaches were common among women 78% (29). The unexpected fear of knowing about hearing status 96% (80) among men and women revealed that majority of participants had suspected some hearing impairment when family members complained about having to speak louder or repeat themselves.

Literature support identifies imbalance in endocrine system linked to emotional disturbance. Researchers [21, 22] remain uncertain about the habituation to stress and posit that repeated exposure to external stimuli can shape adaptive brain plasticity mechanism in response to homotypic challenges when cortical auditory processing areas respond to repeated loud noise.

Study limitations were few including low budget funding, time line for project completion per 10 months Fulbright contract, long delays for obtaining IRB approval to proceed with data collection, and participants who were business owner and could not leave their work to be tested for hearing or feared results.

Participants experienced the physical and emotional effects of persistent noise in form of irritability, anger, nausea, headache, and sleep disturbances. Men 93% (43) mainly reported nervous eating, chewing (gum or tooth picks), and both genders 78% (65) smoked to relieve agitating discomforts (described as auditory disturbance on an aircraft). Participants showed concerns for recent weight gain 51% (42), hypertension 46% (38), and diabetes 54% (45). We assessed participant's hearing, and our measurable indicators and output activities were achieved using audiometer pure tone testing. We found bilateral hearing sensitivity upon assessment by air-conduction audiometric testing at 500–4000 Hz frequencies. Of those tested 40% (33), there were 30% (10) who suffered from asymmetrical high-frequency hearing loss and impairment.

Street noise levels were measured by sound level meter (SLM) near participant's home and workplace at 4 intersections on Hamra and Bliss streets. We selected similar time frames and durations to match the WHO study of 1999 for increased accuracy in comparison. Tabulated and analyzed data showed an increase in environmental noise level between 1999 and 2009. The mean average noise standard dBA by the WHO report during 7 am to 6 pm was 55–65, and in 2010 it was 65–75 with a 12% increase in sound dB and 400% increase in noise intensity (Tables 4 and 5).

Table 4: 2010 assessment of street noise in greater Beirut area.

Land use	Noise standard dBA		
	Morning*	Noon**	Afternoon***
Hamra-1 intersection next to Costa Coffee	65–75	65–75	60–70
Hamra-2 intersection at Red Shoe	65–75	60–70	60–70
Hamra-3 intersection Abou Taleb at Sadat	65–75	60–70	65–75
Bliss—in front of Penrose Gate	60–70	60–70	60–70

*7:00 a.m. to 9 a.m., **12 p.m. to 2 p.m., ***4p.m. to 6 p.m.

Table 5: Lebanese ambient noise limits for intensity in commercial areas.

Comparison	Mean average of noise standard dBA
1999 WHO-Study	55–65*
2010 IFI-Study	62-72* (12% sound dB and 400% increase in noise intensity)

*7:00 a.m. to 6:00 p.m.

3. Discussion

As discovered, Lebanese cope with persistent noise in various forms such as smoking, consuming strong coffee, and sweets. To describe caffeine effects on stress response associated with noise, researchers [22] have reported that high doses of caffeine, a psychoactive substance, can activate hypothalamus-pituitary-adrenal axis (HPA), and low doses of caffeine can restrict some of the stress responses by HPA axis. Also, elevated stress due to loud noise was assessed [23] to find how noise influenced adrenocorticotropic hormone (ACTH) and corticosterone levels in animals with and without caffeine intake. Plasma ACTH and corticosterone levels peaked 30 minutes after exposure to noise and rapidly declined when noise was eliminated. Then low-dose caffeine at 2 mg/kg was injected to find a significant increase in plasma corticosterone and ACTH levels within 30 minutes and return to baseline after 60 minutes. When higher doses of caffeine (30 mg/kg and higher) were injected, the hormone levels increased and lasted for at least 2 hours in response to loud noise.

In this study participants experienced various noise-related physical responses. Researchers [6, 22, 23] showed perceived threat from loud noise on HPA axis and the release of ACTH as corticosterone. Exposure to noise at night in acoustic chambers using various intensities showed elevated plasma ACTH and corticosterone at 85 dBA. Many regions of the brain showed negative response to noise due to audiogenic stress which provoked HPA axis with life-threatening responses.

We found participants expressing rage and frustration by honking and shouting when they could not control noise exposure. Similarly, an investigation [24] of 10 healthy human volunteers who were exposed to loud noise at 100 dB under controllable and uncontrollable conditions on two separate days revealed noteworthy results. Participants self-rated their responses, and both groups reported a higher sense of helplessness, lack of control, tension, stress, unhappiness, anxiety, and depression. There was a greater HPA axis response higher plasma adrenocorticotropic hormone levels and increased levels of sympathetic nervous system electrodermal activity among those exposed to uncontrollable noise [22–24]. Therefore, losing control over aversive stimulus can negatively affect mood and overall health.

This study with literature support highlights many aspects of noise influence on health. The long-term exposure to the environmental noise can pose a threat to health by triggering responses from neuroendocrine and autonomic nervous system.

4. Conclusion

In a nonspecific and unrecognized way, noise can generate an unsettling level of stress with profound influence on general health. Upon our initial approach, Lebanese seemed fully aware and yet resigned toward noise problem. Common thread for adaptation to noise in this study was reported as a series of unhealthy habits and public expression of anger and rage by shouting and honking. Noise and uninvited sounds [25] adversely influence physical and psychological health. Lebanese men and women exposed to chronic noise and tested showed hearing loss at high frequency range, and those who could not attend testing sessions due to long work hours expressed fear of hearing impairment according to family members' complaints for having to speak louder or repeat themselves.

In the United States, nearly 10 million adults and 5.2 million children suffer from irreversible noise-related hearing impairment, and 30 millions are at risk for daily exposure to dangerous levels of noise. The noise-related health effects are often ignored and yet significant such as hypertension, tachycardia and elevated cortisol levels, and stress [9, 12, 24].

Finally, our results showed that environmental sound dB had increased by 12% and sound intensity by 400% above the maximum standard level when compared to the WHO report of 1999 which confirms noise as an increasingly recognized global problem with consequential effects on life quality. This study was an attempt to bring awareness to how noise could affect hearing and over time influence daily behavior leading to systemic diseases. Although this study included seemingly healthy young adults (ages 18–38), we still found them at risk for non-age-related hearing loss. Potential for temporary or permanent loss of hearing among children and young adults warrants greater focus on public education and awareness on noise hazards.

Acknowledgments

This study was funded by an educational grant from Isaam Fares Institute, an entity established to support Public Policy and International Affairs and an affiliate of the American University of Beirut in Lebanon. Credit and gratitude are extended to the research team members Dr. Marc K. Bassim, Co-PI, Faculty of Medicine, Dr. Maya Abou Zeid, Co-PI, Faculty of Transportation Engineering, Mrs. Mary Arevian, Co-PI and our graduate research assistants, Fatima Dirany and Rasha Shehadi in nursing and Sherif Maktabi from Engineering. Our deepest gratitude is offered to Dean H.A.S. Huijer at HSON for her administrative support and encouragements and to Mr. Rami Khuri, Director of the Isaam Fares Institute, and his excellent team.

References

[1] E. El Zir, S. Mansour, P. Salameh, and R. Chahine, "Environmental noise in Beirut, smoking and age are combined risk factors for hearing impairment," *Eastern Mediterranean Health Journal*, vol. 14, no. 4, pp. 888–896, 2008.

[2] S. I. Korfali and M. Massoud, "Assessment of community noise problem in Greater Beirut Area, Lebanon," *Environmental Monitoring and Assessment*, vol. 84, no. 3, pp. 203–218, 2003.

[3] D. Shepherd, D. Welch, K. N. Dirks, and R. Mathews, "Exploring the relationship between noise sensitivity, annoyance and health-related quality of life in a sample of adults exposed to environmental noise," *International Journal of Environmental Research and Public Health*, vol. 7, no. 10, pp. 3579–3594, 2010.

[4] D. Schreckenberg, M. Meis, C. Kahl, C. Peschel, and T. Eikmann, "Aircraft noise and quality of life around frankfurt airport," *International Journal of Environmental Research and Public Health*, vol. 7, no. 9, pp. 3382–3405, 2010.

[5] H. Ising and B. Kruppa, "Health effects caused by noise: evidence in the literature from the past 25 years," *Noise and Health*, vol. 6, no. 22, pp. 5–13, 2004.

[6] B. Gitanjali and R. Dhamodharan, "Effect of occupational noise on the nocturnal sleep architecture of healthy subjects," *Indian Journal of Physiology and Pharmacology*, vol. 48, no. 1, pp. 65–72, 2004.

[7] WHO (World Health Organization), *Averting the Three Outriders of the Transport Apocalypse: Road Accidents, Air and Noise Pollution*, Press Release WHO/57, Geneva, Switzerland, 1998.

[8] G. W. Evans, "The Built Environment and Mental Health," *Journal of Urban Health*, vol. 80, no. 4, pp. 536–555, 2003.

[9] M. Stewart, J. Scherer, and M. E. Lehman, "Perceived effects of high frequency hearing loss in a farming population," *Journal of the American Academy of Audiology*, vol. 14, no. 2, pp. 100–108, 2003.

[10] A. L. Bronzaft, "The effect of a noise abatement program on reading ability," *Journal of Environmental Psychology*, vol. 1, no. 3, pp. 215–222, 1981.

[11] USEPA (United States Environmental Protection Agency), *Noise Effects Handbook*, USEPA, Office of Noise Abatement and Control, EPA 500-9-82-106, 1981.

[12] W. Babish, "Epidemiological studies of cardiovascular effects of noise," in *Advances in Noise, Biological Effects*, D. Prasher and I. Luxon, Eds., vol. 1, pp. 312–327, Whurr Publishers, 1998.

[13] USEPA (United States Environmental Protection Agency), "Information on Levels of Environmental Noise requisite to Protect Public Health and Welfare with an adequate Margin of Safety," EPA/ONAC 550/9-74-004, 1974.

[14] WHO (World Health Organization), *Guidelines for Community Noise*, WHO-Expert Task Force Meeting, London, UK, 1999.

[15] Lebanese MOE (Ministry of Environment), Resolution No. 1/52, Official Gazette issue No. 45, 12/9/1996, 1996.

[16] P. Freire, *Pedagogy of the Oppressed*, M. B. Ramos translation, Continuum, New York, NY, USA, 1999.

[17] J. P. Spradley, *The Ethnographic Interview*, Harcourt Brace Jovanovich College Publishers, Fort Worth, Tex, USA, 1979.

[18] D. F. Polit and B. P. Hungler, *Nursing Research: Principles and Methods*, Lippincott Williams & Wilkins, Philadelphia, Pa, USA, 6th edition, 1999.

[19] G. Bluhm, E. Nordling, and N. Berglind, "Road traffic noise and annoyance—an increasing environmental health problem," *Noise and Health*, vol. 6, no. 24, pp. 43–49, 2004.

[20] E. Daniel, "Noise and hearing loss: a review," *Journal of School Health*, vol. 77, no. 5, pp. 225–231, 2007.
[21] H. E. W. Day, C. V. Masini, and S. Campeau, "Reversible inactivation of the auditory thalamus disrupts HPA axis habituation to repeated loud noise stress exposures," *Brain Research*, vol. 1276, pp. 123–130, 2009.
[22] M. D. Patz, H. E. W. Day, A. Burow, and S. Campeau, "Modulation of the hypothalamo-pituitary-adrenocortical axis by caffeine," *Psychoneuroendocrinology*, vol. 31, no. 4, pp. 493–500, 2006.
[23] A. Burow, H. E. W. Day, and S. Campeau, "A detailed characterization of loud noise stress: intensity analysis of hypothalamo-pituitary-adrenocortical axis and brain activation," *Brain Research*, vol. 1062, no. 1-2, pp. 63–73, 2005.
[24] A. Breier, M. Albus, D. Pickar, T. P. Zahn, O. M. Wolkowitz, and S. M. Paul, "Controllable and uncontrollable stress in humans: alterations in mood and neuroendocrine and psychophysiological function," *American Journal of Psychiatry*, vol. 144, no. 11, pp. 1419–1425, 1987.
[25] M. D. Seidman and R. T. Standring, "Noise and quality of life," *International Journal of Environmental Research and Public Health*, vol. 7, no. 10, pp. 3730–3738, 2010.

Permissions

The contributors of this book come from diverse backgrounds, making this book a truly international effort. This book will bring forth new frontiers with its revolutionizing research information and detailed analysis of the nascent developments around the world.

We would like to thank all the contributing authors for lending their expertise to make the book truly unique. They have played a crucial role in the development of this book. Without their invaluable contributions this book wouldn't have been possible. They have made vital efforts to compile up to date information on the varied aspects of this subject to make this book a valuable addition to the collection of many professionals and students.

This book was conceptualized with the vision of imparting up-to-date information and advanced data in this field. To ensure the same, a matchless editorial board was set up. Every individual on the board went through rigorous rounds of assessment to prove their worth. After which they invested a large part of their time researching and compiling the most relevant data for our readers. Conferences and sessions were held from time to time between the editorial board and the contributing authors to present the data in the most comprehensible form. The editorial team has worked tirelessly to provide valuable and valid information to help people across the globe.

Every chapter published in this book has been scrutinized by our experts. Their significance has been extensively debated. The topics covered herein carry significant findings which will fuel the growth of the discipline. They may even be implemented as practical applications or may be referred to as a beginning point for another development. Chapters in this book were first published by Hindawi Publishing Corporation; hereby published with permission under the Creative Commons Attribution License or equivalent.

The editorial board has been involved in producing this book since its inception. They have spent rigorous hours researching and exploring the diverse topics which have resulted in the successful publishing of this book. They have passed on their knowledge of decades through this book. To expedite this challenging task, the publisher supported the team at every step. A small team of assistant editors was also appointed to further simplify the editing procedure and attain best results for the readers.

Our editorial team has been hand-picked from every corner of the world. Their multi-ethnicity adds dynamic inputs to the discussions which result in innovative outcomes. These outcomes are then further discussed with the researchers and contributors who give their valuable feedback and opinion regarding the same. The feedback is then collaborated with the researches and they are edited in a comprehensive manner to aid the understanding of the subject.

Apart from the editorial board, the designing team has also invested a significant amount of their time in understanding the subject and creating the most relevant covers. They scrutinized every image to scout for the most suitable representation of the subject and create an appropriate cover for the book.

The publishing team has been involved in this book since its early stages. They were actively engaged in every process, be it collecting the data, connecting with the contributors or procuring relevant information. The team has been an ardent support to the editorial, designing and production team. Their endless efforts to recruit the best for this project, has resulted in the accomplishment of this book. They are a veteran in the field of academics and their pool of knowledge is as vast as their experience in printing. Their expertise and guidance has proved useful at every step. Their uncompromising quality standards have made this book an exceptional effort. Their encouragement from time to time has been an inspiration for everyone.

The publisher and the editorial board hope that this book will prove to be a valuable piece of knowledge for researchers, students, practitioners and scholars across the globe.

List of Contributors

Susan R. Davis
Federal Occupational Health, Department of Health and Human Services, 4550 Montgomery Avenue, Suite 950, Bethesda, MD 20814, USA

Xuguang Tao, Edward J. Bernacki and Amy S. Alfriend
Division of Occupational and Environmental Medicine, Department of Medicine, Johns Hopkins University School of Medicine, 615 N. Wolfe Street, Baltimore, MD 21205, USA

Kris Rogers, Erika E. Bohn-Goldbaum, Philayrath Phongsavan and Adrian E. Bauman
Prevention Research Collaboration, School of Public Health, The University of Sydney, NSW2006, Australia

Dafna Merom
School of Science and Health, University of Western Sydney, Camperdown Campus, NSW, Australia

Venugopal Kamalesh
IMPACT Strategic Research Centre, School of Medicine, Deakin University, VIC, Australia

Dean Cooley and Scott Pedersen
University of Tasmania, Faculty of Education, Launceston, TAS 7248, Australia

Michele Cordioli
Department of Bio-Sciences, University of Parma, Parco Area delle Scienze 11/a, 43124 Parma, Italy
Regional Reference Centre Environment & Health, Regional Agency for Environmental Protection in Emilia-Romagna, Via Begarelli 13, 41121 Modena, Italy

Andrea Ranzi and Paolo Lauriola
Regional Reference Centre Environment & Health, Regional Agency for Environmental Protection in Emilia-Romagna, Via Begarelli 13, 41121 Modena, Italy

Giulio A. De Leo
Hopkins Marine Station and Woods Institute for the Environment, Stanford University, 120 Oceanview Boulevard, Pacific Grove, CA 93950, USA

Marie Kruse
Centre for Applied Health Technology Assessment, University of Southern Denmark, J.B. Winsløwsvej 9B 1, 5000 Odense C, Denmark
The Danish Institute for Health Services Research, Dampfærgevej 27–29, 2100 Copenhagen, Denmark

Bjørn Sætterstrøm and Jan Sørensen
Centre for Applied Health Technology Assessment, University of Southern Denmark, J.B. Winsløwsvej 9B 1, 5000 Odense C, Denmark

Jakob Bønløkke
Section of Environmental and Occupational Health, Institute of Public Health, Aarhus University, Bartholins Alle 2, 8000 Aarhus C, Denmark

Henrik Brønnum-Hansen
Institute of Public Health, University of Copenhagen, Øster Farimagsgade 5, 1014 Copenhagen, Denmark

Esben Meulengracht Flachs
National Institute of Public Health, University of Southern Denmark, Øster Farimagsgade 5, 1014 Copenhagen, Denmark

Bethany Elliott and Deepthi Jayatilaka
Population and Public Health, Provincial Health Services Authority, Vancouver, Canada V6Z 2H3

Contessa Brown
Heiltsuk Nation, Bella Bella, Canada V0T 1Z0

Leslie Varley
Aboriginal Health, Provincial Health Services Authority, Vancouver, Canada V5Z 4C2

Kitty K. Corbett
Faculty of Health Science, Simon Fraser University, Burnaby, Canada V5A 1S6

Amir M. Abdelzaher, Helena M. Solo-Gabriele and Matthew C. Phillips
NSF NIEHS Oceans and Human Health Center, University of Miami, Miami, FL 33149, USA
Department of Civil, Architectural, and Environmental Engineering, University of Miami, Coral Gables, FL 33146-0630, USA

Samir M. Elmir
NSF NIEHS Oceans and Human Health Center, University of Miami, Miami, FL 33149, USA
Miami-Dade County Health Department, Miami, FL 33056, USA

Lora E. Fleming
NSF NIEHS Oceans and Human Health Center, University of Miami, Miami, FL 33149, USA
Department of Epidemiology & Public Health and Marine Biology & Fisheries, University of Miami, Miami, FL 33136, USA
European Centre for Environment and Human Health, University of Exeter Medical School, Truro, Cornwall TR1 3HD, UK

Yu Wenjin
Key Laboratory of Meteorological Disaster of Ministry of Education, Nanjing University of Information & Technology, Nanjing 210044, China
Hohai University, Key Laboratory of Coastal Disaster, Nanjing 210093, China

Zou Xinqing
Ministry of Education Key Laboratory for Coast and Islands Development, Nanjing University, Nanjing 210093, China

Rachel Sacks, Micaela H. Coady, Ijeoma G. Mbamalu, Michael Johns and Susan M. Kansagra
Bureau of Chronic Disease Prevention and Tobacco Control, New York City Department of Health and Mental Hygiene, CN-18, Queens, NY 11101, USA

Melinda J. Ickes
Department of Kinesiology and Health Promotion, University of Kentucky, 111 Seaton Building, Lexington, KY 40506, USA

Manoj Sharma
Department of Health Promotion & Education, University of Cincinnati, Teachers College 527 C, P.O. Box 210068, Cincinnati, OH 45221, USA
Department of Public Health, University of Cincinnati, Teachers College 527 C, P.O. Box 210068, Cincinnati, OH 45221, USA

Panos Panagos, Marc Van Liedekerke, Yusuf Yigini and Luca Montanarella
European Commission, Joint Research Centre, Institute for Environment and Sustainability, Via E. Fermi 2749, 21027 Ispra, Italy

Melissa Bopp and Alyssa N. Norton
Department of Kinesiology, The Pennsylvania State University, University Park, PA 16802, USA

Tanis J. Hastmann
Department of Physical Education, Exercise Science and Wellness, the University of North Dakota, Grand Forks, ND 58202, USA

Yohannes Worku
Department of Civil Engineering, Faculty of Engineering, Tshwane University of Technology, Private Bag X680, Pretoria 0001, South Africa

Mammo Muchie
Faculty of Economics and Finance, Institute for Economic Research on Innovation (IERI), Tshwane University of Technology, Private Bag X680, Pretoria 0001, South Africa

Brian G. Luckett
Epidemiology Program, School of Public Health, Louisiana State University Health Sciences Center, 2020 Gravier Street, 3rd Floor, New Orleans, LA 70112, USA
Department of Global Community Health and Behavioral Sciences, School of Public Health and Tropical Medicine, Tulane University, 1440 Canal Street, Suite 2300, New Orleans, LA 70112, USA

L. Joseph Su
Epidemiology Program, School of Public Health, Louisiana State University Health Sciences Center, 2020 Gravier Street, 3rd Floor, New Orleans, LA 70112, USA
Epidemiology and Genomics Research Program, Division of Cancer Control and Population Sciences, National Cancer Institute, 6130 Executive Boulevard, Room 5140, MSC 7393, Bethesda, MD 20892, USA

Jennifer C. Rood
Clinical Chemistry Core, Pennington Biomedical Research Center, 6400 Perkins Road, Baton Rouge, LA 70808, USA

Elizabeth T. H. Fontham
Epidemiology Program, School of Public Health, Louisiana State University Health Sciences Center, 2020 Gravier Street, 3rd Floor, New Orleans, LA 70112, USA

Margaret E. Sears
Children's Hospital of Eastern Ontario Research Institute, Ottawa, ON, Canada K1H 8L1
Clinical Epidemiology, Ottawa Hospital Research Institute, Ottawa, ON, Canada K1Y 4E9

Kathleen J. Kerr and Riina I. Bray
Environmental Health Clinic, Women's College Hospital, Toronto, ON, Canada M5S 1B2
Department of Family and Community Medicine, University of Toronto, Toronto, ON, Canada M5T 1W7

Stephen J. Genuis
Faculty of Medicine, University of Alberta, 2935-66 Street, Edmonton, AB, Canada T6K 4C1

Sanjay Beesoon
Department of Laboratory Medicine, University of Alberta, Edmonton, AB, Canada T6G 2B7

Detlef Birkholz
Environmental Division, ALS Laboratory Group, Edmonton AB, Canada T6E 5C1

Rebecca A. Lobo
Department of Family Medicine, University of Alberta, Edmonton, AB, Canada T6G 2C8

Fatma G. Huffman, Joan A. Vaccaro, Joel C. Exebio, Gustavo G. Zarini, Timothy Katz and Zisca Dixon
Department of Dietetics and Nutrition, Robert Stempel College of Public Health and Social Work, Florida International University, AHC1-435, Miami, FL 33199, USA

Vivian W. Siu
Population Research Center and Institute of Metropolitan Studies, Portland State University, P.O. Box 751, Portland, OR 97207, USA

William E. Lambert and Rongwei Fu
Department of Public Health and Preventive Medicine, Oregon Health & Science University, 3181 SW Sam Jackson Park Road, Mail Code CB 669, Portland, OR 97239, USA

Teresa A. Hillier
Kaiser Permanente Center for Health Research, Northwest/Hawaii, 3800 N. Interstate Avenue, Portland, OR 97227, USA

Mark Bosworth
Metro Data Resource Center, 600 NE Grand Avenue, Portland, OR 97232, USA

Yvonne L. Michael
Department of Epidemiology and Biostatistics, Drexel University School of Public Health, 1505 Race Street, MS 1033, Philadelphia, PA 19102, USA

Diego Saporta
Associates in ENT & Allergy, PA 470 North Aveue, Elizabeth, NJ 07208, USA

Monica H. Swahn, Lindsay Gressard, Jane B. Palmier, Huang Yao and Melissa Haberlen
Institute of Public Health, Georgia State University, P.O. Box 3995, Atlanta, GA 30302-3995, USA

Marjaneh M. Fooladi
Council for International Exchange of Scholars, A Division of the Institute of International Education, 3007 Tilden Street NW, Suite 5-L, Washington, DC 20008, USA
College of Nursing, Florida State University, Vivian M. Duxbury Hall, 98 Varsity Way, P.O. Box 3064310, Tallahassee, FL 32306-4310, USA
School of Nursing, American University of Beirut, P.O. Box 11-0236, Riad El Solh, Beirut 1107 2020, Lebanon